Praise for Zita West

FROM PROFESSIONALS:

'I really believe that good psychological and emotional support is essential for women at all steps of assisted fertility. I have seen the work that Zita West and her multi-disciplinary team do and how women benefit at all stages of the IVF process.'
Mr Mohamed Taranissi, Medical Director of The Assisted Reproduction & Gynaecology Centre (ARGC)

'Infertility and its treatment are inevitably stressful for both partners in a relationship. We know that supportive therapies can make a big difference to treatment and can help people cope with the emotional rollercoaster they find themselves on. Zita's book will be a great help and should be recommended to potential patients at an early stage in their investigation and treatment.'
Professor William Ledger, Professor of Obstetrics and Gynaecology and Head of Unit, University of Sheffield

'While medicine offers an opportunity, IVF technology itself does, I believe, need the help of both partners to be in the healthiest state of body and mind to achieve its most effective success. Zita West has been pioneering this approach with thousands of patients for many years to significant effect; and her skills, knowledge and methods are an important adjunct to the IVF process.'
Professor Simon Fishel, Managing Director of the CARE Fertility Group and Professor of Human Reproduction

'Zita puts the humanity back into IVF-assisted conception and lets patients take some ownership of their IVF journey. Her approach is both holistic and patient-focused, rather than technology-driven. Zita really listens to what patients want and then helps them get what they need.'
Alan Thornhill, Scientific Director at the London Bridge Fertility, Gynaecology and Genetics Centre, London

'Zita West offers a unique service to couples who are preparing for pregnancy. Her fully integrated approach encourages couples to optimise their reproductive health through nutrition and acupuncture while ensuring that they get the best medical care at the same time.'
Sheryl Homa, clinical embryologist and scientist

'The utilisation of ultrasound scanning as part of conventional clinical gynaecological managements has been well documented. Zita West is one of the leaders in extending the role of ultrasound to support a more natural, complementary approach to the treatment of fertility issues in particular. She has promoted the value of ultrasound scanning in providing tremendous reassurance for her patients in addition to its impact in terms of influencing their treatment itself.'
Mr Bill Smith, Ultrasound Specialist, Clinical Diagnostic Services

'Our experience of supporting patients and providing them with information in order to empower them on their journey through infertility is that of a huge interest in complementary therapy and of taking control. Patients want to be involved in their care – Zita offers that involvement. Zita has embraced the fact that it is vital that there is a partnership between complementary therapy and clinical treatment working together to improve that journey for patients.'
Clare Lewis-Jones MBE, Chief Executive, Infertility Network UK

FROM CLIENTS:

'Zita and her team changed our lives. I am certain that without her ability to pull together all the different strands of our problem and suggest positive steps to deal with them as well as to provide a warm and nurturing environment in which to do this, our little girl would not be here. She gave us reason to be hopeful again which is so important in achieving a successful pregnancy.'

Ellen Reilly

'I cannot recommend the Zita West Clinic highly enough. They have given me excellent and unique treatment, support and advice throughout the journey to parenthood and my long-awaited pregnancy. They are a genuinely caring and professional team who are completely committed personally to their clients.'

Nancy Calcroft

Zita West's
Guide to
Fertility
and
Assisted
Conception

Essential advice on preparing your body for IVF and other fertility treatments

ᐯermilion
LONDON

1 3 5 7 9 10 8 6 4 2

Published in 2010 by Vermilion, an imprint of Ebury Publishing
Ebury Publishing is a Random House Group company

The Random House Group Limited Reg. No. 954009

Addresses for companies within the Random House Group can be found at
www.rbooks.co.uk

A CIP catalogue record for this book is available from the British Library

The Random House Group Limited supports The Forest Stewardship Council
(FSC), the leading international forest certification organisation. All our titles that
are printed on Greenpeace approved FSC certified paper carry the FSC logo.
Our paper procurement policy can be found at www.rbooks.co.uk/environment

Designed and set by seagulls.net

Printed and bound in the UK by CPI Mackays, Chatham ME5 8TD

ISBN 9780091929343

Copies are available at special rates for bulk orders. Contact the sales
development team on 020 7840 8487 for more information.

To buy books by your favourite authors and register for offers, visit
www.rbooks.co.uk

The information in this book has been compiled by way of general guidance in
relation to the specific subjects addressed, but is not a substitute and not to be
relied on for medical, healthcare, pharmaceutical or other professional advice on
specific circumstances and in specific locations. Please consult your GP before
changing, stopping or starting any medical treatment. So far as the author is aware
the information given is correct and up to date as at January 2010. Practice, laws
and regulations all change, and the reader should obtain up-to-date professional
advice on any such issues. The author and publishers disclaim, as far as the law
allows, any liability arising directly or indirectly from the use, or misuse,
of the information contained in this book.

This book is dedicated to all the wonderful people who have shared their stories, their diaries and some of their most intimate thoughts, and to every one of you facing the challenges of an uncertain road ahead – may your future be fulfilling.

Contents

Acknowledgements

This book, like so many fertility journeys, has required assistance along the way from a team of highly dedicated individuals. It is hard to know where to start, but I would like to say the greatest thanks to Jane Knight who has provided her unique combination of knowledge on fertility facts and counselling with her supportive friendship and academic rigour to help bring this book to fruition. My special thanks go to my whole team, but especially to: Anita O'Neill, for her midwifery input, enduring support and friendship; Claire Norrish for PR and Judy Davies for typing and organising me; Liz and Melody for their tireless efforts juggling my clinic diary; to my team of acupuncturists, especially Eva Stecz for the acupuncture section, Suzanne Dykes, Mette Heinz, Star Gifford and Lora McFarlane; Melanie Brown for the nutrition section and Isabelle Obert who makes food fun; Dr Sheryl Homa for her invaluable support with the male programme and for writing the male fertility chapters; Josephine Cerqua and Julie Shaw; and finally Brian Astley for his support.

My sincere thanks go to the fertility specialists from all disciplines whom I interviewed for the book and so generously contributed their expert knowledge. Many are leading professors and doctors indeed, but temporarily stripping them of their titles and 'in order of appearance': Allan Pacey, Bill Smith, Anthony Hirsh, Sam Dawkins, Debra Bloor, Clare Lewis-Jones, Eleanor Wharf, Alan Thornhill, Simon Fishel, Tim Child, David Barad, Nick Panay, George Ndukwe, Mohamed Taranissi, Yau Thum, Raj Rai, Laura Witjens, Lena Korea, Hossam Abdalla, Ian Craft, Tarek El-Toukhy, William Ledger, Paul Serhal and Geoffrey Sher. With special thanks to Sam, George, Yau and Tarek for their precious time validating the text.

Finally, to Julia Kellaway my editor at Vermilion for her amazing support throughout; Sarah Bennie PR at Vermilion; Jan Wilson my life-long friend; Sofie West my daughter; Tim Frankell and Fiona Rogers for helping to proofread; Yvonne Williamson and Barbara Vessyer for typing. Last but by no means least, my husband Rob for his enduring support and son Jack for the images; and for everyone else who has contributed in any way. This book may have had a natural conception, but it has benefited enormously from a highly assisted delivery. I owe my gratitude to one and all who have made this possible.

Introduction

I have been a midwife for 30 years, specialising in fertility for about the last 15 years. My holistic approach combines a medical background, which is the bedrock of the work that I do, with training in acupuncture and nutritional therapies.

I am very fortunate to have access to many of the top doctors working in reproductive health and assisted fertility. I have learnt so much from them over the years and I am hugely grateful for their contributions throughout this book. You will find here interviews with many high-profile doctors. IVF is a very exact science, but it is also an art – and as such there are many different perspectives on how to maximise the use of this science. Indeed, some doctors are seen to be pushing the boundaries in their pioneering areas of research and therefore there will always be areas of controversy. This is one of the things that makes this such an exciting field to work in. Throughout this book, I have endeavoured to indicate where there is clear evidence, where there are areas of debate or controversy and where I am expressing my own personal opinion. You will also find case studies throughout the book. These are generally a mix of different scenarios and all names and identifying features have been changed.

At my clinic in London we see over 1,000 couples a year. The Zita West Clinic is a large, successful integrated reproductive health practice, combining both medical and complementary care. We have much experience in helping couples who are finding it difficult to get pregnant to conceive successfully. We firmly believe that the best results come from considering both partners' health and wellness, and that the more the human body is in balance – physically, nutritionally and emotionally – the better the reproductive process is likely to work. My aim at the clinic is for each client to feel truly listened to and supported, having gained the treatment, guidance, knowledge and belief necessary to achieve optimal reproductive health, balance and wellbeing. I want you to be able to experience this from reading this book.

My Approach

I see my approach as looking at the specific needs of the individual and the couple, and helping couples form a focused, planned approach. One question I always ask myself when I have a couple in the room is, 'What is stopping this couple from conceiving?' I ask couples to fill in a detailed questionnaire together about their fertility and lifestyle. Sometimes it highlights things they haven't thought about before as possible reasons why they have not been able to get pregnant. I would much prefer couples to get pregnant naturally rather than go down a route of IVF too early without looking at every aspect of their lives.

The following questions will give you an idea of the sort of areas I address with couples:

- Are you having regular sex: at least two or three times a week?
- Are you aware of your fertile time?
- Are you usually together around your fertile time?
- Are you overweight or underweight?
- Are you on any medication?

- Have you changed your lifestyle in any way, such as cutting down on alcohol or giving up cigarettes?
- What is your work/life balance like – are you overstretching yourself or working too hard?
- How are your energy reserves? If low, are you building them up?
- Are you sleeping well?
- Do you have some hobbies? Do you have time to unwind and relax?
- What is your relationship like with your partner?

Other questions I always ask myself are: 'What is the true potential for this couple? How can I help them? What can I change? What can they change to make a difference?' Very often this highlights issues at the root of the relationship, which I will discuss in Chapter 6. I also ask myself where the couple's stress is coming from. Is it physical, emotional/mental or spiritual? Many of the women I see have been so 'medicalised' that their spirits are depleted. It is very useful to ask yourself what is going on in your life. Where are the blocks to conceiving? What is the dynamic of your relationship? So many couples are emotionally blocked in their relationship without realising it. And some couples use sex as a subconscious currency, causing many resentments to kick in. Does this sound familiar at all? Again, we'll talk more about this in Chapter 6.

One of the questions I am asked frequently by couples is when they should begin IVF treatment. This is difficult to answer because it will depend on many factors, age being the main one. I sometimes think couples have unrealistic expectations – 'We'll do IVF and it will work.' I have always believed there is an awful lot that can be done to help the subconscious, which can often result in a woman becoming pregnant naturally. It is important to explore as many low-tech ways to conceive as possible before starting IVF treatment.

On average it takes 12–18 months to conceive. If you are a woman over about 38, there is a fine line in terms of how long you can afford to keep trying naturally without moving down an IVF route. However, there are no hard and fast rules related to age – chronological age does not necessarily reflect ovarian age and each individual will be very different. I never want people to turn to IVF as a first resort unless there are known factors preventing natural conception, such as blocked tubes, or serious problems with the sperm. I usually give older women three or four months to help them make some lifestyle changes in relation to diet, emotional wellbeing, fitness and sex. Only then do I consider recommending IVF treatment.

How to Use this Book

You may be just starting off and need reassurance, have underlying problems that need addressing, or you may have been trying for a while and are about to go down an assisted conception route. You could have been through IVF and need help deciding where to go and what to do next. I want this book to help you no matter what stage you are at.

There is so much information available for couples trying to conceive: from the internet, friends, magazines, newspapers, television and so on. However, this can sometimes be rather confusing. One of the things we specialise in at the clinic is fertility awareness education – giving couples the time to really understand how fertility works. A German study clearly showed that an understanding of fertility awareness increases the pregnancy rate for couples planning pregnancy. Rather than opt straight for IVF, you may want to consider an educational approach for a limited time first. I hope Part 1 of this book will help you do this. Start by working through the fertility checklist in Chapter 1. You need to consider all aspects of your life. Every one of us has an area of weakness that can be improved upon.

In my initial consultation with couples five key areas I look at are: medical; lifestyle; nutrition; emotional and psychological support; and stress reduction. I make sure they have had all the relevant medical tests, so we will look at reproductive medical health in Chapters 2 and 3. Chapter 4 looks at lifestyle factors. As you read this book, you'll see that 'lifestyle' isn't just about how much alcohol you drink or how many cigarettes you smoke; it's about your relationship, about how you live your life, looking at the whole picture. Very often that involves work/life balance and the stresses and strains of everyday living.

Our emotions and psychological wellbeing have a big impact on fertility (Chapter 5). This is a sensitive area for many couples because it involves their relationship and what has happened to them in the past. We have developed a Manage Your Mind programme to help women deal emotionally and psychologically with issues surrounding conception and IVF treatment. Diet and nutrition are the focus of Chapter 7, where I explain how you can improve your reproductive health through what you eat.

The remaining chapters in the book focus on the questions I get asked the most about IVF: how to get through a cycle; the protocols involved; and understanding the process and tests. But, more importantly, these chapters will also help you to manage your mind and prepare for IVF.

Over the years I have been very fortunate to work with many top IVF doctors. They have been a great help to many of our clients, and having access to them is crucial to the work I do. I have interviewed many of them for this book to get their views of what makes IVF successful.

Implementing and integrating complementary therapies, and visualisation and stress reduction through the use of therapies such as hypnotherapy, breathing techniques and cognitive behaviour therapies, is a large part of the work that we do. With my background as an acupuncturist, this is a very prevalent part of the work at the clinic. Using holistic approaches to complement care helps many couples and our clients feel enormous benefit from a planned, focused approach. What we specialise in is 'pulling all of the strands together' within a time-frame and taking the pressure off. I hope that this book helps you feel that you have a plan and a way forward.

Part 1

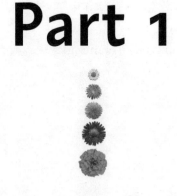

Understanding Your Fertility

Chapter 1

Assessing Your Fertility

Before you start reading the rest of this book, work through this chapter. It contains advice on steps to take before trying to conceive, as well as questions about your health and lifestyle. This chapter is relevant to all couples who wish to conceive, no matter what stage they are at. Answering the questions, and ticking the boxes in the checklists, will help you get the most from the chapters that follow.

Your Fertility Checklist

The checklists in this section will help you build up a picture of your current fertility. Working through them will enable you to pinpoint areas where you can make simple changes, such as to your lifestyle. It will also highlight any aspects of your health that might require investigation.

Before You Conceive (for women)

Are you immune to rubella?	Yes	No
Is your cervical smear up to date?	Yes	No
Are you aware of the importance of folic acid?	Yes	No
Have you had a recent sexual health check-up?	Yes	No

Check Your Rubella Immunity

A woman's immunity to rubella (German measles) is checked with a blood test. Even if you had rubella as a child, or had the injection at school, this does not necessarily mean that you still have enough immunity now. If you are found not to be immune (no antibodies) you will usually be given a rubella booster and will be advised to strictly avoid getting pregnant for at least a month. If you are not immune to rubella and pick up the infection in early pregnancy, it can cause miscarriage or serious congenital abnormalities. I see many women who don't know their status – so if in doubt get it checked out.

Have a Cervical Smear

Smears are done only every three years on the NHS but are also available privately (for about £85 in 2010). The reason to have your smear before conceiving is because it is much easier to treat any abnormal cells when you are not pregnant.

Take Folic Acid

The Department of Health advises women to take folic acid at least three months before conceiving to prevent neural tube defects, such as spina bifida, in the baby. Most multi-vitamins and minerals contain folic acid. It can also be bought over the counter on its own. The recommended dose if you are trying to conceive is 400 micrograms daily. If you are taking medication for epilepsy, or you have any other existing medical condition, you may need a higher dose so check with your GP. Folic acid supplements should be continued for the first 12 weeks of pregnancy.

Check Your Sexual Health

Sexual health is vitally important though it sometimes still holds a stigma. You don't have to have 'slept around' to have picked up an infection, and just as you have routine check-ups with a dentist, the same should apply to sexual health. Infections can be treated easily but any infection you don't know about can damage your future fertility.

Sexually transmitted infections often have few, or even no symptoms, so the damage they cause may go unnoticed until a couple tries for children. Chlamydia, in particular, is on the increase. In 10 per cent of cases it causes enough damage to the fallopian tubes to render a woman infertile, yet has no visible symptoms. It can affect male fertility too. Gonorrhoea, as with chlamydia, can cause infertility in men and women – it blocks the fallopian tubes and, in men, the vas deferens, which carries sperm.

Extra tests might include mycoplasma and ureaplasma (see pages 227 and 279–280). These are not done routinely on the NHS but can have an impact on your fertility, especially if you are going through IVF.

Sexual health clinics are located in many local hospitals or health centres. NHS Direct or the FPA (Family Planning Association) will have further information on how to access these clinics (see Resources). You will usually need to phone and make an appointment. The tests are usually done using swabs or by taking urine samples. Standard tests include the following:

- chlamydia
- gonorrhoea
- syphilis
- HIV
- thrush
- bacterial vaginosis (gardnerella)
- trichomonas
- genital herpes
- genital warts
- pubic lice and scabies

Pre-conception Extra

I believe in taking a good multi-vitamin/mineral supplement designed for fertility plus omega 3 fatty acids (DHA or docosa-hexaenoic acid) prior to conceiving as an all-round insurance policy. The reason for this is that you need to build up your stores of vital vitamins and minerals. Your baby doesn't rely on what you eat on any one day – he or she will rely on your stores of these essential nutrients.

Age

Age is a defining factor – for women and, to a much lesser extent, for men – when it comes to fertility treatment. It is useful to know the age your mother was when she had her menopause (last period) as fertility stops up to 10 years before the last period. Subtract 10 from your mother's menopausal age and that will give you a very rough guide to when your fertility may be seriously compromised. If your mother had an early menopause (before 45) you may have a similar pattern. Generally, women have to wait a year to 18 months before anything will be done on the NHS, but if you are 35 or over and you have been having regular sex (three times a week) for at least six months, then I think you should go to your GP and have all the necessary tests – and so should your partner. Guidelines from NICE (National Institute for Health and Clinical Excellence) recommend referral for investigation earlier if the woman is over 35 (rather than waiting a year). It is important to realise that IVF cannot fully compensate for lost years of fertility.

I believe there is a lot that older women can do to maximise their chances of conception. It's easy to feel bombarded with a list of things that aren't going to happen because you are older. You still have a 'fertile window' of five to six days each month, so frequent sex is vital. Eggs respond to the environment and there are so many lifestyle factors that can have an impact on them. Chapter 2 gives more details on the particular issues facing women, and Chapter 3 looks at those faced by men.

Menstrual Cycle (for women)

Do you have any of the following:	Yes	No
Painful periods?		
Heavy periods?		
Any recent changes in cycle length?		
Irregular cycles?		
Short cycles?		
Any bleeding between periods?		
No periods at all?		

If your periods are very painful and you are taking a lot of painkillers, this may be an indication of an underlying factor, such as endometriosis, and will need further investigation.

If your periods are heavy there could be an underlying factor such as fibroids. Again, this will need further investigation. You should also ask your GP to test you for anaemia.

If your periods have suddenly changed in length, this can be because you are stressed or travelling a lot, or it can mean a hormonal shift. This will depend on how old you are. It may be a cause for concern if they have been very regular and then become irregular, much shorter or longer or stop altogether.

Any bleeding between periods should be investigated. There could be an underlying infection, such as chlamydia, or a hormone imbalance. At worst, it could indicate very early stages of cervical or other gynaecological cancers. It's always important to get checked out if there are any irregularities in your cycle – a doctor is always happier to reassure you that all is well than to allow a serious condition to be missed. A cervical smear is essential.

If your periods have stopped completely there could be many reasons behind this. You may be exercising too much or underweight, or perhaps you have only recently come off the Pill. It could also mean premature ovarian failure (premature menopause) for some women.

All of these issues will be discussed later in this book (see Chapter 9).

The Male Factor (for men)

Answer yes or no to the following:	Yes	No
Any problems with getting or maintaining an erection?		
Any problems with ejaculation?		
Any operations to your testicles or other pelvic surgery?		

	Yes	No
Any lumps in the testicular area?		
Any injury to the testicles?		
Have you fathered a child before?		
Have you had a vasectomy?		
Any sexually transmitted infections?		
Have you had a recent sexual health check-up?		
Are you on any medication?		
Any urinary symptoms?		
Have you had testicular cancer?		

For more about how these factors can affect your fertility, and what you can do to help yourself, see Chapter 3.

Lifestyle Factors

Answer the following:	Woman			Man		
	Yes	No	Details	Yes	No	Details
Are you overweight?						
Are you underweight?						
Do you drink caffeine? If so, how many cups a week?						
Do you drink alcohol? If so, how many units a week?						
Do you smoke? If so, how many a day?						
Do you use recreational drugs?						
Are you taking any medication? Painkillers?						
Anti-inflammatories?						

	Woman			Man		
	Yes	No	Details	Yes	No	Details
Steroids?						
Blood pressure pills?						
Antibiotics?						
Have you stopped taking the contraceptive pill in the last year?				N/A	N/A	N/A

For more about how these lifestyle factors affect your fertility, see Chapter 4.

Work and Stress

	Woman	Man
Consider:	Hours per day	Hours per day
Number of Hours Worked		
Relaxation Time		

Many couples work really long hours without enough relaxation time. Try and look at ways you can create a better work/life balance. This is important if you're trying for a baby (see Chapter 4 for more on this).

Sex

	Woman		Man	
	Yes	No	Yes	No
Are you having sex at the fertile time?				
Are you having enough sex?				
Are you both still enjoying sex?				

For more about how these factors can affect your fertility, and what you can do to help yourself, see Chapter 6.

Possible Medical Problems

If you have a pre-existing medical condition or a history of serious illness, such as heart problems or cancer, then do discuss your intentions to conceive with your GP or specialist. In some situations you may need to change medication or be alert for potential difficulties either prior to or during pregnancy.

The checklist overleaf is for women to complete. Please don't panic if any of the following apply to you, but they need to be considered or ruled out as part of any pre-conception checklist. All these conditions can be treated and stabilised to improve your chances of getting pregnant.

Please tick appropriate boxes:	Yes	No
Thyroid problems?		
Diabetes ?		
Anaemia?		
Endometriosis?		
Polycystic ovary syndrome (PCOS)?		
Fibroids?		
Previous ectopic pregnancy?		
Abdominal surgery?		
Auto-immune disease in the family?		

For more about possible medical problems, see Chapter 9.

Being aware of your fertility means understanding how it works, what is normal for you and when to seek medical help. The remaining chapters in Part 1 are designed to equip you with the knowledge to maximise your chances of natural conception.

Chapter 2

A Woman's Fertility

My interest in a woman's fertility and fertility awareness started many years ago when I read Fertility Nurse Specialist/Counsellor Jane Knight's book *Fertility*. I have worked with Jane for the last seven years and have interviewed her for this chapter, so here we really speak as one voice.

First of all we need to consider what we mean by 'fertility'. We are really talking about the combined fertility of the couple. Although a man's sperm has the potential to live for up to seven days inside a woman's body, the average sperm survival is around two to three days. A woman's egg lives for a maximum of 24 hours. This is why it is so important to shift the whole focus away from ovulation. To optimise conception, we must give the sperm a chance. Sex three to four times a week, especially around your fertile time, ensures there is enough sperm in the reproductive tract ready for when the egg is released.

During each menstrual cycle, a woman has a fertile time – or window – of about six days. This lasts from five days before ovulation, during which time sperm are able to survive in the fertile secretions in a woman's cervix, to the day of ovulation itself. It is not possible, or necessary, to predict precisely when ovulation will occur; rather, couples need to be aware of the full width of the fertile time.

Understanding Female Anatomy

The main organs responsible for reproduction are the brain, ovaries, fallopian tubes, womb and cervix:

- Brain – for good hormone release and overall control.
- Ovaries – for egg production and production of the hormones oestrogen and progesterone. The two ovaries are small – about the size of an almond.
- Fallopian tubes – these are lined with very fine hair-like structures (cilia) that assist the egg when it is released at ovulation. They move it along the tube and provide a place in the outer third of the tube for fertilisation to take place.
- Womb (uterus) – one of the strongest muscles in the body, the womb has to stretch to accommodate a developing pregnancy and is approximately the size of a pear. The womb lining is called the endometrium and fluctuates during each menstrual cycle, shedding when a woman has her period.
- Cervix – the lowest third of the womb which protrudes down into the vagina and is sometimes called the neck of the womb. The cervix is where the secretions are formed in order to allow the sperm to swim up into the womb and to the fallopian tubes.

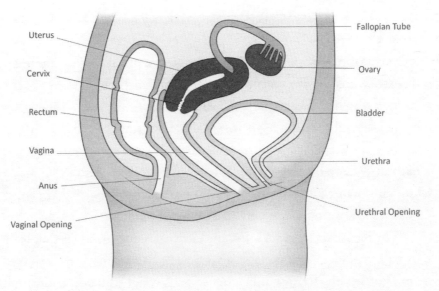

Uterus

Cervix

Rectum

Vagina

Anus

Vaginal Opening

Fallopian Tube

Ovary

Bladder

Urethra

Urethral Opening

What is a Retroverted Uterus?

A lot of women get worried if they have heard they have a retro-verted uterus. The most common position for the uterus is anteverted (as above), which means that the uterus lies at an angle of about 90 degrees to the vagina with the cervix (neck of the womb) in a forward-pointing position, angled ready for the sperm. However, about 1 in 5 women have a retroverted uterus which means that the main part of the uterus tilts backwards and the cervix points upwards, which may make it harder for the sperm to reach the cervix. Provided the uterus is naturally in the retroverted (backward tilting) position, it is unlikely to cause a problem. However, if the uterus has become fixed in a retroverted position due to adhesions (scarring), pelvic infections or endometriosis, then this may be more of a problem.

The Menstrual Cycle

So much of my work is to do with helping women understand their menstrual cycles and become more aware of their fertility. Many women who have been on the Pill since they were 16 or 17 and do not come off until they are in their mid-30s have no idea what a normal cycle is for them. It's important to have a basic understanding of a natural cycle to optimise your chances of conceiving naturally; and if you go down the IVF route you will understand what is happening both naturally and artificially in a cycle.

The menstrual cycle is a complex interplay of hormones that have to be in balance each cycle so that an egg can be matured, released and, potentially, fertilised. Factors such as weight, stress, medication and diet can affect the menstrual cycle, and periods can sometimes become irregular or stop altogether. A menstrual cycle can be anything from about 24 to 35 days or more.

The menstrual cycle starts on the first day of a woman's period. Women get confused about this, often counting the start of the cycle as when they get slight blood spotting, but Day 1 of the cycle is the first day of the fresh, red bleed. If there is any pinkish or brown spotting, then that belongs to the end of the previous cycle.

A woman's period can last between two and six days, or even longer. After that, most women will be aware of a time when they feel relatively dry at the vaginal lips. This is when the cervix is quite tightly closed with a thick, sticky plug of secretions that prevents sperm from getting through. During this part of the cycle, sperm are left in the acidic vagina, and they will be killed off within a matter of hours.

A woman then begins to notice she no longer feels dry, but is aware of a slight stickiness or sees a white or opaque secretion. These fertile secretions nourish the sperm, forming channels to enable them to swim up and giving them energy on their journey. Some strong sperm may manage to get through at this stage.

The Follicular Phase

The follicular phase is the first half of the cycle – from the first day of a period to the day of ovulation – and its length will vary from woman to woman and even from one cycle to the next. During this phase, very small fluid-filled sacs called follicles begin to develop in the ovaries. Under instruction from the hypothalamus gland in the brain, follicle stimulating hormone (FSH) is released from the pituitary gland into the bloodstream to stimulate the selected follicles to grow. One follicle will grow faster than the others in a natural cycle to become the dominant one. In IVF, the idea is to produce lots of follicles all of the same size, so FSH will be given in larger doses via injections to make this happen. The ovarian follicles start to produce oestrogen, increasing each day until it reaches a peak prior to ovulation. FSH production is shut down and a surge of luteinising hormone (LH) is released triggering ovulation – the release of an egg (ovum). After ovulation the corpus luteum is formed from the remains of the dominant follicle and progesterone is released. The follicles that are not destined to ovulate will eventually decrease in size and degenerate in a natural cycle. This dialogue continues between the brain and the ovaries.

Factors Needed for Conception

- Healthy egg released at ovulation
- Healthy sperm
- Sex at the fertile time
- Fertilisation
- Implantation

As the body produces more and more oestrogen, the secretions become noticeably wetter, more slippery, clearer (more transparent) and sometimes quite stretchy. These highly fertile secretions nourish the sperm and encourage them to swim through the cervix. They may last for a matter of hours or up to several days. The last day that these wet secretions are present is often known as the peak day, and this is generally around the time of ovulation.

The two key hormones which influence the cervical secretions are the ovarian hormones oestrogen and progesterone. Oestrogen is the dominant hormone in the first half of the cycle, leading up to ovulation and essentially opens the cervix and makes its secretions wetter and more sperm-friendly. The progesterone which is produced after ovulation is designed to form a thick sticky plug preventing sperm from getting through the cervix. So, in effect the cervix acts like a gateway – oestrogen causes the cervix to soften and open up and the fertile

Maintaining Hormonal Balance

There are many reasons for hormone imbalances. If you are not getting pregnant naturally, blood tests can be done on certain days of your cycle which will pick up these imbalances (see Chapter 9).

Factors that can affect the hormonal balance include:

- Age (see pages 41–43): oestrogen production declines as women get older.
- Body weight: as oestrogen is stored in body fat, being under- or overweight can affect the hormone balance and cause problems with ovulation, so maintaining a healthy weight or body mass index is important.
- Excessive exercise will reduce the levels of circulating oestrogen – the ratio of body fat to lean mass is important.
- Smoking can affect the body's ability to use oestrogen efficiently.
- Stress, anxiety and environmental factors affect hormonal balance.

secretions allow the sperm to swim through the cervix, providing the right conditions to help them survive and wait for the egg to be released.

The Luteal Phase

The luteal phase is the second half of the cycle, from ovulation to the next period. Once ovulation has taken place, the follicle collapses and is called the corpus luteum or 'yellow body'. The corpus luteum then starts to produce the hormone progesterone. Progesterone will encourage the womb lining to thicken, close the cervix and thicken the secretions to prevent any further sperm from getting through.

If the egg is not fertilised, progesterone levels drop and the womb lining is shed as a period after 10–16 days. When the level of progesterone reaches a certain low point, the brain will start to release FSH and the cycle begins again. After the peak day (the last day of the wetter secretions), a woman usually notices that the secretions become thicker and whiter again or she becomes dry. This stays fairly consistent until the start of the next period. If the egg is fertilised by a sperm, the fertilised egg will then implant – there will be no period and pregnancy will have started.

The luteal phase needs to last at least 10 days for the implantation process to be completed. An interval of less than 10 days can be a reason for a delay in conceiving. Many women worry that they don't have enough days in the second half of their cycle. Clinicians tend to be divided about the significance of the luteal phase and the impact of progesterone levels. As a general rule if there is a problem in the second half of the cycle, it is not likely to be helpful simply to give extra progesterone to supplement the luteal phase. This is because the problem is likely to originate before ovulation.

I often liken this to shopping for eggs in a supermarket. You might say that a really good-quality egg is a large egg, which may be free range, barn-reared or whatever; but you can also get much smaller, lower-grade eggs – it is still an egg and would make an omelette, but you may not get the quality or the richness of colour. So if a woman is producing a 'good-quality', 'juicy' egg, it will tend to produce a better corpus luteum (collapsed follicle), which in turn produces a higher level of progesterone to maintain the womb lining in the second half of the cycle.

If the level of progesterone does not reach a certain height or starts to drop off towards the end of the cycle, a woman may notice a few days of blood spotting before her proper period starts. If the progesterone level is checked and is not high enough then an ovulation stimulation or boosting drug such as clomiphene (Clomid) may be given to enhance the first half of the cycle, which in turn boosts the progesterone. Some women have acupuncture to try and balance the hormones and regulate the cycle. As ever, it is important that any treatment is done within a certain time-frame. If there are any concerns about unusual bleeding or spotting, it is important to discuss them with your doctor first.

Cycle Variability

It is a myth that women have menstrual cycles of 28 days. The vast majority of women will have some variability. If cycles vary by fewer than seven days then they are still considered to be regular. However, if there is more than a week's variability, then the cycles are said to be irregular. Many variations are possible:

- As women get older, cycles often become shorter for a while.
- A shorter luteal phase (see above) may result in a shorter cycle overall.
- Sometimes ovulation will be delayed followed by a shorter luteal phase, giving a fairly normal-length cycle.

- The overall cycle length may be quite long despite a short luteal phase.

Working out Your Fertile Time

If you have an idea of the length of your cycles over the past six to twelve months you can use a simple calculation to work out your fertile time. Look at your cycle lengths, find the longest and shortest cycles, then subtract 20 from the shortest one and 10 from the longest one. This gives you the potential fertile time.

For example, if over the last six months your cycles have been 28, 26, 31, 25, 32 and 31 days, the shortest cycle is 25 days and the longest cycle is 32 days. So taking 20 from 25 gives you the first fertile day as Day 5. Then subtracting 10 from 32 gives you Day 22 as your last fertile day, so you would be potentially fertile from Day 5 to Day 22.

Your potential fertile time – based on the history of your previous cycles – is therefore quite wide. If you were going to have a short cycle you could possibly conceive from having sex as early as Day 5 in this example, and if you were going to have a longer cycle, your fertile time may extend to as late as Day 22. Calculations based on cycle length will always give a very wide potential fertile time, but within that range, the changes in cervical secretions will give you a more accurate estimate of the fertile time for that particular cycle.

If your cycles are very consistent – say always 31 days in length – then you can use the same calculation to define your fertile time. The more regular your cycles, the more consistent your fertile time will be. Again, changes in cervical secretions will give a more accurate estimation of the fertile time.

If a woman has a very short cycle, there will usually still be about five days when sperm will be able to survive, nourished by the fertile cervical secretions. It is really important that women who have short cycles are having sex from very early on in the cycle. Many women with short cycles will notice that they have fertile secretions during or towards the end of their period. Sperm are quite capable of surviving if there are any secretions, even if there is still some bleeding. As ever, it is really important to get the sperm there ahead of the game – they will survive happily in the recesses of the cervix. The sperm actually need to spend some time in the cervix to go through a process called capacitation before they are capable of fertilising the egg. It is almost as if they have to recover from the first part of their journey and need time to spruce themselves up before they set off to meet the egg.

Some women, particularly women with polycystic ovaries, may have quite a bit of variability in the length of their cycles. Their cycles may be a combination of long, short and average lengths. This can make it more difficult to target sex, particularly if either partner travels with work. Where cycles are very variable, ovulation predictor kits and monitors may not really help and can give false readings. Although it may not always be manageable, the best way to optimise conception is to try and have sex every couple of days.

Alert!

Any change in your periods should be reported to your GP. Although this is generally of no consequence, it may be a sign of an infection, a gynaecological problem, or even a very early sign of gynaecological cancer, so any unusual bleeding or spotting should be fully investigated by your doctor. This is likely to include a cervical smear re-check and a screen for infections such as chlamydia.

All about Ovulation

Many women have concerns about ovulation. Ovulation is a cryptic, hidden event in women. There are only three ways to be sure you are ovulating:

1. being pregnant
2. an ultrasound scan showing a collapsed egg follicle
3. a blood test showing a raised level of progesterone in the second half of the cycle

Other signs and symptoms just reflect changes in hormone levels. Even an ovulation predictor kit is simply reflecting a surge in luteinising hormone (LH), predicting that ovulation is likely to happen within about 36 hours. If the LH test is positive, it is a very good sign but it is not conclusive proof that an egg has been released. A fertility monitor which measures urinary oestrogen and LH provides information about the full fertile window so may be more useful, and some women find them useful to confirm their own observations. Remember that essentially there are only two things most couples need to get pregnant: time (and it often takes a while) and plenty of sex. So, if the sperm are to stand a chance, then you need a 'top-up' of fresh healthy swimmers every couple of days. (This is generally something that men feel naturally convinced about while women still search for the enigmatic egg!)

Women *can* ovulate twice in a cycle – this would be the case with non-identical twins. However, a second ovulation will always occur within 24 hours of the first one. Sometimes women think they are ovulating for a second time later in their cycle if they see more fertile secretions but these are purely a reflection of hormone levels. If hormones are fluctuating a little, there may be more than one patch of cervical secretions, and women are often aware of some quite fertile-looking secretions just before a period starts.

It is quite normal for women to have occasional cycles where they don't ovulate at all – sometimes known as anovulatory cycles. This may happen quite randomly and tends to become more common as women get older. One of the reasons for declining fertility is the reduced number of cycles where ovulation happens over a year. Severe stress can also inhibit ovulation, as can serious weight loss. It is also quite normal for women not to ovulate at times when fertility is suppressed, such as during breast-feeding, and sometimes for a while after a miscarriage or after stopping hormonal contraception, particularly the longer-acting methods such as depot injections.

Sometimes a woman will be aware of the signs of fertility suggesting approaching ovulation but then the period will arrive sooner than expected. This indicates a short luteal phase (see page 25). Unless there are at least 10 days between ovulation (around the last day of wetter secretions) and the next period, there may not be enough time for a fertilised egg to implant. Although it is very common for women not to ovulate occasionally or to have the odd short luteal phase, if this is happening persistently it is a good idea to see your doctor who could arrange some blood tests such as a progesterone test to confirm ovulation.

If a progesterone test result comes back saying you have not ovulated, it just means you didn't ovulate in that particular cycle; it is worth repeating the test to see if that was an unusual cycle. It can also be difficult to get the progesterone test timed accurately, particularly if you have irregular cycles. It is often called the 'Day 21 progesterone test' as it needs to be taken around the 21st day in a typical 28-day cycle. It should more accurately be called a 'mid-luteal phase' progesterone test as it needs to be taken about a week after your peak day of secretions (last day of wetness). To check it has been taken at about the right time, you should have your period about a

Changes Through the Menstrual Cycle

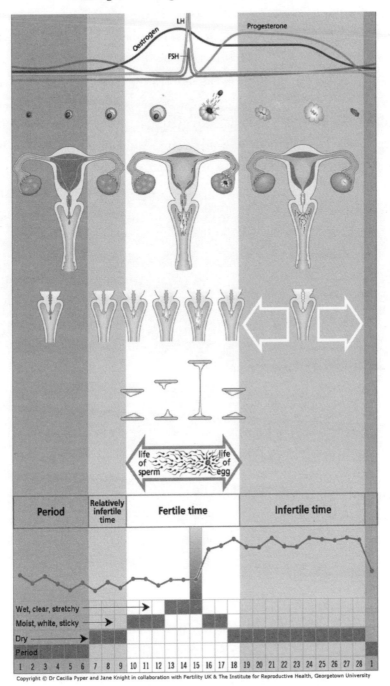

Copyright © Dr Cecilia Pyper and Jane Knight in collaboration with Fertility UK & The Institute for Reproductive Health, Georgetown University

week after the test is done. If the test is not properly timed it will give a false reading, so will need to be redone.

Getting a period doesn't necessarily mean that ovulation has happened. A period, which is the endometrium or womb lining being shed, simply mirrors a fall in the level of the hormone progesterone. Even if you are not ovulating, you will have a certain level of progesterone in your body, and at some stage it is almost as if the womb lining gets tired of hanging on any longer and breaks down. Consider for a moment what happens during cycles where a woman is taking the combined contraceptive pill and ovulation is suppressed; when she stops the Pill, usually at the end of the packet, she will get a 'period' a few days later – this is sometimes known as a 'hormone withdrawal bleed' because that is what it really is. It is not a 'true' period. This is basically what is happening during a cycle where ovulation has not occurred.

Taking Your Temperature

If you are trying to get pregnant, taking your temperature is not at all helpful in targeting sex. This is because the waking temperature doesn't rise to the higher level until about 24 hours after ovulation, by which time the egg would have disintegrated and it is too late. There is no value in trying to time sex to just before the temperature goes up either, because you can have no idea when that will be. You should also forget about anything you have read about a dip in temperature signifying ovulation as this is not reliable.

There may occasionally be times when an accurately taken waking temperature might help identify cyclic disturbances. For example, it might give a more objective idea of the length of the second half of the cycle. As discussed above, the luteal phase needs to be at least 10 days to ensure there is enough time for implantation.

I would never recommend taking temperatures for more than two or three cycles as this is enough to identify any abnormalities.

Many factors can disturb the waking temperature, including getting up later, a late night, alcohol, travel, illness and various medications such as paracetamol. If a temperature reading is to be of any value at all, it is important that women use the correct type of thermometer – usually an accurate digital thermometer – and take the temperature orally and consistently. The recordings should be made on a legible chart with the appropriate grid. (Downloadable fertility charts are available and you can find a list of fertility awareness practitioners at Fertility UK, see Resources.)

So as a general rule, forget all about thermometers – you really don't need any more gadgets or things interrupting the mood! Remember, research clearly shows that your body is giving you the best sign of all in the changes in cervical secretions. I know that some of you will have been taking your temperature, especially if you are seeing an acupuncturist as it may be part of their treatment plan. Doing so for a couple of months is fine but not for longer periods. It makes some of the woman I see really obsessive and focuses their attention on trying all of the time.

Facts about Vaginal Secretions

These secretions are simply a reflection of changing hormone levels. Don't obsess about them.

- Seeing or feeling any type of secretion at the vaginal entrance means that the oestrogen levels are rising and the cervix has opened a little, producing a wetter secretion, and is allowing the sperm to swim through.

- Some women say they notice wetter, transparent secretions just before a period starts. This is not likely to be fertile, but is simply due to the progesterone level dropping a little, allowing the oestrogen level to rise slightly.

- Young women tend to notice a lot more secretions, but as we get older the amount and quality of secretions decreases. A healthy cervix will still be producing secretions, even if you are less aware of them at the vaginal opening.

- It is worth considering whether you are doing anything that may be drying up the secretions. For example, thongs can be quite drying as they are in continuous contact with the vaginal area, so I generally suggest women avoid wearing thongs completely, or save them for 'special occasions'. Similarly, tampons can be very drying so use them only on the heavier flow days. Use the minimal absorbency to manage the flow. On lighter flow or spotting days, use a pad. Never use a tampon 'just in case' a period starts. Tampons are designed to absorb fluid – just try putting one into a glass of water. If there is no blood flow to be absorbed, the tampon will absorb all the natural moisture from the cervix and the vaginal walls, causing a drying effect. It is very common for women to report increased dryness, soreness or 'thrush' just after a period, and especially after sex, as the drying effect and then the friction can cause minor abrasions in the vaginal walls.

- Some of you may have read that expectorant cough mixtures can increase cervical secretions. A research study in the early 1980s looked at the effect of the ingredient guaiphenesin on improving the amount and quality of cervical secretions. However, this is not something I would recommend unless under medical supervision. Some cough mixtures contain other ingredients that have been linked to birth defects, so it is really important *not* to self-medicate when trying for a baby.

Sexual Positions

I hear endless tales of women with their bottoms raised on pillows, legs elevated up the wall, or hanging by their toes from the chandelier in order to avoid losing a lot of the sperm after sex. This is a common anxiety but is really not necessary and can be pretty off-putting for most men! Bodies have some amazing tricks. First, the seminal fluid (semen) is ejaculated with a lot of force. I have no idea who managed to measure this, but apparently seminal fluid is ejaculated at 28mph. When the fluid is first ejaculated it is a greyish white colour and is pretty sticky stuff – it is designed to stick to the cervix. Within a matter of a few minutes it liquefies. During this process the sperm are released to swim upwards, so all that is lost from the vagina in the 'flow back' is a lot of the fluid and a few dead or dying sperm. There should be a good supply of the strong healthy swimmers on their way. So do lie flat after sex for about 10–15 minutes, but you don't need to do any gymnastics to hang on to the sperm.

Some couples who enjoy a 'woman on top' position express anxiety about losing the seminal fluid and will often forgo pleasure in an effort to try and hang on to the sperm. If you both enjoy this position then do continue; after orgasm, you can both turn together so that the woman is then left flat on her back for a few minutes. When a woman is lying on her back, the natural angle of the vagina helps to keep the pool of sperm in contact with the cervix to give them the best chance.

- If cervical secretions are present at the same time as the period or just as the bleeding is getting lighter, it is likely that this will be a shorter cycle and your body is preparing for an earlier ovulation. The key thing here is not to wait for any magical day based on numbers, pee sticks or anything else. If your body is telling you that you have fertile secretions, don't ignore it. It is giving you all the clues to when the conditions are right for the sperm to survive!

- Cervical secretions can be affected by some drugs. Antihistamines may have a drying effect. After stopping hormones such as the contraceptive pill, the secretions may be disturbed for a while and may show fewer fertile characteristics. Fertility drugs such as clomiphene may help to boost ovulation, but they tend to reduce the amount of secretions. Conditions such as cervical erosion can also disrupt the normal pattern, often producing copious amounts of wetter secretions.

Alert!

Any woman who notices a change in her usual pattern of secretions should see her doctor. It is a good idea to have a full sexual health check-up at your local GU (genito-urinary) clinic when you are trying to conceive. It is also important to make sure that your smear is up to date because it is harder to treat any abnormalities of the cervix while you are pregnant.

Lubricants and Gels

Ideally, couples should avoid the use of additional lubricants, focusing more on intimacy and foreplay. However, sex often becomes rushed or mechanical after trying for a baby for a while. If extra lubrication is needed, it is important to realise that virtually all oil-based and water-based lubricants reduce sperm motility (movement). One of the worst things for sperm is saliva because it contains digestive enzymes that have a very damaging effect – so go carefully with oral sex around the fertile time. A research study published in the medical journal *Fertility and Sterility* found that the relatively new lubricant, Preseed, has no significantly adverse effect on sperm.

Can You Influence the Sex of the Baby?

Case Study

We have two boys and are desperate to have a sister for them. I'm now 38 and worried about my age. I'm also worried about the gap – I don't want a huge gap between the siblings. I hate the fact that all my friends seem to have girls really easily and my life doesn't seem complete without a daughter. I'm trying everything to conceive a girl: having sex before ovulation, trying to have shallow penetration, avoid having an orgasm, eating acidic foods and even douching with lemon juice, and I'm getting more distraught each month when it's not happening. I just feel that if I have a daughter it would be great to do things together.

Many couples ask about the chances of influencing the baby's sex prior to conception. This may be for cultural reasons, personal preference or family balancing. There is plenty of well-intentioned advice in the public domain, but the evidence for natural techniques for choosing the desired sex is seriously lacking.

The chances of having a child of the desired sex are 50:50. The sex of the baby is determined at the moment of fertilisation, depending on the type of sex chromosome provided by the sperm. The egg contains 22 chromosomes plus one X sex chromosome. The sperm contains 22 chromosomes plus either an X or Y chromosome. An XX embryo will be a girl and an XY embryo will be a boy.

So: X egg + X sperm = XX girl; X egg + Y sperm = XY boy.

Much of the popular literature is based on work done in the 1960s which looked at the swimming ability and stamina of sperm and contact with an acid or alkaline vaginal environment. Y-bearing (male) sperm are lighter and swim faster than the heavier X-bearing (female) sperm. It was thought that intercourse closer to ovulation increased the chances of a boy and intercourse very early in the fertile time increased the chances of a girl. This study is frequently quoted and the theory behind it is perpetuated. However, a very small study from over 40 years ago is not evidence-based research. Since that time there has been much research interest in natural sex selection and many well-conducted prospective studies looking at the probability of conception on different days of the cycle, showing conflicting results. The bottom line on this topic is that we fully endorse the FPA (Family Planning Association) statement: 'To date, there is no reliable scientific evidence to support claims made for choosing the sex of the baby, such as when you have sex, sexual positions or diet.'

Sadly, we often see couples who have been trying to conceive unsuccessfully for a while and then rather shyly admit that they have been limiting intercourse in an endeavour to have a baby of their desired sex – all this has done is delayed conception considerably – and this can have serious consequences especially for older women.

Self-insemination

It is not uncommon for couples who are feeling pressured to conceive, to experience temporary sexual difficulties and some couples find self-insemination helpful. This involves collecting a sample of sperm through masturbation and placing it high into the woman's vagina –

Case Study

Jim and Jo had a very good relationship, including a fulfilling sex life. Owing to a chronic condition requiring medication, however, Jim was rarely able to get an erection sufficient to achieve penetration. He recognised that there was a psychological element to it too, and felt he was letting Jo down. They were considering assisted conception and wanted to discuss referral for IUI (intrauterine insemination). As Jo was in her early 30s and they had been trying to conceive for only a few months, Jane Knight discussed trying self-insemination for three to six months first, which would be less stressful and medicalised. Jane explained the practicalities of self-insemination and ways to identify Jo's fertile time. As her cycles were longer than average (over 35 days), it was important for her to recognise that the changes in her cervical secretions would occur later in her cycle but still give her a clear indication of her fertile time. Jo conceived on their second cycle using self-insemination. They were thrilled – for them the ability to use self-insemination as a backup if Jim did not get an erection actually allowed him to relax so that he was able to have full intercourse on several occasions. They were delighted to have got pregnant without medical intervention and at no additional cost.

simulating intercourse. Self-insemination is also used by many lesbian couples. The main practical considerations with self-insemination are identifying the fertile time accurately (see page 27) and handling the sperm correctly.

The seminal fluid can easily be collected by ejaculation into a clean pot. Immediately after ejaculation, the seminal fluid will be quite thick, but within 10–15 minutes it will liquefy and is then easier to suck up into a syringe. You can buy packs of 10ml plastic syringes from most chemists or online. It is best to use a new syringe for each insemination. Try to place the seminal fluid as close to your cervix (neck of the womb) as possible. This gives the sperm a head-start. To keep the seminal fluid in place long enough for the sperm to swim through the cervix, stay flat for about 20 minutes afterwards. You will inevitably lose some of the residual seminal fluid, but this is simply the remainder of the fluid and a few dead and dying sperm. The active sperm – the strong swimmers – will already be well on their way through the cervix at this stage, so don't be concerned about this 'flow-back'. You will increase your chances of pregnancy by doing at least two, and preferably three to five, inseminations during your cycle, targeting the most fertile time.

A word of caution about self-insemination: when clinics are doing IUI (intrauterine insemination) for single or lesbian women, donor sperm is always quarantined for six months to ensure it is free from infections such as HIV. The regulations behind sperm donation are very strict, and both the donor and the recipient will be expected to attend counselling to consider the implications of the donation for themselves, their family and any child born as a result of the dona-tion. If you do not have a regular partner and are considering self-insemination using a male friend, for example, you are poten-tially exposing yourself (and a future baby) to the risk of infections including HIV, so it is really important to ensure that the donor has had a full sexual health screen. Remember, though, that even if he has a clean bill of health today, this is not necessarily enough – all infec-tions have an incubation period so if he has picked up an infection in the previous few months, it will not yet show up on any screening test. This is where trust is a major issue (for both of you).

A Woman's Age

A woman's chronological age is the key factor determining her fertility potential. Women are born with their full supply of eggs and so their ovarian reserve is pre-determined at birth. There is also a possible genetic link, so it is useful to know how old your mother was when she had her menopause. The word 'menopause' literally means cessation of periods and the key issue here is that fertility stops up to 10 years before the last period. So, if your mother had her last period at 51 (the average age for menopause) then she would very likely have been unable to conceive after about 41. Clearly this is a very general figure and there will be many variables. If, of course, you were trying to avoid getting pregnant then it would be important to use contraception for one to two years after your last period, depending on your age, to avoid any risk of unintended pregnancy. This dichotomy causes great confusion.

There are a number of tests available that can assess a woman's ovarian reserve and fertility potential (see pages 47 and 48, and Chapter 9).

25 to 34

Women aged 25 to 34 generally come to my clinic for a pre-conception or fertility health check; they need guidance and reassurance that everything is okay. The majority have just come off the Pill and need a greater understanding of their menstrual cycles and fertility. Further investigations may be needed, such as blood tests and scans, depending on the individual and their history. This group is sometimes not taken seriously by doctors and told to go away and try for a year or so. The fact that they are young is a good thing, but equally they have chosen to have their babies early and should be taken seriously. Women younger than 25 who are having trouble conceiving can often have an even more difficult time getting heard. Of course they have time on their side, but the waiting can still be very difficult.

35 to 44

Women aged 35 to 44 don't need to be told that their age is a factor. The majority of women I see haven't 'left it too late'; they just haven't met anybody or been in the right situation for a pregnancy to happen. Women differ biologically: one woman at 40 could have the eggs of a woman of 35, and another woman at 35 could have the eggs of a 40-year-old. We know that there is a decline in egg quality at around 37 years. Despite women looking so fantastic today for their age, their eggs are still ageing. Many women look at me and say, 'Well, I look so young for my age that my eggs must be in good shape too,' but that, sadly, is simply not the case.

When women are older, their cycles are likely to be more irregular, and ovulation occurs less frequently. There is reduced blood supply, reduced quality and quantity of secretions, possibly less frequent intercourse and increased vaginal dryness. There is also an increased rate of miscarriage. This is why women should not waste time. I always try to get women to think ahead about how many children they want. If it is two, you should be starting much earlier if you can, especially if your mother had an early menopause. If you are over 35, make sure you have seen your GP. I do a lot of work with this group of women. They need to feel that they are being proactive and doing everything they can to make it happen.

If you have been trying for six months or longer you should move on to investigations. It is very important that you put yourselves in the hands of someone who will look at all aspects of your lifestyle and fertility. I see and support many women over 40 and help them to optimise their chances naturally and with IVF.

45 and Older

Some women will get pregnant at 45, but the numbers are very, very few, and the miscarriage rate is extremely high. There is, however, a good chance of a woman this age getting pregnant if she uses egg donation using a younger woman's eggs. Many women do this very successfully (see page 451).

Home Tests for Fertility

There is a range of fertility tests which can now be done at home for women and men. While this may be a good thing, the downside is that a negative result can cause unnecessary anxiety. The positive side to home testing is that it can make you take action sooner rather than later. Bear in mind, though, that these tests cannot rule out underlying problems; they only tell you part of the picture.

Ovulation Predictor Kits

The most commonly used home tests are ovulation predictor kits. These kits detect a surge in luteinising hormone (see page 29), giving a positive reading when this is above a critical threshold. Usually there will be a series of negative tests and then one or two days of positive tests (when the hormone level is high) followed by more negative tests. The problem with ovulation predictor kits is that they identify only a very short window of fertility. Although they may pinpoint the two days with the highest probability of conception, limiting sex to those days potentially reduces your chances of conceiving. This is because the fertile window lasts from five days before ovulation to the day of ovulation itself, so in effect you are potentially losing out on chances on these other days.

Ovulation normally occurs about 36 hours after a surge in luteinising hormone. However, not all women will be able to identify a pre-ovulation surge. It is very short-lived and, as the tests are done only every 24 hours, it is possible to miss the surge if it occurs between one test and the next. Some kits only have five test sticks, while others have seven which may give a better chance of detecting the surge. Some women with hormone imbalances, such as PCOS (see pages 176 and 251), may have high background levels of luteinising hormone so these tests may only give positive results and will not be reliable. If you do one of these tests and never get a negative result, see your doctor for further investigations.

Women often get very confused by the ovulation predictor tests. A surge in luteinising hormone does not necessarily mean that ovulation will follow. LH is a trigger hormone, and the trigger may not necessarily fire the desired response of maturing and releasing the egg, so although it is a good sign to see an LH surge it does not prove that ovulation occurred.

Fertility Monitors – to Identify the Fertile Time

The Clearblue fertility monitor is a hand-held battery-powered personal monitor combined with disposable urine test sticks which tracks two hormones, oestrogen and LH. It is more useful because it is designed to identify the full width of the fertile window. The monitor tells you which days to use the test sticks and then records the information. It provides information on low, high or peak days of fertility on a digital screen. A Clearblue survey of 2,000 women revealed that two out of three women in the UK don't recognise that there is only a very short window of fertility, wrongly believing that they can get pregnant at any time of the cycle. Some women will find a fertility monitor useful if they are unable to identify their own natural signs of fertility, but the downside is the initial cost of the monitor and ongoing cost of test sticks.

Other 'Gizmos'

There are a multitude of fertility gizmos widely available to help women to find their fertile time. Sadly, many women often feel compelled to buy these things in a quest to get pregnant. The main thing to remember is that many of these gadgets have not been subjected to rigorous clinical trials and so their reliability should always be questioned.

There are a number of computerised thermometers on the market which rely on a daily temperature reading. However, as discussed earlier, the temperature rise is not observable until at least 24 hours after ovulation, by which time it is usually too late for conception. Although some of these products may have useful features, clear displays and sometimes a means to input other data such as changes in cervical secretions, they are still working on secondary indicators and don't really do anything that you could not do with an ordinary digital thermometer and a paper graph.

There is a new fertility monitor which uses a sensor (stick-on patch) which continually measures your body temperature. It then uses a hand-held reader to read the data from the patch. The information regarding your fertility level is read from the reader or, as with other devices, can be input into your computer.

Some home kits analyse saliva. This works on the principle that saliva has similar properties to cervical secretions producing a 'ferning' effect when dried and viewed through a microscope. Historically, the ferning effect was used in fertility clinics as part of the investigation process, providing a kind of cervical scoring system, but this is rarely used now as more sophisticated testing and scans are available.

It is important to realise that these saliva tests have not been subjected to clinical trials and cannot reliably identify the fertile time. In one study, published in *The Lancet*, 10 men all tested positive for ovulation with the use of a saliva test. So, I think this really speaks for itself.

You will always read lots of 'success stories' for the various gizmos, but if you are aware of your own fertility indicators, it is debatable whether they add anything to your own assessment which is cost-free. One of the most common mistakes women make when trying to conceive is to focus purely on their own cycle and try and pinpoint the time of ovulation. Remember, it is frequent sex with fresh healthy sperm that is the key to achieving conception. If you turn your bedroom into a laboratory and wait for the tests to go positive you are not only potentially missing out on the full fertile window, but you are not doing yourself, or your relationship, any favours.

Hair Analysis – for Testing for 'Fitness to Conceive'

Hair analysis involves the chemical testing of a sample of hair. It is widely used in forensic science and for testing for illicit drug use, because hair retains substances long after they would have been eliminated from the urine or bloodstream. The use of hair mineral analysis testing for environmental toxins in fertility is controversial. Although some complementary therapists may use these tests, it is not something that we use at the clinic. Indeed, we frequently see women who have had their hair analysed through another clinic or even through a postal service. They are often very anxious and confused when they get the results back. Hair is not a reliable substance to analyse as it is affected by so many different things, such as hair dye, chlorine and pollution.

Home Tests for Checking Female Hormone Levels (and Sperm)

Over-the-counter tests are available to test female hormones such as FSH. A urine test is usually done on Day 3 of the cycle and the results show a single red line if the test is normal (below 10) and a second red line if the test is abnormal (above 10). Although you may be reassured by a normal reading, it is really important to remember that this test is for a single hormone only and there are many other factors that can affect your chances of pregnancy, such as blocked tubes (see Chapter 9). Even if the test result is normal, women over 35 should not delay in seeking medical help. It is also important to realise that many IVF clinics will not treat women with an FSH above 10, so the threshold for this test is very low, and it is possible for your level to read 'normal' when in fact it is critically close to 10.

Some test kits include a male test which is a very basic test checking the concentration of motile sperm (see page 270). We often see men who have tested negative with such a test and then want to go on and do a more comprehensive test, so the test may initiate further action, but I have concerns about men (and women) feeling falsely reassured by these home testing kits.

Home Tests for Predicting Ovarian Reserve

PlanAhead is a mail order service developed by Professor William Ledger at Sheffield University, where you get a blood sample taken by your GP or practice nurse, then send it off to a lab. Your results are sent to you by post within 21 days. The test kit checks for FSH, AMH (see overleaf and Chapter 11) and another hormone called Inhibin B. Together these hormone profiles are plotted on a graph against the average ovarian reserve for your age. As ever, this can be very reassuring if your results indicate all is well, but remember it does not test for any other causes of fertility delays. If the result shows that you have an issue with your ovarian reserve, it can be really useful to do this test as a wake-up call that you may need to investigate further. There is a helpline attached to this service, which is designed to support women with low results and to discuss the next steps. You must have stopped taking the Pill for at least a month before doing this test and, if you have PCOS (see pages 176 and 251), the results might not be accurate.

Fertility MOT

We increasingly see women at the clinic who want to do a Fertility 'MOT' to get an idea of their fertility potential. This is often women around 30-plus who feel that having a family is really important for them, but they may not have found the right man. A key part of our MOT service is the Anti-mullerian Hormone (AMH) Test and possibly an antral follicle count.

Anti-mullerian Hormone (AMH) Test

AMH is a substance produced by the ovaries. The level of AMH correlates to ovarian reserve, which declines with age. This test can be used in combination with an ultrasound scan measuring antral follicles (see opposite). IVF clinics are now using this test to give them an idea about how a woman will respond to IVF treatment and how many eggs she is likely to produce. This test tells us about the egg reserves but not the quality.

- An AMH test does not give an indication about whether or not a woman is ovulating or whether her tubes are patent (clear/open).
- If you are on the Pill you will need to allow at least one cycle after stopping the Pill before taking an AMH test.
- The main use of AMH testing is as a predictor of how well a woman is likely to respond to IVF drugs, and many clinics are now using this test in this way. Although it may give some indication of your natural fertility potential, there has not been enough research into this and we have seen women with extremely low levels (almost off the bottom of the scale) getting pregnant naturally. As ever, the woman's chronological age is still the most significant factor.

Antral Follicle Count

This is an ultrasound scanning test. Antral follicles are small resting follicles on the ovary, about 2–8mm in diameter. The antral follicle count can be used, alongside the AMH blood test (see above), to estimate your ovarian reserve. The number of follicles you have on both ovaries is indicative of your ovarian reserve. So, the more visible follicles, the more eggs you are likely to have. This test, used alongside the AMH test, also gives a useful indication of how well you are likely to respond to IVF treatment.

The level of testing which is included as part of a Fertility MOT check can vary from finding out your egg reserve and, if you have a partner testing his sperm, to ultrasound scans, having your tubes checked and a full sexual health screen. I think it is important to consider your individual circumstances and remember that for every test there is a result. If you have not got a partner and the test comes back low it can feel very dismal and send you into a panic. Also, your result may be really good, but that doesn't rule out any underlying problems that may happen later on: it only tells you part of the picture. Having said this, I understand that many women do want to get an idea of their fertility potential.

A good Fertility MOT or Health Check should also include discussion about the relevance of:
- A blood test to check for rubella (German measles) antibodies
- Cervical smear
- Fertility infection screen
- Blood pressure and urine test
- The importance of folic acid to prevent neural tube defects such as spina bifida
- Good nutrition to optimise the health of a future baby

The crucial thing about doing any fertility test is that you may need support in interpreting the results and planning the way forward. For some women it may be appropriate to consider prioritising pregnancy, even consider egg freezing or moving to a more assisted route sooner rather than later.

So far this chapter has focused on normal fertility and optimising conception for couples trying to conceive their first baby. But at times couples will conceive very easily (often unintentionally or when least expecting it) and may then have difficulties getting pregnant again. The following section focuses on issues which are relevant for couples with secondary fertility problems.

Secondary Fertility Problems

Many women who have had one baby find it difficult to get pregnant the second time around. This topic is rarely discussed in either social or medical circles. Victoria Lambert vividly described the emotional pain of secondary infertility in her article 'One is not enough' (*Telegraph Magazine*, 4 April 2009). She writes very sensitively about the huge guilt behind wanting another child when other women can only dream of having one:

> 'For those of us who suffer – and we are a growing number – it is a very real and devastating condition. Typically we feel guilty that our one, always beloved child, is not enough. We feel frustrated at our own bodies and relationships because something we achieved once cannot be repeated.'

If you have one child you seem to be surrounded by other mothers with double buggies, you may have a toddler who is demanding a baby brother or sister. Other people may ask you when you are going to have your next one, or make insensitive comments about the negative impact of having an only child. Most women do not expect any sympathy or understanding from family or friends as they feel they should be content with the child they have.

Women usually have an idea of how many children they want. Whether this is two, four or more children, that is their choice and they should not be judged. Some women feel that there is another baby 'waiting to come', and cannot rest or feel settled unless that happens. The need to provide a sibling for their existing child can be very strong. There can be a sense of not wanting the child to grow up alone, and a real fear of the child being left alone after their own death. This might be of particular concern for women who were an only child themselves and have had to cope with the intense isolation of the loss of a parent.

I try to help women with the concept of 'the gap'. So many women feel anxious about the age gap and are concerned about having more than two or three years between children. The concept of what constitutes a family and desirable child spacing is often fundamental to the way we are brought up, and this often needs to be explored. It may help to talk to a fertility counsellor to try and sort out some of your emotions about the need for a second child and your anticipated sense of fulfilment.

Many couples who conceived easily the first time will be quite shocked when they have difficulties conceiving again. It can be even more difficult if you have intentionally delayed the second child expecting it to happen again pretty quickly. Sadly, age is often the biggest factor. Women who are older (in their mid-30s) when they have their first baby really need to get on and have a second baby within a reasonable time-frame.

Secondary Infertility Checklist

	Yes	No
Has anything changed significantly, medically or health-wise, since your first child?		
Have you completely stopped breast-feeding and have your breasts returned to normal (see below)?		
Have your cycles changed since your first child?		
Has your weight changed considerably since you conceived before?		
Have you seen your doctor for tests (see below)?		

Initial Tests

Your doctor can organise tests to help identify why you are not conceiving. He or she can check your hormones to see if you are ovulating. You might also consider an AMH test (see page 48). Blood tests can rule out thyroid problems (see page 247) or anaemia (see page 250). A pelvic scan can also be useful as infections are not uncommon following the birth of the first child. The scan will also check for other problems such as fibroids (see page 258). After your partner has had a sperm test, your doctor might also want to check your tubes. A sperm test is really important, even if your partner has recently fathered a child, as sperm parameters can change very dramatically, sometimes without any warning signs, such as serious illness.

Return of Fertility after Childbirth and Breast-feeding

- The breast-feeding hormone prolactin suppresses ovulation.
- It can take a while for full ovulatory cycles to return after breast-feeding.
- A 'period' does not necessarily confirm that ovulation is occurring.
- If you are trying for a second or subsequent baby and are still breast-feeding, even small amounts, then you may need to stop feeding completely.
- The breasts should return to normal – feeling soft again with no leakage.
- If you still notice any leakage from your breasts, then do see your doctor as this could be reducing your fertility potential.
- Remember, any breast stimulation – even from a partner – will encourage the hormonal changes leading to milk production, so avoid any breast stimulation to allow the breasts time to dry up completely.

How You Can Help Yourself Conceive Again

Start with a big bit of paper. Make a plan of the changes you can make over the next three months. These could include:

- making quality time for each other
- trying to get back to the fun sex you were having before the baby came along
- planning evenings out together – and maybe a weekend away (without the baby!)
- finishing work earlier
- finding something you can do to relax, such as a weekly massage, facial or acupuncture session
- making time to nourish yourself and eat well

Try and look for the positive things in your life first rather than focusing on possible medical issues. If you are not pregnant after three to six months of passionate sex and making some positive changes in your life, then start to look at some of the other medical tests and, if necessary, consider a more assisted route.

It is not uncommon for couples to need assistance with a second pregnancy, sometimes in the form of IVF. Going through an IVF cycle (see Chapter 12) can be difficult with a small child around, so it is really important to think through the logistics of this. You will need appropriate childcare so you can be as calm and rested as possible while going through a cycle.

Chapter 3

A Man's Fertility

Introduction by Zita West

I am indebted to Dr Sheryl Homa for writing this chapter. Sheryl is a clinical embryologist and scientist who heads up the male fertility programme at the Zita West Clinic. Here she echoes the voices of so many men: 'What about the boys?' It is recognised that there is a male factor involved in up to half of fertility problems and yet male reproductive health is often under-investigated. As Sheryl writes, she tends to see it 'from the bloke's side', but here she clearly demonstrates that although male fertility has been revolutionised by ICSI (intracytoplasmic sperm injection, see page 336), there is more to it than simply counting the number of wriggling sperm.

Male infertility represents one of the largest known causes of infertility. We are now aware that almost 50 per cent of all cases of infertility are associated with a male factor. Many people find this fact surprising as, throughout the generations, we have been led to believe that fertility is a 'woman's problem'. This myth is still perpetuated in some circles by clinicians and patients alike, which can make it difficult to identify the cause of the problem and for men to accept it and deal with it when it has been recognised.

Many men discount the need for investigating themselves. I believe one reason for this is that some men are secretly terrified that there may be a problem and that they will not be able to deal with the consequences. However, burying your head in the sand will not make the problem go away – it is far better to be proactive because it may be the only way you will achieve a pregnancy with your partner. Other reasons are based on the misconception that a man who has fathered a child before has already proven his fertility. Although he has obviously proved his fertility at the time of those conceptions, circumstances may well have changed since then, and his sperm quality may have significantly deteriorated.

It is important to have a diagnosis early on so that you can get on with the process of trying to improve your reproductive health as soon as possible (see Chapter 10) and do not waste any precious time. The good news is that with the state-of-the-art treatments currently available, even the most severe cases of male fertility can often be treated quite effectively, whereas in the past these men could only resort to sperm donation.

Causes of Male Infertility

Poor Sperm Quality

The single most important factor determining a man's fertility potential is the production of healthy sperm. In order to impregnate a woman naturally, a man needs to produce sperm that are capable of finding their way to the egg and fertilising it when it gets there. To do this, sperm need to be produced in sufficient numbers and quality. If the production of healthy sperm is compromised in any way, then this may affect fertility. While in the majority of cases, the cause of poor sperm quality is not known (idiopathic), more and more evidence is coming to light to show that there are plenty of ways in which sperm quality may be improved.

Defective sperm may be due to inherited conditions, defects that are present at birth, a hormone imbalance, damage to the testicles or lower abdomen, exposure to harmful chemicals or drugs and a poor lifestyle. We often hear that there is nothing much that can be done for male infertility. While it is true that a man cannot change his genetic constitution or repair damage to the testicular region, some medical conditions can be treated. This is why I believe men with a fertility problem should be assessed by a specialist andrologist or a urologist with an interest in fertility before they are sent off for IVF treatment (see interview with Mr Hirsh, page 69).

All men can certainly address their lifestyle, which may be the only cause of infertility in some cases. Even if there are factors that cannot be corrected, you should not be making a bad situation worse by compromising your sperm further with a poor lifestyle. Doing all you can to try to improve your sperm health may make all the difference to being able to father a child naturally.

Do not give up if you are diagnosed as 'infertile'. This term is not strictly correct, as it implies that you are unable to achieve a pregnancy with your partner. This is true only for men who are actually sterile, that is, men who cannot produce any sperm at all. Men who have poor sperm quality are really 'subfertile' – in other words, they are less likely to achieve a natural pregnancy with their partner. Obviously, the worse your sperm quality, the less likely pregnancy is to occur; and realistically, if your sperm are exceptionally poor, your chances of a natural pregnancy may be negligible.

Physical Abnormalities

Sometimes structural blockages occur. These obstructions can be present from birth (congenital) such as absence of the vas deferens, which are the tubes that carry the sperm out of the testicles. Sometimes, obstructions may develop later in life, such as from an infection. Another congenital physical defect is undescended testicles, which may result in permanent damage to them if not corrected by surgery early on. Hypospadias is a congenital condition where the opening of the urethra is on the underside of the penis instead of at the end. This quite rare condition can occasionally cause infertility because it is more difficult to deposit the sperm high up in the vagina. It is easily corrected by surgery.

Varicocoele

One of the most common anatomical defects is varicocoele, a group of dilated or varicose veins in the scrotum. Some varicocoeles are more prominent than others. They slow down the flow of blood around the testicle, causing the temperature of the testicle to rise and thus creating problems with sperm formation. Not all men with varicocoele are infertile. However, if you have poor sperm quality and you have a varicocoele it is quite likely that this is a major cause of your problems. Some clinics use surgery to correct varicocoele, but because the benefits are controversial, it is not always recommended and men may be advised to go direct to IVF or ICSI.

Infection

There is increasing evidence that infection can have a considerable impact on male fertility. Infection may trigger immunological infertility and cause oxidative stress (see Chapter 10) which then results in poor sperm function and sperm DNA damage. This in turn decreases your partner's chances of conception and increases the rate of miscarriage. In extreme cases, it can permanently damage the reproductive system and cause obstruction. Importantly, infections in men can cause infertility in their partners if transmitted (see more on infections in Chapter 10).

Prostatitis

Prostatitis is an inflammation of the prostate gland. It is quite common – as many as one in two men will have prostate problems at some point in their life – and it may affect fertility because of infection and inflammation. Cells produced as part of an inflammatory process may cause free radical damage to the sperm (see Oxidative Stress, page 282). Symptoms include increased urination, discomfort and aches and pains in the testicles. The condition needs to be treated by a specialist urologist.

Erectile Dysfunction

Erectile dysfunction refers to problems in achieving and sustaining an erection. There are many causes of erectile dysfunction: physical, structural, medical (such as diabetes) and psychological. Stress is a common culprit. When men are feeling stressed, their testosterone levels can drop, affecting their ability to maintain an erection. Pressure and stress can therefore have a major impact on a couple's sex life, and the severity of the problem depends on the root cause. Some younger men take Viagra while trying for a baby, a drug that was designed for older men with erection problems. They need reassurance that the problem is common and transient and, once the pressure is off, their libido and erectile function will return. I often find that,

Case Study

Alice and Simon had never had a very active sex life but were happy together. Alice was 38 and they had been trying for a baby for 18 months. They found that the pressure of trying for a baby was really affecting the sex that they were having. Even with the use of Viagra they were achieving sex only about twice a month around the fertile time. They had gone for couples counselling and to Relate to try and sort out their sexual problems. Simon had issues from his childhood that he found hard to discuss openly. He felt a failure and that he had let down his wife because he couldn't fully communicate his feelings. He was also starting to fail at work because he felt she might leave him as they couldn't have a baby.

This couple needed the pressure taking off them. They had spent long enough trying to sort out their sex life, which was a really deep issue. The options we came up with were to try intrauterine insemination (IUI) for a couple of months and then move on to IVF. Sometimes you have to be realistic about what couples can achieve. In this case, moving to IVF and so not wasting valuable fertile time trying to sort out their sex life was the best option.

with guidance, couples are able to work out the issues around sex and how they can best help one another. There are many reasons for resorting to Viagra. Some sexual or performance issues go deeper than others and will need expert help or psychosexual counselling.

Although Viagra has been found to improve sperm motility it also affects the way the egg is fertilised. Studies on mice showed that fewer eggs were fertilised when Viagra was used. If you are taking Viagra look at why you are taking it and what the pressures are for you both. Is one of you pressuring the other in terms of having sex? Discuss ways in which you could get the intimacy back into your relationship. If you are having sexual difficulties, try to work out if they are temporary and linked with trying for a baby. If they are, talk about how you can take the pressure off one another. If they are not, seek help or consider an assisted conception route. I am a realist. Some things you can't fix easily, and if the lack of sex is not improving over time then it will be very difficult to conceive.

Sperm and Age

One of the most common misunderstandings is the role of age in male fertility. While we are all very much aware of the effect of age on female fertility, we do not always know that age can have consequences for men. Although a normal fertile man may be producing sperm throughout his life, the quality of that sperm has been shown to be compromised the older he becomes. Researchers who studied over 12,000 couples undergoing fertility treatment found that if the man was over 35 the chances of conception were more challenging. If he was over 40 they were significantly delayed. The study also found that the rate of miscarriage was higher. As a man ages, his sperm production is affected by a number of factors, including changing hormone levels. Genetic abnormalities in sperm become more common, and sperm numbers and function generally decline. Older men are more prone to developing unrelated medical conditions where either the condition, or the treatment for it, affects the quality of his sperm.

Understanding Male Anatomy

To get the best out of your reproductive system, it often helps to find out how it functions so that you know what to expect from it. Sometimes, your worries may be unfounded, and discovering a few simple facts about the way in which your reproductive system works may put your mind at ease.

Male Hormones

The hormones that control the male reproductive system are produced by glands in the brain. Follicle stimulating hormone (FSH) and luteinising hormone (LH) are produced by the pituitary gland in both males and females but have very different effects. In women, they act on the ovaries, stimulating follicle growth and the production of oestrogen, while in men they act on the testicles, stimulating the production of testosterone and sperm development. In a man the production of these hormones should remain relatively constant, resulting in a continuous supply of sperm.

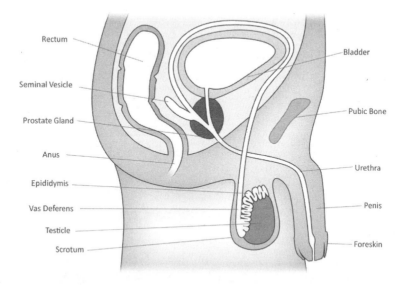

Sperm Development

The testicles (testes) are the two male reproductive glands enclosed in the scrotum. Sperm development occurs in the seminiferous tubules within the testicles. To begin with, the immature round germ cells divide, followed by a halving of the chromosome number. Continued development involves elongation of the cell, the formation of the tail and completion of the acrosome cap which constitutes about half of the head in a normal sperm. The sperm then travel into the epididymis (the coiled tubules) at the top of the scrotum where they complete their maturation, acquiring the ability to fertilise the egg. Finally, they start to move into the vas deferens, waiting to be ejaculated. It takes approximately 64 days for a mature sperm to develop from an immature sperm cell, and another 10–14 days to pass through the epididymis ready for ejaculation. Each day, some 100 million sperm are made in each human testicle, and each ejaculation releases on average around 200 million sperm.

Sperm Structure

- **Head** – this contains the genetic material (DNA). Forty to seventy per cent of the head region is covered by a cap called the acrosome. The contents of the acrosome are required for penetrating the egg.
- **Mid-piece** – this contains the energy for the sperm to move.
- **Tail** – this propels the sperm forward.

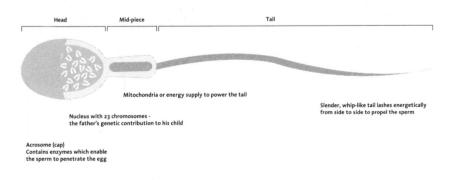

Head   Mid-piece   Tail

Mitochondria or energy supply to power the tail

Nucleus with 23 chromosomes -
the father's genetic contribution to his child

Slender, whip-like tail lashes energetically
from side to side to propel the sperm

Acrosome (cap)
Contains enzymes which enable
the sperm to penetrate the egg

Male Accessory Glands

The male accessory glands are the seminal vesicles and the prostate. At ejaculation, they expel a large amount of fluid to push the sperm through the urethra. The very first drop (2–5 per cent) of the ejaculate comes from the testicles and is the richest in sperm. This is followed by fluids from the seminal vesicles, which constitute around 65 per cent of the semen and provide fructose, the main energy source for the sperm. The last part of the ejaculate comes from the prostate. This is rich in zinc, which is required for sperm function and stabilisation of sperm DNA, the genetic material in the sperm. Prostatic fluid also contains prostaglandins which stimulate the vagina to contract at ejaculation, helping the sperm to move towards the cervix.

The pH balance of the seminal fluid (semen) is alkaline, around 7.2–8.0, which allows the sperm to function at its best. It is vital that the male accessory glands remain healthy because the fluid they produce is so important to normal sperm function. For example, an infection in either of these glands can significantly affect the quality of the semen and subsequent quality of the sperm.

Many men worry about the amount of semen they produce but the amount does not necessarily indicate whether the sperm count is high or low. On average, men produce an ejaculate of around 2–5ml. This is only a half to one teaspoonful. Men are usually surprised by this as they imagine they are producing considerably more fluid.

Ejaculation

Between 50 and 500 million sperm may be deposited in the vagina at ejaculation. The sperm then move through the semen towards the cervix. Here they have to navigate their way through the cervical mucus (secretions). This acts as a plug at the entrance to the womb for a large part of a woman's cycle. The sperm can only pass into the womb if the cervical mucus is of a thin, watery consistency, at an alkaline pH, and is not 'hostile' to the sperm. Only about 0.1 per cent of sperm ever make it through the cervical mucus.

Once they get to the womb, the sperm then have to find their way to the fallopian tubes. Most are lost in the complex glands in the cervix or the wall of the womb along the way, with only a hundred or so ever arriving at their destination. Obviously, the sperm have to be fit and healthy to make it, and the larger the number at ejaculation, the better. If sperm motility is poor or if counts are very low, then it is going to be extremely difficult for sperm to reach the egg. Sperm may take only a few minutes to reach the fallopian tubes after intercourse, but will quite happily survive here for several days.

Fertilisation

For fertilisation to take place, the sperm has to be able to recognise the egg and bind to it. When the sperm attaches to the egg, the acrosome cap opens up and substances are released which dissolve a hole through the egg surface. The sperm is then able to deposit its genetic material (DNA) into the egg. Sperm that have an abnormal shape may not be able to recognise the egg. Some sperm do not have a proper acrosomal cap, and therefore cannot get into the egg (see more on sperm shape – morphology – in Chapter 10).

Common Questions about Sperm

- *Does the amount of semen you produce affect fertility?*
Not necessarily. It is not the amount of fluid that matters. The important thing is the number and quality of the sperm within the semen. On the other hand, if the volume is consistently very low (less than 1.5ml) it may indicate an underlying problem with the male accessory glands which may need investigation.

• *Can I become infertile after having a successful vasectomy reversal?*
Yes. According to your surgeon, a 'successful' reversal means producing sperm again in your ejaculate. However, the tubes that were unblocked during the reversal to allow sperm through can close up again with time. Furthermore, any surgery to the testicles might cause the body to produce sperm antibodies, resulting in immunological infertility (see Chapter 10). For these reasons, it is always a good idea to try to freeze sperm produced after a vasectomy reversal, just in case.

• *Should we save up sperm?*
No. Sperm do not live forever, and will start to die off in the epididymis if they are not ejaculated. If you abstain from sex for long periods of time, the proportion of dead sperm will increase. As these decay, they will release toxins into the epididymis which will harm the fresh sperm moving in. Having sex at least three times a week, if possible, is a good insurance policy. If you can't have sex regularly for any reason, don't save the sperm up but masturbate to keep it moving. Many of the couples I see do not have sex in the second half of the woman's cycle; that can really make a difference to their chances of success because if the sperm are not kept moving the quality deteriorates. The only time you will be guided around having or not having sex is when you are going through IVF (see Chapter 12).

Case Study

Every month, John and Gemma had sex once when she finished her period and then nothing for days until she thought it was her fertile time. Once I explained the consequences and they changed this to making love on a regular basis, they achieved a pregnancy after three months.

- *Why do we have to make love more than once around the fertile time?*

Healthy sperm last several days inside the woman during the fertile window, but the egg lives for only 24 hours when it is ovulated. Because you cannot know exactly when your partner ovulates, you need to ensure there are plenty of sperm in the fallopian tubes to fertilise the egg when it is released.

Alert!

- Any urinary symptoms, such as pain on urination, pain at ejaculation or lower abdominal pain, could be a sign of infection. It is always a good idea to check yourself out with a full sexual health screen.
- Men should regularly examine themselves for lumps in the testicles and report any unusual lumps or pain to their GP. The top part of the testicles (the epididymis) can feel quite lumpy. This is quite normal – get to know what feels normal for you.

Zita's Tips for Improving Male Fertility

- Eat breakfast. You need a big breakfast in the morning for energy; otherwise the body is in survival mode where making healthy sperm is not a priority.
- Avoid high-protein diets. Sperm need to be nourished on their journey to the egg and protected from the acidic environment of the woman's vagina. High-protein diets will make the sperm very acidic.
- Try acupuncture. Some studies (although small) have shown that it may help with motility (movement) of the sperm.

How to Increase Chances of Conception in Your Partner

1. The good news first – have lots of sex. Forget about the big focus on her 'fertile' time. You need to be having sex at least every two or three days. You do *not* need to 'save up the sperm'. The key thing is to make sure there is a good supply of fresh, healthy sperm at the ready. You can have a break at the end of her cycle after her most fertile time is over, but if you have a long gap (more than five days) without ejaculating, the sperm quality may start to decline, and it takes at least two ejaculations to clear out the old sperm. So if you or your partner prefer not to have intercourse during her period, just make sure you keep the supply going.

2. Give up smoking – it can affect the count, motility and shape of the sperm, but most importantly, it damages the sperm DNA and passes on a risk of cancer to your child.

3. Avoid recreational drugs, as these can affect sperm quality.

4. Keep alcohol to a minimum – try and give up the beer and keep to just an occasional glass of wine; red is best for its antioxidants. Alcohol affects sperm DNA and can increase both the time it takes to conceive and the risk of miscarriage.

5. Keep your caffeine intake down. This includes fizzy drinks such as colas. Caffeine affects sperm quality and can increase genetic damage in sperm.

6. Do not over-exercise – this can divert testosterone away from your testicles and your sperm count will drop.

7. Keep your testicles cool – sperm development occurs at temperatures three to four degrees cooler than body temperature, but this does *not* mean keeping a bottle of iced water between your legs!

8. Eat well – include lots of vegetables and fruit in your diet and take a good multi-vitamin and mineral supplement.
9. Arrange a sexual health check-up.
10. Have your sperm checked at an accredited andrology lab (see Chapter 10).
11. Reduce your stress levels.
12. Support your partner – remember you're in this together!

Interview with Mr Anthony Hirsh, a surgeon specialising in male fertility disorders

Anthony Hirsh is a Consultant in Andrology to Whipps Cross and Homerton Hospitals London and Bourn Hall Clinic Cambridge, and is Honorary Senior Lecturer at Guy's and St Thomas' Hospitals. He was a member of the Development Group for the NICE Fertility Guidelines in 2004.

How important is the male factor in fertility?
Abnormal semen quality is the largest single cause of human sub-fertility. I feel it is important that sub-fertile men are seen, examined and appropriately tested – they are not just sperm providers, they are also patients. We need to ensure the man ejaculates frequently – couples need to make love every couple of days throughout the woman's cycle for their best chance of conceiving naturally. We should help men to improve their lifestyle, and exclude any infections or testicular problems (such as lumps which could include early tumours). If a comprehensive sperm test is normal, he is more likely to be okay.

If a man has impaired semen quality, even a very low count, the couple could still conceive naturally if their trying time is under a year and intercourse is frequent, provided his partner is fertile.

If a man has borderline semen parameters, I screen for a low grade infection and, in some cases, antibiotics can tip the balance to favour an earlier conception. Some 10 per cent of men have inflammation of the prostate gland (prostatitis) causing pain or urinary symptoms that may also require treatment.

What is the cause of male factor infertility?

We don't know in most cases. I am on the lookout for the 2 per cent we can cure, who have a sperm blockage, deficiency of pituitary hormones or retrograde ejaculation, where semen passes backwards into the bladder during intercourse. Most sub-fertile men have a reduced sperm count, with weaker movement (motility) and abnormal structure (morphology). So the delay in conception is not just about sperm numbers, it is likely to be a quality issue we call 'sperm dysfunction', reducing the sperm's ability to fertilise the egg.

There are many possible causes of sperm dysfunction but we don't always know why. Lifestyle may seriously affect sperm, although it doesn't always affect normal sperm producers – one of my patients drank a bottle of whisky a day and his sperm count was 200 million! But if the count is low this is more sensitive to lifestyle factors. If the count is zero (azoospermia) due to testicular failure, stopping alcohol for three months leads to live sperm re-appearing in the semen in 5–10 per cent of men and can avoid an operation to extract sperm. So I will always recommend stopping alcohol as a first measure. Smoking and obesity have also been shown to have adverse effects on male fertility.

Can antioxidants help sperm quality?

There is emerging evidence. Antioxidants (usually vitamins E and C, and selenium) may improve the sperm quality and increase the chance of natural or assisted conception. I use antioxidants in my practice if the semen quality is poor. Antioxidants remove oxygen molecules (free radicals) that damage sperm and particularly sperm DNA. However, sperm do need some free radicals to trigger their ability to move and fertilise the egg, so the antioxidant dosage for treatment needs to be appropriate.

In your experience, have you noticed any changes in the sperm results of your patients?
Thirty years ago it wasn't unusual to see sperm counts of 120 to 150 million. Counts have come down over the years, but not necessarily men's fertility potential. We suspect this reduction may be due to environmental oestrogens and there is scientific proof of this from some countries. However, it is also possible we are more accurate at counting sperm today due to improved technical methods.

How much do you feel male sub-fertility is related to genetics?
Sub-fertility affects 5 per cent of men and it is usually a sperm problem. I do not feel it is genetic in most cases, as we might then have an epidemic of male infertility and it could not then be passed down the generations. Only about 8 per cent of the men who have severely low sperm counts will have Y chromosome deletions. This is where tiny areas of the Y (male) chromosome are missing. These missing areas contain the genes that code for sperm development. Some men are poor sperm producers with slightly smaller testes, but usually no indication of a genetic cause or a disease process and they are unlikely to develop testosterone deficiency. Any transient sexual problems are mostly due to anxiety but, as ever, it is important that this is appropriately investigated as there are also physical causes for sexual difficulties.

Where do you see male factor fertility going in the next five to ten years?
I see much work in the future into antioxidants and sperm DNA damage. If we look back, around 30 years, when the same proportion

of sub-fertile men (2 per cent) was curable, the vast majority of infertile couples required donor sperm insemination (DI) to conceive. DI is now only required for the 1 in 200 couples where the man has no sperm. We now refer couples with male factor sub-fertility for ICSI so they can have their own biological children. But we are still no closer to understanding the causes of male fertility problems in most cases. We require new sperm function tests to determine whether male sub-fertility is likely to be increasing.

Chapter 4

Could Your Lifestyle Be Affecting Your Fertility?

Fertility is a whole-body event. Couples trying for a baby are usually aware that some of their lifestyle choices may affect their chances of conception or a successful IVF outcome. However, lifestyle is not only about what you eat, drink and smoke; it covers everything. It's about the work/life balance, sleep, stress and diet, and the dynamic of your relationship: all can have negative impacts on the body by causing stress. Lifestyle is one area that causes a lot of tension between couples and can put pressure on the relationship.

Work/Life Balance

The work/life balance comes up more and more in consultations. This balance can be elusive, especially when couples are going through, or preparing for, IVF. So many of the women I see are building their careers. If they are in their late 30s or early 40s then they are usually career women at the top of the ladder with their diaries booked out weeks or months in advance. If your partner is also busy then diary co-ordinating becomes a huge issue. Often, part of our work includes just helping couples to plan things in a bite-sized, manageable way. It is important to look at the overall picture for each couple and to show them how they can seize back some time to feel ready for what lies ahead. Many women don't seem to have time or space in their lives for a baby.

When one of my clients gets pregnant after trying for a while, I always ask the couple what they thought made the difference. Many tell me that they simply slowed down, relaxed and made more time for themselves.

Stress

Trying for a baby naturally or having IVF treatment can be an emotionally draining experience. On top of this, coping with the normal stresses and strains of everyday life can be difficult and tiring, and get you down on every level. Many of the couples I see work long hours and are low in energy. Others have the added pressure of major upheavals, such as moving house or having building work done. A large part of my work with couples involves building up their reserves and conserving their energy, helping them to achieve a good work/life balance.

The menstrual cycle is a complex interplay of hormones; all need to be released at the right level at the right time to produce a healthy, mature egg. When the body has additional psychological and emotional stress it influences the production of hormones. Long-term stress raises levels of the stress hormones, including cortisol, which interfere with the reproductive hormones. The hormone prolactin, also raised with stress, can suppress ovulation and can create a loss of libido in women. The body's automatic 'fight or flight' response to stress is to go into survival mode; reproductive processes are effectively superfluous as they consume too much energy, so blood flow is directed away from the pelvic organs to more vital areas for survival.

I am frequently asked, 'Will my IVF not work because I am stressed?' Or 'Will stress stop me getting pregnant?' Although I do think that stress causes difficulties conceiving, you can learn to let go by practising relaxation techniques. At the clinic we use relaxation training, hypnotherapy, visualisation and breathing techniques. We also have a Manage Your Mind programme which may include cognitive behavioural therapy.

Feeling anxious and stressed about getting pregnant or whether IVF will work can exacerbate life's day-to-day stresses. Messages from the hypothalamus affect the autonomic nervous system, which is in two parts:

- the sympathetic nervous system: when you are stressed this kicks into action and increases cortisol – one of the stress hormones – which affects the ovaries and reproduction.
- the parasympathetic nervous system: when you are feeling calm, relaxed and in control this is turned on. This state of calm is more conducive to helping you reduce your FSH levels, for example (see page 23). Getting the parasympathetic nervous system into action requires practise of relaxation techniques.

'Man Stress'

When a couple is trying for a baby or going through IVF treatment, the man tends to invest a huge amount of energy into reassuring his partner that everything will be okay. Sometimes it can be difficult for men to express their own feelings as they worry about saying the wrong thing and upsetting their partner.

If a man is under pressure or stress, it will affect his hormones. Levels of the hormones needed for sperm production can be reduced (for more on male hormones, see Chapter 3). For many men – under strict orders to time sex to the 'right' time and in the 'right' position – there will be the inevitable 'performance anxiety' at some stage, which is actually a lot more common than people think. The additional problem of not being able to get or maintain an erection, or having difficulty ejaculating because of the pressure, is usually short-lived, but some men may need help to get through it (see Chapter 3).

'Woman Stress'

The worst thing you can say to a woman who is trying for a baby or going through IVF is, 'You are too stressed. Relax and it will happen.' It is next to impossible to relax when going through the uncertainty of IVF. Negative thoughts and emotions, such as guilt, worry and fear, are buried in our subconscious minds and do cause stress, especially when trying for a baby. Women question every single thing about themselves: 'Why, why, why isn't it working?' 'Is it because I did this?' 'Is it because I had a cup of coffee?' I often find that while women are great at sorting out the home and finances and so on, they find it more difficult to manage their emotions. They also tend to exercise to wind down, and while exercise is good and can help to reduce stress levels, it is not the same as true relaxation as you are still active.

IVF treatment can be incredibly stressful – going to consultations, waiting for scans, having bloods taken, hearing bad news, trying to work and live your life. Some studies show that if women are really stressed it can affect the outcome of IVF, but the jury is still out on this, as in other studies stress did not appear to impact IVF outcome.

Reading this I don't want you to panic: the answer is to practise, practise, practise relaxation techniques (see below).

Reducing Stress

Dealing with stress is a personal thing, but when the key stressor is fertility, there are some specific techniques I find useful (see Chapter 5). Women who are not conceiving or who receive poor test results experience a lot of anxiety. Many feel their lives are on hold, and that once they have got through the next cycle they will start to relax and

---

Get the Balance Right – Finding the Middle Ground

Most couples I see have done everything they can to try for a baby. For some, the main struggle is about balance and moderation: trying not to let their wish for a baby take over their lives. For example, in some couples the woman restricts her diet in the belief that this will help her fertility. I've seen women who deny themselves all treats, cutting out wheat, dairy, sugar – everything! Sometimes her partner joins her, which often makes them both miserable; and if he doesn't do anything to change his diet, this can cause friction and arguments. Couples sometimes stop going out to eat because they are frightened that the restaurant food might contain too much salt or other 'banned' ingredients. Friendships are often compromised when couples decide not to mix with friends who have babies. Such attitudes may sound extreme but I commonly encounter them in couples. I am not here to judge but I do want to offer support and advice and help couples change their lives for the better. Sometimes a couple needs to relax, to have a meal out and a glass of wine without feeling guilty, especially if they have been trying for a long time.

do something different. Many also feel that they have to learn to relax to get pregnant. I try to encourage them to let go on some level because that's when the shift happens for so many of the women I see. We look at diet and use techniques including visualisation and acupuncture (see Chapter 8), which has been shown to help release feel-good endorphins and increase blood flow to the pelvic organs.

I often ask clients what they do to relax. Watching television, exercising and having a bath are popular responses. Total relaxation – being able to stop and calm the mind – is a skill you have to learn. You also need to conserve energy – mentally, physically and emotionally. Relaxation counteracts negative feelings, thoughts and emotions, all of which can play havoc with reproductive hormones. Practising a relaxation technique for just 20 minutes a day will have huge benefits of feeling in control, deeply relaxed and achieving better hormonal balance.

Weight

Weighing too much, or too little, can interrupt normal menstrual cycles and disrupt or stop ovulation. Male fertility is also affected by body weight (see Chapter 7).

Being Overweight

Some studies have shown a link between being overweight and a decrease in IVF success rates. Many people find it difficult to access the right dietary information and, in their haste to lose weight, often put themselves on unhealthy regimes. There are important dietary protocols to follow with IVF and so sensitive, careful and skilled management is essential (see Chapter 7).

When a woman is overweight, excess oestrogen is stored in the fat cells. This causes hormonal imbalances that can interfere with ovulation. Being overweight is now known to be a risk factor for infertility, unsuccessful IVF cycles, miscarriage and problems in pregnancy, such as high blood pressure (pre-eclampsia) or diabetes. It can also elevate the mother's chances of needing a Caesarean section. Weight gain can indicate an underlying problem, such as thyroid or other endocrine (hormone) disorders, such as PCOS (see pages 176 and 251). The dangers of being overweight extend to a woman's baby as well. In fact, many IVF clinics will not allow a client to undertake an IVF cycle unless they have a body mass index (BMI) of below 30.

Body Mass Index (BMI)

To work out your BMI, take your height in metres squared and divide it by your weight in kilograms, or use an online BMI calculator.

Research has shown that women with a BMI higher than 25 have more problems with ovulation. It is important to remember that only small changes are needed to improve the chances of becoming pregnant. If you are overweight, a loss of 5–10 per cent can get you ovulating again.

It is also important for men who are overweight to lose excess pounds. Excess weight can affect male reproduction because a process carried out in fat cells, called aromatisation, can convert testosterone to oestrogen and affect sperm count. Even a slightly overweight man, with a BMI of more than 25, will have a 22 per cent lower sperm count. A study published in 2006 of more than 2,000 American farmers and their wives showed that fertility levels declined as BMI increased.

Moreover, obesity can lead to the development of an apron of fat around the genital area which can cause overheating of the testicles, potentially reducing sperm numbers. A sedentary lifestyle may also be a factor in semen quality so walking as much as possible, using stairs instead of lifts and incorporating some form of regular exercise may be beneficial (see below).

Being Underweight

Being underweight can also affect your health and fertility. If you are underweight, the body senses famine and the reproductive system shuts down. Underweight women might not have enough oestrogen in the body for ovulation to occur. Studies have shown that even small changes in body weight (being 5–10 per cent below ideal body weight) may be associated with alterations in the menstrual cycle and infertility, as well as causing a lack of bone density. In fact, 50 per cent of women with a BMI of 19 or below have severe menstrual irregularities. Underweight men – those with a body mass index (BMI) of less than 20 – have substantially lower fertility than men of a normal weight.

Exercise

It is important that you maintain a healthy level of exercise. Many people I see are either doing too much or too little exercise. When trying for a baby, women often don't know how much exercise they should be doing and how often. I commonly hear things like 'I used to enjoy running but I don't want to do it any more in case it's stopping me from getting pregnant'. If you enjoy running and have a certain level of fitness, keep it up. The only time I advise women to take a break is when they are actually going through an IVF cycle, which can be tiring: during the down-regulation process very often you can feel exhausted. During the stimulation part of the IVF process, the body needs all the energy it can get in order to grow plenty of follicles.

More studies need to be done in this area. The safe limit seems to be 30 minutes a day. If you are not exercising at all then build up to doing cardiovascular exercise for 30 minutes a day. If you are overweight and have PCOS (see pages 176 and 251) you will need to increase the amount you exercise to get your body fat levels into the normal range and optimise your hormonal balance.

It is important that you do exercise you enjoy, such as walking, swimming, jogging, playing tennis or badminton. It shouldn't be seen as too much of a chore because this won't help with motivation.

Benefits of Exercise

- Reduces stress levels
- Regulates blood sugar
- Promotes good blood circulation to the reproductive organs
- Lifts mood

Men and Exercise

Professor Diana Vaamonde found that high-intensity training by male triathletes significantly diminished the quality of their sperm. There appeared to be a direct correlation between intensive exercise, especially cycling, and sperm quality: the more time and distance covered the worse the sperm quality became. This could be due to localised heat, friction with the testicles against the saddle, free radical damage or compression of the penile arteries. We are not really talking here about a 30-minute cycle to work and back – the benefits of exercise generally outweigh the risks – but for men on bikes, make sure you wear padded shorts and have a good saddle with a groove or gap to reduce pressure. Male athletes should avoid high-protein diets as they are very acidic; sperm need to be nourished on their journey to reach the egg and protected from the acidic environment of the woman's vagina.

> ## — Alert! —
>
> To optimise sperm production, testicles need to be about 3 degrees centigrade below normal body temperature. So, lay off jacuzzis, steam rooms, tight boxer shorts and marathon running, i.e. avoid excessive or prolonged exposure to heat. Heat effectively 'fries' your sperm. One study showed that the heat generated by laptop processors increases scrotal temperature, and another study of taxi drivers (prolonged sitting) showed similar results.

Caffeine

Caffeine, alcohol and recreational drugs are the constant niggles that couples have between them if one partner is doing one, or all, of the above. Caffeine is an energy booster and mood enhancer that makes you feel more alert and stimulated. If you suddenly remove it from your diet you get withdrawal symptoms, such as headaches and feeling a bit jittery. Caffeine intake is a real concern for many women – it may well lower their chances of conceiving naturally or going through IVF successfully – but there is a lot of conflicting advice regarding safe levels. Caffeine also raises the risk of miscarriage, although how much is too much is still unclear. A study by the US National Institute of Child Health and Human Development published in *The New England Journal of Medicine* found that women who drank five or more caffeinated drinks a day were more than twice as likely to miscarry than those who drank less. Research also suggests caffeine may magnify the negative effects of alcohol.

The total caffeine content of the average mug of coffee will vary and remember that caffeine is present in tea and chocolate, and also in drinks like cola and energy drinks. It is also often added to many over-the-counter pain killers. If you have a high caffeine intake it is really important to cut down, but do it slowly over a few days to reduce the negative side effects, such as headaches. I don't want you to feel you have to cut out all caffeine but do try to cut down as much as you can. We generally advise balance – a cup of tea a day is fine, and maybe have a cup of coffee at the weekend if you would enjoy one, but not if you are doing IVF (see page 159).

Prescription Drugs

If you take any prescription drugs, talk to your doctor and get advice about reducing or changing them. The following have been known to reduce fertility:

- Pain medications, such as non-steroidal anti-inflammatory drugs (NSAIDs)
- Some antibiotics
- Some antidepressants
- Hormone treatments
- Chemotherapy

Recreational Drugs

Street drugs, including cocaine, heroin and ecstasy, have all been shown to have dramatic adverse effects on fertility. Long-term use of these drugs can lead to permanent reproductive problems and could prevent you from becoming pregnant. Women who use these drugs can have problems with ovulation and irregular periods. Their reserve of eggs may also be affected.

Men who smoke marijuana tend to have lower sperm counts, less seminal fluid and sperm that swim abnormally. This is one of the biggest obstacles I come up against with men. A glass of wine or the occasional beer is okay but no cigarettes (see below) and no marijuana – no compromise. It's only for a couple of months – see it like a project. Studies show that THC, the active ingredient of cannabis, messes up the timing in sperm. Usually, sperm start to swim furiously as they approach the egg but in cannabis users the sperm make a dash for the line too soon.

Men who use cocaine, heroin and ecstasy often suffer from:

- reduced libido
- abnormally shaped sperm
- poor sperm count

Smoking

Many studies show that cigarette smoking has an impact on fertility:

- Smokers take longer to conceive.
- Smoking harms the ovaries.
- Smoking accelerates the loss of eggs.

- Smoking can bring the menopause forward by several years.
- Cigarettes interfere with oestrogen production.
- Smoking lowers sperm count and impairs sperm shape and function.

If a woman smokes, her eggs are prone to genetic abnormalities. Smoking is also linked to an increased risk of miscarriage and ectopic pregnancy due to the cilia (short hair-like structures) in the fallopian tubes being affected. If you are pregnant and smoke you are more likely to have a low-birth-weight or premature baby. Smoking can deplete the body of vital nutrients, such as vitamin C, zinc and antioxidants. Vitamin C deficiency causes a reduction in progesterone; lack of zinc contributes to fertility problems and low birth weight.

Smoking while going through IVF treatment reduces the chances of success. Studies have shown that female smokers require higher doses of IVF drugs to stimulate their ovaries. They have lower oestradiol levels, and fewer oocytes (eggs) collected. Smokers have more cancelled cycles, lower implantation rates and higher rates of unsuccessful fertilisation. Add to that the increased miscarriage rate and there are more than enough reasons to stub out that cigarette. This goes for men as well as women. Some IVF clinics will not treat smokers as their chances of success will be so low.

The great thing about the body is that it is always trying to get the balance back. Studies by the American Society for Reproduction show that couples who stop smoking for at least two months before starting IVF significantly increase their chances of conception. If you need help to give up smoking, your GP is likely to have a smoking cessation clinic or you could try hypnotherapy, acupuncture or meditation. There are also organisations, such as QUIT, that can help (see Resources).

Alcohol

When it comes to alcohol, there is so much conflicting advice for couples trying to conceive and there is much we don't understand about the impact of alcohol on conception. There are two issues: the first is the potential effect on the unborn child, and the second is possible delay in time to pregnancy or reduced chances of IVF success.

One of the most frequent questions I'm asked is: 'How much is safe to drink?' The answer is we don't know. There is no known safe limit with alcohol when you are trying for a baby. The alcohol molecule is small enough to pass from mother to baby as early as two weeks after conception. We can feel the effects of tiny alcohol molecules slowly passing through membranes whenever we drink alcohol. Alcohol can affect the development of all cells and organs, but the developing foetal brain is very vulnerable causing a whole range of alcohol-related damage. The effects of foetal alcohol spectrum disorder on a child vary from a slight loss of IQ to learning difficulties and behavioural problems, through to serious brain damage and other organ damage. For this reason, a very strict no-alcohol policy is advisable during pregnancy.

Ideally you should consider not having any alcohol at all when trying to conceive – treating your body the way that you would during pregnancy. If you knew for sure that you would be pregnant in three months, then that may be achievable, but the reality is that for so many women it takes considerably longer and you really need to get on and enjoy life. If part of that fun is having a social life and a drink with friends, then maintaining that aspect of normality can easily do you a power of good as long as you don't drink to excess.

NICE guidelines recommend 1–2 units 1–2 times a week if you want to drink at all when planning pregnancy and no binges. I advise couples to drink fewer than six units a week if possible – spread over the week – and to have two evenings a week without alcohol. Some women find a good compromise by avoiding alcohol completely in

Case Study

Sarah and Jim have done two rounds of IVF – both have been unsuccessful. Jim has a low sperm count and poor morphology and they have had to have ICSI (see page 336). Jim likes to go out to the pub on Fridays with his mates and can easily get through a bottle of wine and four or five pints of beer. He also smokes socially. In the last four months there have been three weddings and stag nights. Sarah is getting increasingly tense and they are having lots of rows as she feels she is doing everything to prepare for IVF and Jim is doing nothing.

Jim: 'It's all starting to really get me down. The doctor said I only need one sperm and that I can drink. I'm not an alcoholic but Sarah makes me feel I'm the worst person in the world and wants me to stop everything. When we're out I hate seeing her glare at me from the other side of the room, then we argue all the way home.'

Sarah: 'I am doing everything humanly possible. I want the next IVF to work so much and feel that we have to make changes. I was happy to go out drinking in the past and felt I could do both, but for the next round I want to feel that we have both tried.'

Zita: 'Your next cycle of IVF is in three months. Jim – what are you prepared to cut down on to help Sarah?'

Jim: 'I will cut it down to 10 units and stop smoking if Sarah doesn't nag or mention anything to me about what I have had to drink. I feel the more she nags me the more I want to drink and smoke. It isn't just about the alcohol; it's everything – "Take the vitamins, don't have a cup of coffee, don't eat bacon sandwiches ... We have to do this, we have to do that, we should do this ..."'

Tips for Cutting Down

1. Decide together what your weekly alcohol limit will be.
2. If you are an 'all or nothing' person, the best way forward might be to cut out alcohol completely for a couple of months.
3. Decide which evenings in the week you are not going to drink.
4. Accept there will be occasions, such as weddings and family gatherings, when you will probably go over your limit, but don't beat yourself up or let it lead to an argument.
5. Persevere: once you get into the habit of drinking less, it gets easier.

the second half of their cycle when there is a possibility that they could be pregnant and then being a bit more relaxed about it in the first few days of the cycle. We often see women who go into panic mode because they realise they are pregnant and had just had a celebration night out. It is very easy to get things out of perspective here so relax – it is highly unlikely that it has done any damage. Just get yourself back on track again and enjoy your pregnancy.

Couples having IVF are advised not to drink alcohol during treatment and for around 4–6 weeks before. A recent study has shown that having half a bottle of wine the week before IVF can reduce your chances of success. I try to give couples realistic advice so, although studies show that it will take less time to get pregnant if you drink no alcohol at all, this isn't an option for everyone, particularly when it takes longer than expected to conceive.

Every couple is different when it comes to drinking. I encourage honesty and am not at all judgemental about what I am told. Indeed, I would rather a man or a woman cut down from drinking 50 units a week to 15 than make no changes at all, and for those 15 units to be spread out over the week rather than in a single night. It is estimated that it takes the liver about an hour to detoxify every unit of alcohol, so binge drinking puts a huge strain on the liver.

Friction can occur when one partner is drinking and the other has given up. This is the case for so many couples – the tyranny of the 'should' and 'have to'. There is compromise to be had. Sitting a couple down and being able to see how they can move forward together to reach their goal is very rewarding and possible in most cases.

Also, the way couples drink differs. Men tend to binge drink more: they don't have a drink all week and then go on a bender at the weekend; again, this can cause tension in the relationship. If his sperm is good, a man often feels he doesn't have to make any lifestyle changes, but alcohol can affect sperm by increasing the amount of free radical damage (see Chapter 7).

> A recent American study (Harvard Medical School) found that men and women who drank the equivalent of more than 6 units of alcohol a week significantly reduced their chances of IVF success. White wine for women and beer for men had a particularly bad effect.

Hormone Disruptors

More and more evidence is emerging about hormone disruptors in our environment. The press often label them 'gender-bending' chemicals due to the effects they have on reproductive health. Blood taken from placentas has shown that many babies are being exposed to endocrine disruptor hormones in the womb. Environmental toxins also have an effect on the immune system.

Hormones are produced by the endocrine system and released into the bloodstream where they affect the endocrine glands: the ovaries, testicles, thyroid, pancreas and so on. Hormone disruptors are not naturally found in the body and they interfere with the production, release and transport of naturally occurring hormones by mimicking them and binding to natural hormone receptors. We are exposed to them through our environment and household products, such as cosmetics, cleaning materials and garden pesticides. Although you cannot wrap yourself in cotton wool you can limit your exposure.

Lifestyle

Trying Naturally

The difficulty women and men have when trying naturally is that they don't know how long it is going to take to conceive. Three months is manageable to cut things out, but a year is much harder. If you are too harsh on yourself you are likely to fall off the wagon.

- Cut out cigarettes and recreational drugs – a must!
- Limit caffeine to the odd cup of coffee.
- Limit alcohol to 6 units a week.
- Exercise regularly.
- Take a multi-vitamin and mineral supplement, plus omega 3.

When Going Through IVF

Your Body

- Start preparing 4–6 weeks prior to treatment, three months if possible.
- Lose weight or, if you're underweight, gain weight.

- Exercise at least three times a week before you start your IVF cycle.
- Cut out alcohol, caffeine and cigarettes.
- Eat a diet rich in antioxidants.
- Take a multi-vitamin and mineral supplement, plus omega 3.

Your Mind
- Do 15–20 minutes of visualisation a day.
- Plan your diary and pay attention to time management.
- Use stress-reduction techniques (see page 104).
- Try acupuncture.

Part 2

Getting Ready:
Preparing Your Mind and Body for Pregnancy

Chapter 5

Managing Your Mind

The mind–body connection is so important to fertility. Getting pregnant is not just about having sex at the 'right' time or going through the motions of IVF; the mind can have a very powerful influence on the whole process of conception. Negative thoughts, emotions and behaviours can lead to increased anxiety and depression, getting in the way of your goal of conceiving.

Women are great multi-taskers: we manage our finances, home and work, but often managing our minds and emotions is one of the biggest challenges for women going through fertility and IVF. A positive mind–body connection, I believe, is the key to conceiving, no matter what stage of the process you are at.

If you knew you were going to be pregnant in three months, or that after your second round of IVF you would be pregnant, you would be fine, but dealing with uncertainty is so hard. I believe that there is a deep connection between the mind, the body and the spirit, especially in the group of clients I see. My team and I have devised a positive mind–body programme that helps with emotional and psychological support using tools and skill sets that help you to relax and feel more in control.

What do I mean by mind, body and spirit or the mind–body connection? So many couples are medicalised and in a process of tests and investigations for IVF; but this bio-medical model just focuses on hormones, tubes and the uterus. The emotional, psychological and holistic approaches for that couple are not always looked at. I believe that mind/body is the key in many cases in helping a woman connect to her body through mind/body work. When your mind can conceive your body will follow and this is what this chapter will help you to do.

I believe that women need to have the confidence to trust the wisdom of their bodies. Many have lost the ability to connect to their bodies. Trying for a baby may be the first time in your life when you haven't felt in control of your destiny. Remember, though, that you do have control over what you choose to do and which route you take. What you are missing is the certainty of whether and when pregnancy will happen.

Can you identify with any of these statements?

- 'I need help to stay positive.'
- 'I feel out of control.'
- 'I am getting over-anxious.'
- 'I have never failed at anything until now.'
- 'I need help to manage my stress.'
- 'I know I am a perfectionist by nature.'
- 'Maybe I don't deserve to have a child.'
- 'I don't want to have any regrets.'
- 'We need help to make the right decision.'
- 'The clock is ticking.'
- 'IVF won't work for me.'
- 'I've had such a lucky life. This is the one thing that will evade me.'

This chapter will help you to understand your mindset. If you need to learn to let go it will show you how to challenge your negative beliefs. There are strategies to help you cope positively with the rigours of fertility investigations and treatment, and to maximise your fertility potential.

The Mind

The Subconscious Mind

The mind is often likened to an iceberg: imagine the tip of the iceberg (the part above sea level) as the 5 per cent which is the conscious mind or our awareness, and the other 95 per cent is the subconscious mind (the part of the iceberg below sea level). The subconscious (or unconscious) mind covers all the mental processes that are operating outside of immediate conscious awareness. The subconscious mind contains our learned experiences, such as memories, instincts and intuition. Cognitive neuro-imaging shows us that the subconscious part of the mind is much more powerful than the conscious part. The patterns we repeat from our past come from the subconscious mind, as do, I believe, emotional blocks about fertility. For example, if you had a termination in the past and still feel guilty about it, or if as a child you were told you were worthless or you had low self-esteem, these feelings will play themselves out time and time again in your life.

Some women trying for a baby say: 'I wish I could put out of my mind the fact that I'm trying so hard.' Sometimes it is indeed essential to do just this. Reproductive processes are largely unconscious activities – from the sexual response right through to conception and pregnancy. Think about the last time you tried to remember someone's name or the name of a place – the more you struggled to think of it, the more the name evaded you; and of course as soon as you stopped thinking about it, the name popped into your mind. You had been trying to use your conscious mind to perform what is essentially an unconscious task. Nearly every woman I come across who has been trying to conceive and has had an unsuccessful IVF cycle or miscarriage will unconsciously start to think negatively.

So many women have deep anxieties, often unexpressed at a conscious level, that can create anxiety about conception or ongoing pregnancy. If you are trying to conceive, and there is no identified physical obstacle to conception, the more you can distract yourself by absorbing yourself in other activities the better. Even if it feels phoney at first, force yourself to do other things to take your mind off trying for a baby. Learn a language (with a promise to yourself to have a holiday there later); start a course; play that old instrument which is gathering dust; tend your garden – the more stuff you can do outdoors the better. When women come back to the clinic, call or email to say they are pregnant, we ask, 'So what changed?' Often they say they had stopped thinking about getting pregnant; they had 'taken their eye off the ball' and made the trying less trying.

Some women feel real inner conflict. One part of them is going through all the motions of preparing for conception: eating correctly, not drinking or smoking, cutting out caffeine, exercising, staying healthy; then another part of their mind is saying, 'Why are we doing all this when I'm questioning whether I really want a baby?' or 'It won't work anyway.' Some women may genuinely feel that they do not want a baby, or certainly not at the time their biological clock or social pressure is saying they should; while for other women playing down the importance of the baby can be a protective mechanism – in case it does not happen.

Negative Beliefs

Negativity is the biggest mindset issue I deal with every day. Women are so beaten down, many to the point of exhaustion, with what they perceive as failing. It is not always easy to keep negative feelings at bay when trying for a baby. I work with women every day who are finding it difficult to cope positively with the emotional upheaval, uncertainty and feelings of failure they are experiencing, whether trying naturally or through IVF treatment. Past or present experiences can also create blocks that prevent a woman from achieving the optimal mindset for conception to take place. Such blocks include:

- Past terminations: women sometimes feel they have missed their opportunity to have a baby.
- Childhood experiences: women who feel they were mothered badly worry about how they will be as mothers. This can be compounded if they have a poor, or no, relationship with their mother.
- The loss of a parent (see overleaf).
- Sexual or physical abuse: this affects the self-esteem of many women and their belief that they will have a baby.
- Relationship difficulties: new relationships can be challenging, as can ex-partners, leading to stress and problems with self-esteem.

When couples are going through IVF treatment, they can become removed from the mind–body connection that I believe is fundamental to fertility. Tests and investigations focus on the 'mechanics' – such as hormones, tubes and sperm count – yet a high percentage of couples having IVF have no identifiable physical problem, and fall into the 'unexplained' group. What may be missing is a more holistic approach to couples' needs, looking at the emotional and psychological picture as well as the physical one.

Coping with the Loss of a Parent

Many women and men who have lost a parent will experience mixed emotions when trying to conceive. If you have been close to a parent, you may feel very alone at this time. You will be aware of how natural it would be to tell them about your plans to conceive, of any difficulties you are experiencing or of your decision to move to IVF.

There can be a strong sense of not being able to make a connection between past and future generations. It can be helpful to create something tangible to remind you and your future children of your parent. For example, you could save special childhood recipes (grandma's delicious chocolate cake) or keep a bottle of your mother's perfume. For some women and men who have lost a parent, it may be good to consider writing a letter to them. This is a way to voice your innermost thoughts about how their loss may now be affecting you as you move on with your life and contemplate starting your own family.

Dealing with Uncertainty

Uncertainty is the hardest factor for so many couples going through IVF treatment. Some feel that their lives are on hold but it is important not to let that happen. Women who have come through the process one way or another often say they regret putting their lives on hold for years. So many women give up absolutely everything – they stop socialising, having the odd drink, mixing with family. This narrows their world and affects them on every single level, compromising their sense of fun and general wellbeing. The hardest thing for most women is finding the middle ground and not punishing themselves.

Uncertainty is a vicious circle, leading to anxiety, worry and fear, and fear is one of the most paralysing emotions. As well as the fear of pregnancy not happening, people have other everyday anxieties: fear of drugs, clinics or doctors; fear of their relationship ending (see

Chapter 6). Fear is a common emotion among women experiencing fertility problems. They may be frightened by the idea of never being able to have a child. Irrational fears and phobias often become more troublesome at times of stress. They can be triggered, for example, by disappointing results during the IVF process.

The worst thing you can do is withdraw. Try and build in some pleasures and treats for yourself. Use distractions; do things you haven't done for a while that you enjoy; take the pressure off yourself. Living with uncertainty is like a huge weight; it uses all of your energy and is absolutely exhausting. Live from day to day. Have a positive thought when you wake up about how you are going to see that day.

Challenging Negative Messages

Negative messages, especially from figures of authority such as doctors, filter through every cell of your body. If, as a young woman, a doctor tells you: 'You are likely to have problems conceiving when you get older,' this can have a devastating effect, subconsciously crushing your hopes of motherhood; or if a man has had a very authoritarian father, it may affect his sexuality and his belief about his ability to father a child. Negative feelings can lead to anxiety about sex and the belief that it's not really worth having sex. Similarly, any traumatic events from the past, such as an abortion (often from years back), repeated unsuccessful attempts at IVF or recurrent miscarriages can create feelings of negativity and despair.

Many of the older women I treat arrive at my doorstep absolutely traumatised by a consultation they've had where they've been told that their eggs are too old, the quality is no good, they are not responding to IVF drugs or they are never going to have a baby. That negativity can block them on absolutely every level. Negative messages – particularly when delivered by a person in authority – can

How Women Perceive Their Bodies

The way women perceive their bodies is fascinating. So many women have negative views about low egg reserve, a poor womb lining, a small ovary, and even that IVF won't work. When I ask them to describe their womb or ovaries they tell me: 'I feel I have geriatric eggs', 'I think my womb is shrivelled', 'I see it as grey down there'. Comments like this carry weight for a woman and can cause her to lose confidence in her ability to conceive and shatter her beliefs. Work done by Candace Pert has shown that cells have an emotional response and act on messages sent to them: so positive messages make us happy and negative messages of no hope tell the cells to give up. At the clinic we use art therapy and a mixture of guided visualisation and hypnotherapy to help women to prepare for pregnancy. We spend a lot of time helping women to visualise juicy, plump eggs and a vibrant, fertile-rich womb lining that is ready to conceive. For those going through IVF, we use this to help them visualise healthy eggs, plenty of follicles and also to modulate the immune system (see Chapter 14).

play havoc with your rational mind. I feel that older women get a hard time in the press as well, as if it is their fault that they have left it too late. Many of the women I see just didn't meet the right partner when they were younger, and they are convinced motherhood is never going to happen for them.

Managing Your Emotions

After reading this chapter you may decide to make some positive lifestyle changes to boost your chances of pregnancy. I hope that doing this will make you feel confident. However, trying for a baby is emotionally demanding, and some days will be better than others, so here are a few tips for coping with negative emotions.

1. Look at stress management techniques (see overleaf). We know that high stress levels have an impact on hormones. I believe stress can have a negative influence on IVF due to increased stress hormones surging through the body.

2. Try visualisation. Being able to see pictures or images through techniques that incorporate breathing, meditation or listening to a CD can all help you relax (I have a CD for trying naturally and going through IVF – see page 486).

3. Remove stress triggers such as alcohol, cigarettes and caffeine. Although they may provide temporary respite from a stressful situation, they can really affect mood and give you highs and lows.

4. If you are going through fertility treatment, avoid people who make you feel stressed by their insensitive comments, but do include family and friends who are supportive of you.

5. Look at your relationship. You have got to be together on this. Effective communication is essential. If you are feeling needy then you must tell your partner so that you can support each other.

6. Don't beat yourself up. Get rid of the negative dialogue in your head and decide you are going to change something. Write down how you are feeling and where you can realistically make changes.

7. Get a better work/life balance.

8. Build in treats for yourself.

The Positive Mind Plan

The Mind Plan will help you to consider your situation regarding fertility, but also to look outside the fertility box at other aspects of your life. The Mind Plan starts off by exploring your situation and what you are trying to achieve (in addition to the baby). It then looks at the reality of your current situation and how it is affecting how you feel and your behaviour. It explores any obstacles to making changes and your personal characteristics that might help or hinder you. We use different techniques to achieve this: written work, cognitive behavioural therapy, hypnotherapy, breathing techniques and visualisation. The whole idea of a Positive Mind Plan is to practise these therapies which will help you to cope and elicit a relaxation response. The key part of this is to arrive at a specific plan of action to help you to identify the way forward, including specific tasks and time-frames. The aim is to help you safely explore how you feel and find new tools to regain your strength, improve your self-esteem and mobilise your inner resources – to give you back the control which so often seems to have deserted you.

I will give you a couple of examples of how this type of Mind Plan can be used. One woman described her main goal as to get pregnant, with the key issue of needing to lose weight before being accepted on an IVF programme. Her clinic had told her that she needed to reduce her body mass index (BMI), but had not offered her any support in doing this. She described the reality of her situation as being stressed, overworked and unable to make decisions. She felt her main issues were her weight, stress and a fear of failure. Her mood was anxious and depressed, which made her isolate herself and comfort-eat. Her chief obstacle was her low self-esteem. Her plan included:

1. The support of a nutritionist to get her diet back on track.
2. Changing her way of thinking and behaving.
3. Working on her relationship and intimacy.

She set herself some specific but manageable physical challenges, dug out her old pedometer and bought some smart new trainers. She built in time to wind down after work. Very importantly, she spent some real quality time with her husband, getting back to activities they used to share before the whole fertility thing took over. In no time, she was back in control of her eating; her relationship had improved and she felt confident that her goal was in sight.

Another woman had been trying to conceive for over two years with unexplained infertility, and had just had an unsuccessful IVF cycle. She identified her main problem as being related to the quality of her eggs. She noted down that her body felt old, her thinking was all over the place and she was very frightened of the future. She recognised that she was oversensitive in her reactions. Her specific plan included:

1. Relaxation.
2. Healthy eating.
3. Taking herself less seriously.
4. Starting to play her clarinet again.
5. Having wild sex.

As she was preparing for another IVF cycle she realised that her period was late and she was pregnant. It is hard to know what did the trick, but the wild sex certainly didn't work against them!

Positive Affirmations

List all your negative thoughts about getting pregnant, for example:

- 'The doctor says I have only a 5 per cent chance.'
- 'I have a high FSH.'
- 'I'm worried my partner will leave me if I can't get pregnant.'

Then rewrite the negative messages you have been giving yourself. To make this successful, you need to make the messages positive and write them in the present tense. For example:

- 'I am one of the 5 per cent.'
- 'I am young and healthy and in great nutritional shape.'
- 'My partner loves me and we have a great life together, no matter what.'

Say your positive affirmations out loud convincingly. Then make yourself comfortable, close your eyes and take 10 long, slow, deep breaths, allowing your body to relax more deeply with each out-breath. When you are deeply relaxed, allow the positive affirmation to repeat itself over and over in your subconscious mind, while at the same time picturing yourself living each statement, for example: 'I will be a wonderful mother'; imagine yourself playing with your child.

Visualisation

When women receive negative news about their fertility, or are not getting pregnant and having repeated unsuccessful IVF cycles, visualisation can be very powerful. It is used by Olympic athletes to help them hone their technique. You may have experienced the power of the mind to spur you on to complete an event, to push yourself harder, to pedal to the top of the hill. I use visualisation alongside acupuncture to help women to re-connect with their bodies.

Case Study

Amanda, aged 39, came to me reeling from the shock that her FSH was 39 and her AMH was low, beating herself up about the fact that she hadn't met somebody until later in life and she was never going to get pregnant. She was told that the only route for her was egg donation. She was tearful, stressed and desperate.

I told her I was going to do absolutely everything I could to help improve her chances. So she had a very good nutritional consultation, making sure she was on all the appropriate vitamins and minerals. I used visualisation and meditation to help her focus and connect with her uterus, which she had been unable to do because of the shock, and also to help her change her anxious mindset. I gave her four to five months to do this. She got pregnant naturally and calls it the 'miracle baby'.

Although techniques such as the ones described in the case above will not result in pregnancy for every woman, I believe it is worth doing everything you can to be positive.

Chinese Medicine and the Heart–Uterus Connection

In Chinese medicine the conception vessel meridian follows a straight line and links the heart to the uterus (womb). The heart is the seat of our emotions. If the heart is heavy or blocked through emotional disturbances, the chi (vital energy) cannot flow down to the uterus. I use visualisation techniques to help women make this connection (see Chapter 8).

Meditation

There are many types of meditation. Techniques to help calm your mind can be taught easily and have huge benefits for relaxation. The more you practise the better you become. Research has shown that there are many health benefits to these techniques, such as reduced stress levels, lower blood pressure and a healthier immune system. To benefit from meditation and still the mind you will need to practise for at least 20 minutes a day: practising regularly will help you feel more in control. Many people use prayer as a means of meditation.

Therapeutic Writing

It is often so hard to put feelings into words. Some people find a great release through writing – just allowing the thoughts to flow freely in a totally uninhibited way. This can be particularly helpful if you have been through a difficult time, such as an unsuccessful IVF cycle or a miscarriage. Just allow the emotions out as you write. You may never go back and read it again or, if you do, it is very likely you will then realise just how down you felt at the time and how things have moved on for you.

Try drawing an emotional timeline (a wavy horizontal line) as a first step. This so often highlights very quickly the ups and downs of life. So, for example, a timeline might show a very happy childhood, some bullying at school, parents divorcing, the development of an eating disorder, a relationship breakdown or the death of a parent or a close friend. You will recognise that you may have had other low times or times when you felt particularly vulnerable or out of control. Where you feel on that scale of life's ups and downs can be quite important to establish. A timeline helps to focus on ways to use new or existing resources to make changes to help you manage your current situation.

Hypnotherapy

Hypnotherapy is the process of inducing hypnosis and then making suggestions as a form of therapy. The state of hypnosis is a naturally occurring event during which your body is relaxed and your mind is highly focused. This happens frequently throughout the day, such as when day-dreaming or engrossed in something. If you were reading on a train, for example, you would be aware of other people in the carriage, but you might have 'switched off' from them if absorbed in your book. The term 'highway hypnosis' is often used to describe the state of driving 'on auto-pilot' where the route is so familiar that you are not thinking of where you are going – you are in effect in a trance state. If there was any change along the route, such as a traffic diversion or a cow in the middle of the road, your mind would suddenly be on full alert again and you would respond appropriately. When you are under hypnosis, you are completely in control and aware of your surroundings. Hypnotherapy is completely safe and very effective.

Hypnotherapy can help fertility by encouraging general relaxation and reducing stress. It can boost confidence in your ability to conceive naturally or after a miscarriage, and can also be effective for men who have developed 'performance anxiety' related to the pressures to have sex at the fertile time. Hypnotherapy, including self-hypnosis, is a valuable tool for managing the stresses of an IVF cycle and helping you to let go. It can also help you to visualise what is happening physically in your body and to be able to relax fully during IVF procedures.

All sorts of anxieties and emotional issues from the immediate or distant past can be buried in the subconscious mind. These can act as blocks to fertility. Over a number of sessions, the hypnotherapist can help you reach a deep state of relaxation where the subconscious part of the mind is accessed and positive suggestions are made that release deep-seated fears and anxieties.

Some of the most common issues that can cause subconscious blocks to fertility and conception include past abortions, miscarriages, rape or sexual abuse. Some women will struggle if they are perfectionists or have concerns about their own ability to manage the physical challenges of pregnancy, birth, medical investigations or treatments. For other women there may be fears related to loss of control, loss of independence and earning power or loss of self; concerns about the changing dynamic of their relationship and the transition to parenthood. Difficulties within their relationship or past or perceived issues within the wider family can also create blocks to fertility at a subconscious level.

Recent research from Israel has shown that women who are able to relinquish control and 'let go' are nearly twice as likely to conceive as women who don't adopt this attitude. This is where techniques such as meditation or hypnotherapy can focus on teaching you to 'let go'. In most situations in life, we are accustomed to being in control and 'problem-focused coping' helps us to manage different situations. With fertility problems our usual coping mechanisms are challenged as there are elements outside our control. 'Emotion-focused coping' strategies, which involve humour, relaxation and 'letting go', are beneficial. The researchers believe that women who find it hard to let go spend more time worrying about whether or not they will conceive and this can impact on fertility. So learning to relax and 'let go' is really important and some women manage this better than others.

The Hypnotherapy Session

A typical session would start with you telling the hypnotherapist a little about yourself and your goals and objectives for the session. If it is your first session, the hypnotherapist will then explain how hypnosis works and allay any anxieties. You are then usually invited to make yourself comfortable, either sitting or lying on a couch or reclining chair. The next step is the induction which is the process of taking you safely from normal waking consciousness into the 'hypnotic state'. The hypnotherapist may use a simple countdown from 10 to 1 along with suggestions of relaxation or the use of guided imagery such as a set of steps. This is really a way of helping you to relax your mind and body.

When you are deeply relaxed, the hypnotherapist can make positive suggestions which will be accepted by your subconscious mind. Depending on the situation, there will be a variety of suggestions made at this stage. This could be positive reinforcement about your ability to conceive; reminding your subconscious mind that it does not need to think about conception – it will happen in its own time, so you can simply 'let go' – or opportunities for you to use different guided techniques of self-healing. Where appropriate, there may be other exploratory work related to the past. When going through IVF, a lot of the work will involve visualising your growing follicles and your womb lining – creating a safe nurturing space to receive your embryos. Different techniques may be used including visualising warmth, moving light or energy through your body. Before the hypnotherapist wakes you, he or she gives you more positive suggestions and then usually counts up from 1 to 10 to bring you back to a full state of alertness. You may be invited to discuss some aspects of your experience before you leave.

Many people are unsure whether 'it worked' because they expect something slightly different. You are not asleep during hypnosis. Although your body will feel very relaxed and often quite heavy, you can move around if you need to and make yourself comfortable, exactly as you do when asleep. You will hear every word that is spoken, but your attention may wander at times – and that is fine. You will remember everything that is of any importance for you, and you will only take in positive suggestions which are safe and appropriate to you. Most people say that they feel deeply relaxed after hypnosis – possibly more relaxed than they have ever felt before. Many women later report the biggest benefit as the fact that they have been able to stop thinking about it (getting pregnant) and get on with their lives.

A single session of hypnotherapy can be very beneficial, by helping you to learn to relax and let go. If you are going through IVF, hypnotherapy can help you to visualise very positively the changes through your cycle. One study found that hypnosis effectively doubled the success rates of IVF at the stage of embryo transfer. Twenty-eight per cent of the women who were hypnotised for the embryo transfer became pregnant, compared to 14 per cent of the women in the control group. It is possible that relaxation through hypnosis has a significant effect on relaxing the uterus, allowing an easier transfer procedure and minimising uterine contractions. However, larger studies are required to confirm these findings. (For information on obtaining my relaxation CDs, see page 486.)

Cognitive Behavioural Therapy

Cognitive Behavioural Therapy (CBT) is widely used in the NHS to help with depression and is based on the concept that the way you think about events in your life will influence how you feel about them and consequently how you behave. Many people hold negative core beliefs based on things which may have happened in early life. CBT deals with distorted thought patterns and helps reframe them.

So many of the women I see have lost confidence in their body's ability to perform or to conceive. They feel despair, hopelessness, anger and fear. These emotions are raw and, for some, festering in the subconscious. What a CBT therapist will do is change their mindset to get away from their current thinking and stop these negative feelings and emotions from growing, trying to calm the negative thinking down and giving women the ability not to fight these emotions but to recognise how to deal with them and be able to nourish the good thoughts. We don't just get feelings; they arrive out of our thoughts and emotions. For example, some aspects of worrying are helpful and can stir you into action, but worrying can also increase your anxiety levels. CBT can help you to normalise a difficult emotion, accept it, respond to it and change the way you think about it.

Common thoughts such as 'I can't get pregnant' may be the reality but being able to change the way you think enables you to respond to be able to reach your goal. It is hard on paper to describe how CBT works, but it challenges these negative patterns and restructures your mind to work in a different way, helping you to have an appropriate response and accepting it has to be dealt with and can't be pushed away. This is done by talking to a therapist who asks questions about how and why, for example, you are feeling anxious.

Some of the thinking patterns that CBT works to counteract are:

- Catastrophising: always predicting the worst outcome.
- Over-generalising: assuming that something that happened once will happen again.
- Exaggerating: giving power to negative events and reducing the positive.
- Taking things personally: blaming yourself for events you are not responsible for.
- Emotional reasoning: making mistakes feel like facts ('I feel like a failure so I must be one').
- All-or-nothing thinking: seeing everything as black or white; allowing no shades of grey or middle ground.
- Labelling: 'I'm no good. I don't deserve to conceive.'

Case Study

If Ruth, 35, saw a pregnant woman she felt self pity ('poor me') and her mood would drop. She then felt angry and didn't know how to deal with her anger, so when her husband came home from work she would take it out on him. Everything he did was wrong; he couldn't do or say anything right. He did not know how to deal with this or fix it and would just suggest going straight for IVF, looking for a two-dimensional solution ('Let's fix it now'). But he also couldn't deal with the endless chatter.

Unconsciously Ruth was unaware of what was going on and did not have any strategies to deal with it. Alongside this she was over-researching, over-focusing on the problems, and what we were trying to do with CBT was help her with her unhealthy behaviours which were heightening her distress. What we were dealing with were:

- Low mood
- Anger and frustration

First we had to find out what would help her with her mood. We decided that calling a girlfriend with whom she could let everything off her chest would help. Also starting kick boxing would help her vent the anger and frustration she felt and finally she would keep herself in check an hour before her husband came home so as not to slip into a difficult mood and to have more pleasurable activities in the evening. As a result of feeling so negative with him she would have self-loathing and not taking responsibility and then begging forgiveness and swearing it wouldn't happen again. Her period would come and her negative cycle would be repeated.

Most of the women I see have to deal with fluctuating mood and negativity on a regular basis. CBT helps them to understand how to deal with it and building in some self-help techniques enables them to manage the process. Dealing with uncertainty creates anxiety and can tip you into negative thinking. By changing the way you think you can get the balance back and enjoy positive emotions.

Fertility Counselling
(by Jane Knight, Fertility Counsellor)

The aim of fertility counselling is to help individuals or couples make sense of their situation and the feelings they are experiencing. As a fertility counsellor, I see couples every day who are struggling with the challenges of repeated unsuccessful attempts to achieve pregnancy, to maintain a pregnancy or complete their desired family. Zita has really captured the essence of what so many couples go through at different stages of the fertility process, but she has asked me to add a few words from the perspective of a fertility counsellor. My background is in nursing and midwifery. I have had a special interest in fertility for over 25 years and trained as a fertility counsellor in 1991. My work has increasingly highlighted the real difficulties that so many couples face in their highly pressurised lives – from the time of first considering getting pregnant right through to IVF and beyond.

Do I Need a Counsellor? If So, How Do I Find One?

It is so important that both men and women have someone they can turn to, to talk about their concerns. This may be a partner, a parent, a sibling, a friend or a colleague. It really does not matter, provided you can trust someone and feel comfortable with them – that may be all that is needed. However, so many couples we see either do not feel they have anyone they can confide in, or they really do not want to discuss issues of such an intimate nature. This is where counselling can help. There may be a counsellor you can see at your GP's surgery. If you attend a licensed fertility clinic you can ask to see the clinic counsellor. Fertility counsellors come from varied backgrounds – some are from a nursing or medical background; others are from a social work or psychology background.

You need to feel comfortable with your counsellor and that you are making progress. If you don't feel happy, it may be that their approach doesn't suit you. Counsellors work in many different ways and it may be better for you to find someone else. If you are unhappy with being challenged, bear in mind that this may be what you need to help you sort out your situation. Your IVF clinic will provide access to a fertility counsellor.

What is Fertility Counselling?

Fertility counselling is a process through which individuals and couples have the opportunity to explore their thoughts, feelings and beliefs in order to come to a greater understanding of themselves and their present situation. This can be helpful at all stages, from contemplating pregnancy right the way through to fertility investigations and treatment, IVF, possibly egg donation, and having to come to terms with not having your own child. If you are going through IVF, then your licensed fertility unit is obliged to offer you access to counselling in line with the HFEA Code of Practice.

Couples who are considering using donated gametes or embryos have additional complex issues to consider. Similarly, couples who may be considering surrogacy have even more complex considerations, including the importance of the legal side. As increasing numbers of couples are travelling outside the UK for treatments, appropriate counselling may not be accessible in the country where they are receiving treatment and there may be additional language barriers.

Are Counselling Sessions Confidential?

Whatever you discuss during your counselling session is confidential. No information will be disclosed outside without your specific permission apart from in very exceptional circumstances. These circumstances are: if there is a serious risk of harm coming to you or to someone else; or if you disclose information relevant to a serious crime. In this case the counsellor is obliged to disclose relevant information to the appropriate agency. It is only rarely necessary to do this and the disclosure would be discussed with you.

Art Therapy

At times people are stuck for words to describe their feelings. This is where image work comes in. Creating images uses another part of our brain and allows access to the subconscious mind. This can help to provide a way in which to give shape to difficulties. As children, we all had the capacity to be visually creative, but we have frequently buried this under adult anxieties of 'not being good enough' or being afraid of revealing our true selves. Many people find creating images a helpful way of working, as it helps to focus the attention. We are not talking here about producing works of art; more a means of self-expression – stick men, doodles. Sometimes a picture really can tell a thousand words.

Sometimes it can really help to get out a few pens or paints, or just do a simple doodle with a Biro – simply allow yourself to show how you feel on paper. The more mess you make the better. Just starting to

Case Study

Tom had started having difficulties getting an erection since beginning a relationship with a woman who was keen to have a baby. He, too, was ready to have a child and they usually had great sex. He only had the problem when he was at her flat. When I asked him to show me the woman's room by drawing it, the first thing he drew was a large square, and in the middle of the square was a cat. He had solved his own problem in no time at all. This cat belonged to the woman's ex, and as this guy was not able to house the cat when they split up, the cat stayed and still took up its favourite spot in the middle of the bed. Tom could see that the cat's presence was symbolic of the ex, and was preventing him from having uninhibited sex. Turfing the cat out soon solved his erection problems.

Case Study

Jess desperately wanted a baby but had developed vaginismus (involuntary spasms of the vagina preventing penetration) and was not able to let her partner near her since they had stopped using contraception. Again, I asked her to show me the bedroom with the aid of a few coloured pens. She quietly, but immediately, drew a rectangular shape (which I assumed was the bed) and then a smaller square in the top right-hand corner of the 'bed' (which I assumed might be a pillow) and then she started to sob. Her image had reminded her of a letter – and this was the letter from an ex-boyfriend ending their five-year relationship. She was terrified that trying to conceive with this new partner would end in another relationship split and her body was saying 'No'. Again, once she could see the link and discuss her concerns with her new partner, the 'problem' disappeared.

Case Study

Harry was completely unable to manage his wife's increasing volatility. He felt that an IVF cycle could easily bring their relationship into crisis. When I asked them to allow me to see an argument (on paper) they each drew a very telling image. Harry's was a simple image of walking on eggshells and Sally's image showed a Munch-like scream with Harry cowering. When they were able to see the situation objectively, they arrived at an idea for developing a kind of 'barometer' which Sally could set to try and get across her needs. They acknowledged that whatever Harry did would be wrong because he could not put things right (fix the baby problem). Sally's barometer included things like: 'I just need a hug', 'Leave me to cry alone for a bit', 'Let's just walk till I can talk'. They had developed their own way of communicating at crucial times.

give some of the feelings a physical form can help you to talk about how you feel and to work on it – the knot in your tummy, the empty vessel, the big cloud, the fog, the sad face, the lonely figure, the prickly porcupine. This can help you start to give shape to the problem and often to talk about it more easily – with your partner, a good friend or a counsellor.

Making Your Own Positive Mind Plan

Your own Mind Plan can involve many different things:

1. Action Plan
The plan of action is the most important aspect – keep reviewing your action plan and remember this needs to include lots of things that give

you pleasure as well as all the logistics of any fertility investigations or treatments you may be involved with.

2. Positive Affirmations

Put positive messages out there! Write your positive affirmations down and look at them before you go to bed. These are carefully worded, personal, positive statements that you repeat and need to be in the present tense.

3. Visualisation Techniques

You might want to listen to a CD of guided meditation or practise breathing techniques or yoga. If possible, practise a self-help visualisation or stress-reduction technique for 20 minutes a day.

4. Keep a Journal

Many women find this beneficial for a period of time. It often helps them to work through their emotions.

5. Do Something You Enjoy

Listen to music, go for a walk in the countryside or do something else that you really enjoy.

6. Exercise

Exercise for 30 minutes a day where possible.

7. Therapies

Useful therapies include art therapy (page 117), counselling (page 115), CBT (page 112) and hypnotherapy (page 109). Meditation and breathing techniques are also useful.

Take time to write down the things that are certainties in your life so that you are able to hang on to them. Those certainties may be a loving partner who supports you; friends and family; the certainty that you are going to keep on trying and investigate other avenues; the certainty that you are doing your best. Think of what you would do for somebody who was in a similar situation – and then do it for yourself. This may involve treats, such as a massage.

Managing your mind and connecting with your body and your relationship will give you control over your situation. It's hard to control when you will get pregnant, but you can take control of your thoughts, emotions, mind and body. However, like everything it takes time and practice, but some of the ideas and therapies outlined in this chapter may help you to move forward more positively.

Chapter 6

Your Relationship

Much of the work we do involves looking at the communication between couples and how they are feeling generally. I look for factors that might be having an impact on their ability to conceive. I strongly believe that the dynamic of the couple's relationship holds the key to why some couples may struggle to conceive.

Very rarely are both partners on the same page in terms of when – or if – they feel ready to try for a baby. Age may be quite a significant factor. When partners are of a similar age, then it is more likely that they will both feel ready at around the same time as this generally coincides with the life-stage of friends or siblings. Where the woman is older, she may be feeling much more pressure related to her age; sometimes it is really difficult for a younger man to catch up with her enthusiasm (and biological need) to have a family. It is very common for men to feel they cannot cope with the pace at which a new relationship is moving. They often feel very pressured and some men have even said they feel more like a sperm donor even if the woman's intentions are absolutely genuine. So many men describe how they really want a family but 'not just yet', and can find it very difficult if the woman's age is dictating the pace. This may be made even more difficult if early fertility tests reveal there is a problem. If one partner already has children this can also have an impact. Very often men need a bit of a breather before they get to IVF. At times the situation may be reversed: the man is keen for a baby and the woman is feeling coerced into pregnancy to maintain the relationship.

Fertility counselling can help couples to resolve conflicts related to starting to conceive (see page 115). It is so important that you are both able to talk about your concerns. For example, men might be anxious about having their freedom curtailed; women might worry about the effect motherhood will have on their career. Simply being able to acknowledge some of these concerns goes a long way to starting to solve them and to finding a middle ground where necessary.

Sex and Intimacy

Sex is a huge stumbling block for so many couples: they worry about doing it at the right time, about having an orgasm, sexual positions, depth of penetration, whether the sperm is getting there, and so on. Sex should just happen – and hopefully with a tad of enthusiasm and passion – it is not part of a tick list.

When you are trying for a baby, or if you are going on to IVF, it can seem like there isn't enough time for sex. Intimacy can also go out of the relationship very quickly. Sex is often used as a subconscious currency between couples. Resentments often set in and go very deep. A woman might demand sex during her fertile time, then show no interest in it for the rest of her cycle. The man might feel pressured into knowing every intimate detail of his partner's fertility, and may experience feelings of stress about performing. 'Performance anxiety' (difficulty getting or maintaining an erection or ejaculating) is quite common in the men we see. It tends to be a temporary problem, linked to trying for a baby. Similarly with IVF sex very often stops altogether and leaves many men wanting their old relationship back. I really encourage couples to work hard on their relationship as repeated rounds of IVF can have a major impact.

It is easy to see how the joy and intimacy can go out of a relationship for many couples. The failure to conceive can take over your life if you are not careful because you are influenced by everything around you – by friends who are getting pregnant; friends whose IVF cycles are working; family members asking you why it's not happening.

One of the questions I always ask is: 'How is your relationship coping with trying for a baby?' Very often this gives couples an opportunity to air how they are both feeling. I also ask: 'Are you having any fun in your life?' Very often the answer is 'No'. It depends on how long they have been trying, but so many of the couples I see have spent much of their young lives focused on trying for a baby. It is essential to look at the relationship because you need to get through this process and come out the other end intact. Sadly, many couples don't achieve that.

Resolving Differences

Both men and women can find it difficult to have sex or feel intimate when they are coping with feelings of anger or resentment, when trying naturally or especially when going through IVF. Women, in particular, need to be relaxed and feeling positive towards their partner. The key to making your relationship work is to resolve the small things that happen in your life. Each misunderstanding you have that hurts your feelings is hard to repair, but it makes the relationship worse if you don't resolve it.

Another question I always ask couples is, 'Are you being kind to one another?' This always causes a couple to look at one another. Very often a woman might answer something like:

- 'Well, I am to him, but he is not to me.'
- 'He doesn't want this as much as me.'
- 'It's okay for him – he doesn't have to be prodded and poked.'
- 'I'm the one who has to take all the drugs.'
- 'He's not willing to make any changes.'

Asked the same question a man might reply:

- 'I try but it is never enough.'
- 'I feel helpless because I can't do anything.'
- 'She can't understand that just because I don't go on about it all the time, it doesn't mean that I don't want a baby.'

Case Study

Jason and Jane were barely even together when they came to see me. I asked what happened every day in their relationship and it was humdrum: getting back from work, sitting watching television, barely talking, him going off into another room on his computer. I asked Jane what happened when Jason came home. She said she carried on sitting and watching the television, not getting up to greet him. His interpretation of that was that her mood was heavy and dark: 'She doesn't care that much about me, and she has stopped appreciating me.' There was coldness between the two of them, and they had stopped trying on every level. She had become very indifferent to him, even when they went to bed at night. If he reached out, she was not in the mood and so he saw that as a rejection. She said that she asked him constantly if they could go out for dinner together, but it turned out he was avoiding it because it meant sitting intensely and arguing about when they should do their next IVF cycle. All she wants to do is get another cycle in.

You need to see it from each other's perspective because perceptions can be blown out of all proportion when you are trying for a baby or going through IVF. The woman feels she is doing absolutely everything for the man, who doesn't have to do anything (well, very little, but a rather vital contribution). The man finds it very hard to know how to be with her and to recognise her needs. Being able to communicate is vital. It's when communication breaks down that the relationship breaks down and the pregnancy often doesn't happen.

So many men obviously love their partner and want to do everything they can to help her, but that burning desire to have a child is so strong in a woman it is difficult to understand. When a woman starts off on a fertility journey she absolutely goes for it: she researches and understands everything about vitamins, minerals, clinics, her cycle, IVF and so on. The man, on the other hand, can feel left behind. Women expect them to be very much on board, and to some extent men want this too. However, for many men every single aspect of the process doesn't mean as much to them as it does to women.

A woman often feels she has no control over her situation. Her reaction can be to try and control everything that is going on in her partner's life. For example, it is common for a woman to take control over sex – demanding sex at her fertile time, making her partner rush home from work. She may also try to control the amount he drinks and what he eats.

Tips for Men

As a man you try and do the right thing but I'll let you into a secret: you can *never* do the right thing for a woman! She is going through a very difficult time because this is a big focus in her life. You might feel that nothing you do will ever be right. You can turn round and tell her to relax as much as you like, but she can't hear it and has possibly also lost her natural ability to simply let go. When I am sitting in the consulting room the man will often say to me, 'I've told her everything you say, but she won't hear it from me. She needs to hear it from you.'

As difficult as she is being, as difficult as it is for you, remember that she is hurting emotionally on every level. The one thing a woman wants to say to her man is, 'I'm pregnant!' I do understand that as a man you want to be able to fix it, but this is one thing you can't easily fix. Be kind and reach out to her; even if she is being difficult and rejecting you, what she needs is love and cuddles.

Many men find it hard to cope when there is a problem or issue so they distance themselves. Be patient with her and don't distance yourself or pretend it isn't happening. It's not enough to agree to talk about this for five or ten minutes at the end of the day. Do understand that she has to keep seeking information, even though this is so irritating. Give her some treats; encourage her to socialise and mix with friends, family and people who have babies. Reassure her that you are not going to go off if it doesn't happen for her. This is really big. Communicate how you are really feeling from the heart.

Kindness, warmth and love pay huge dividends for many women. It's not about the big romantic gesture. What makes the difference for women is when their partner is thoughtful: emptying the dishwasher, doing some of the shopping, cooking the odd meal and being spontaneous.

The Male and Female Brain

Women are very emotional beings and their feelings are heightened when they are trying for a baby or going for IVF, especially if they have already had one, or repeated, unsuccessful cycles. A typical male brain tends to be more logical (thankfully) and maintains the sense of reasoning and statistical chance. Many women have to cry to get attention from their man but often he doesn't know how to react; it comes as a bit of a shock and may make him feel uncomfortable.

Men and women have different brain chemistry. Women rely more on serotonin and men on dopamine. Dopamine makes a man feel protective towards his woman. Serotonin makes a woman feel happy, content and able to relax. For a man to produce dopamine he needs to know he is appreciated, loved and accepted for who he is.

At times, many men seem emotionally absent to their women, especially when they get back from work. If a couple has fertility issues, the woman will often want to talk about them as soon as he steps over the doorstep or for quite a long time. However, I think men generally need a bit of time and space on their own to recharge.

Oxytocin, the Feel-good Hormone

Oxytocin has a significant role in childbirth and breast-feeding but is equally important to reduce stress in women and men. A woman can increase her oxytocin levels if she is caring and befriends people. Oxytocin is stimulated when a woman nurtures herself. It is often very hard to encourage women to nurture themselves, however, because they tend to be doing everything for others all the time. I often see that women are not good to themselves, especially when struggling with IVF or not getting pregnant. They berate themselves and stop doing the things they love and enjoy – this doesn't help with their oxytocin level. Physical touch, massage and orgasm help to release oxytocin.

Toxic Relationships

Even the healthiest relationship can be tested by trying for a baby, whether naturally or through IVF. Some couples I see, however, have a 'toxic' relationship. They argue through the whole consultation, and are quite bitter and nasty to one another. When there is such a high level of resentment I often suggest that they need to work on their relationship first if they really want to make a baby together. For many couples, simply airing their differences in front of a fertility or relationship counsellor can help. Often it can take as little as an hour to help you take a step back and see what is going on in your relationship.

A counsellor will help you to explore the nature of your problems and what changes you would each like to see. Counselling helps you to understand why you are struggling with specific problems, what is lacking and how you can create appropriate changes and find the resources to resolve your issues. The key thing is to appreciate the importance of spending time together to strengthen your relationship and to ensure that you are both communicating effectively. At times, no amount of relationship counselling will help a couple to stay together; then the focus is on helping the two people resolve their differences in a healthy manner and to go their separate ways.

Relationship Tips (by Jane Knight, Fertility Counsellor)

The key part of any relationship is how effectively you communicate. At times of stress, clear, honest, open communication is often the first thing to go.

How Well Do You Communicate with Your Partner?
- Do you make time to have a proper conversation?
- Do you think you are a good listener?

- Would a friend say you are a good listener?
- Do you always wait until your partner has finished speaking?
- How often do you interrupt or continue with your own train of thought?
- Do you really acknowledge what your partner has said?
- Can you hear out your partner's viewpoint even if you disagree or it makes you feel uncomfortable?

How to Improve Communication with Your Partner

- Learn to say no to unimportant things so that you can create time together.
- Set aside time to talk when you know you will not be interrupted – this means away from distractions so switch off the television and the BlackBerry!
- Spend quality time together in a relaxing environment – a walk in the woods, a picnic by a lake or a candlelit meal.
- Take it in turns to talk – and really allow the other person their space.
- Own your feelings. Don't blame the other person for the way you are feeling. Tell your partner how a situation has made you feel, or how you might expect to feel about something.
- Don't be destructive and say things you will regret. This can often happen, especially after a few drinks.

Sadly, sometimes going through IVF can bring out the worst in a couple. For others it brings them closer together. Relationships take time to build and can easily be damaged. Rebuilding a relationship takes time, so don't expect a quick fix. If you are struggling, get professional help sooner rather than later. Men generally tend to be more logical and women tend to be more emotional, but essentially we all want the same things out of a relationship – to feel connected, loved, understood and in harmony with each other emotionally.

Case Study

Jasmine and Paul came for a consultation after trying for a baby for two and a half years. It became evident that their relationship was close to ending, and this needed pointing out to them.

Jasmine: 'We have had four unsuccessful IVF attempts. I have some endometriosis, but Paul's sperm count is really low and has poor morphology, and it's really coming between us. He's not prepared to do anything to improve his sperm. He carries on smoking, he carries on drinking and I just feel increasingly frustrated that it's not happening. He also makes it incredibly difficult to have sex when he knows it's my fertile time. I feel he's punishing me by not having sex with me. Apart from IVF this is the only option we have. Can you please tell him he has to stop drinking and smoking cigarettes and marijuana?'

Zita: 'Paul, what are your thoughts about trying for a baby? What do you think is going on?'

Paul: 'We've been married for five years and, if I'm really honest, I never thought my life would turn out like this. I was really excited about getting married to Jasmine and I was looking forward to our life together. Because we were a bit older than average, we started trying for a baby very quickly and it wasn't happening. I don't feel we gave it long enough trying on our own. Within about four months Jasmine became absolutely obsessed, and I found myself in an IVF unit before I could even blink. I had a semen analysis done that was absolutely terrible, and before I knew it the words IVF and ICSI were said. I didn't have time to really think and take it all in. All we had been focusing on was a baby and Jasmine's needs; I didn't feel my needs were met at all. I'm terrified to talk to her and feel I have disappointed her in her quest to have a baby. I do love her very much but she has become a different person. She is anxious, neurotic, totally driven by this whole baby thing, and as a result she has been turning against me and I feel she is drifting away. I hate coming home at the moment because when she has her period I don't know what her reaction is going to be. The more unhappy she becomes, the more she picks on me.'

Jasmine interrupts here and says: 'Yes, but I am doing everything. You are doing nothing. You continue to drink, you are still smoking, and you are still carrying on with marijuana.'

Paul loses it, turns round and says: 'The more you try to stop me doing these things and having some life, the more I will rebel; the more marijuana, the more cigarettes and the more alcohol I will have.'

Zita: 'Do you feel like you are having fun in your lives?'

Tears well up in Paul's eyes and he says: 'I don't feel I am having a life. I feel the fun has completely gone out of my life in the drive for IVF.'

Paul and Jasmine were not ready to start another IVF cycle. What they needed was some time to get close again. Intimacy was sadly lacking in their relationship because they were using so much of their energy to argue and were both very stubborn. For a man to have sex he has to have passion, and the passion had completely gone out of their relationship. This is one of the biggest quandaries I see with couples. The woman cannot understand why her man won't change his lifestyle and give up the things he enjoys when he wants a baby as desperately as she does so she ends up nagging and being critical. There has to be more kindness and understanding within the relationship. Generally, if a man isn't nagged but is let be, he will eventually come round and make the changes of his own accord.

Emotional and psychological blocks, and relationship issues, really can get in the way of conception. Your relationship with your partner holds the key. If you are feeling anger and resentment towards your partner, not enjoying sex and not really 'connecting' but simply existing alongside each other in a vacuum, this passion-starved existence is hardly conducive to making a baby together.

Sadly, as with any major life crisis, fertility problems can cause a real rift in relationships and may even precipitate the end of the relationship. So, really really look at the areas in your relationship that need addressing. I do understand that having fertility issues can blow everything out of proportion for you and take the focus away from what is important. Relationships need nurturing and nourishing to stay together. Sometimes couples cannot see how close they are to pushing their relationship to extremes.

Remember how you felt when you both met and what you loved about one another. If you are having problems, look ahead and consider how you would feel if the relationship ended and he or she was not in your life. Think about the little things you can change to make your relationship better: a walk in the park; getting home early one night during the week. Build on your strengths and support one another.

Chapter 7

Nutrition, Fertility and IVF

Introduction by Zita West

Melanie Brown heads up the nutrition service at the clinic. Mel and I have worked together since I opened the clinic in 2002. We have developed a practical nutritional programme for couples at all stages of pregnancy planning, throughout pregnancy and post-natal recovery. Our philosophy is that good nutrition has to be balanced, easily managed and achievable alongside busy lives. Men and women generally have differing approaches to food; women sometimes have an unhealthy relationship with food, weight and body image. For many couples with delays in conception, food and drink can become another battle-ground. I am hugely grateful for Mel's contribution to this chapter and her scientific, but realistic and fun approach to food.

When you are trying to conceive, the food that you eat is particularly relevant because you are now nourishing the egg and sperm cells that are going to become your baby. These are cells like any other in the human body, and yet in recent years how they are nourished and looked after is largely ignored when considering they have the most important job of all – continuing the species. Even in earliest times both the Greeks and the Romans recognised that alcohol had a damaging effect on conception. Vets and farmers are aware of the benefits of feeding their breeding animals a nutrient-rich diet. In fact, there has probably been more research done on bull sperm than human sperm!

The maturing egg, sperm, endometrium (womb lining) and foetus depend upon vital nutrients for development. If the diet contains too many environmental endocrine-disrupting chemicals, trans-fats, refined sugars, or excessive additives, or is depleted of nutrients, then research shows it can significantly affect an individual's fertility. Moreover, studies are now beginning to show how the health of both the sperm and the egg before they even meet can affect the outcome of the pregnancy and the health of the baby, developing child and even through to adulthood. Studies now are suggesting that even grandparental nutritional status during mid-childhood can be linked to the mortality risk ratio in their grandchildren two generations later. One could say that you can help to programme the future health of your children using pre-conceptual nutritional care.

That is why having a three-month pre-conception window for both partners can really help to prepare you for pregnancy. This is especially so when you are having IVF. There are just more demands made on your body. Normally women release one egg in a cycle; with IVF your ovaries are going to be stimulated to produce many more eggs to increase your chances of conception, and so certain nutrient requirements are increased. Sperm takes approximately 85 days to mature and this is an ideal window of opportunity to make it the very best it can be. If there are egg quality problems and IVF is the best option, then there is more of an incentive to make even better quality sperm. Research is beginning to show that what happens around implantation may determine the future events of a pregnancy such as miscarriage or low birth weight. Therefore building up your stores of essential nutrients is a good insurance policy for pregnancy and the future health of your child. Many of our clients will have specific requirements that need a specialist approach, and possibly blood tests to look at vitamin and mineral needs.

What to eat and what not to eat, to conceive naturally or to go through IVF has become such a complicated issue for so many people. Women have very different attitudes to food than men. We don't see many women who do not have food issues, or concerns about what they should and shouldn't be eating. When it comes to getting pregnant, there are so many emotional links to food for women, and food is used to control various aspects of their lives. Women don't nurture themselves enough. They feel guilty and beat themselves up over a late-night takeaway or a bar of chocolate, often saying to themselves, 'I've been really good this week' or 'I've been really bad this week.' The sad fact is that many women go to extremes, cutting everything out and depleting themselves of vital nutrients. If you knew you were going to be pregnant in three months then yes, you could manage to live like this, but the reality is that it often takes longer and life can easily become really restrictive. For example, many women avoid wheat or dairy products for long periods of time, thereby depleting the body of important nutrients, such as folic acid, calcium, B vitamins and fibre.

The aim of this chapter is to take you through the areas that can really be helped by good nutrition. It is not about being 'good' or 'bad', or on a special diet – it is not meant to be a punishing regime in any way. After all, the human race would have died out a long time ago if that were the case! At the clinic we try to integrate the latest evidence-based nutritional research into our healthy eating plans. We look at the whole person, find out how and what you eat and then make a bespoke plan that is enjoyable and delicious for both partners, and very importantly that fits in with your lifestyle. Remember, food excites our taste buds and is one of life's great pleasures. So, while you're trying to eat correctly, don't lose sight of the fun aspect of food.

Can I Improve My Egg Quality?

Many of our clients are older, and have gone through a number of unsuccessful IVF cycles, and this is a question we are asked every day. The answer has to be that we would say you can improve the environment in which the eggs develop and mature, and that is going to have a beneficial effect on egg quality. It's a bit like growing tomatoes – it all depends on the soil, the feed and the sunshine – think about it being the same for your eggs. Women are having babies later in life and you cannot pick up a newspaper nowadays without reading about the dangers of leaving it too late, the ticking of the biological clock, eggs are too old, and now even sperm are getting old when men get past the age of 35. The ageing process damages all the cells of the body, including eggs. Unstable molecules called free radicals cause cellular destruction and high levels speed up the process of ageing. Some causes are poor nutrition, pollutants such as smoking, and impaired detoxification processes by the body. Eggs need good quality protein for building, essential fatty acids for the outer layer cell membrane, and antioxidants to protect them from damage. In order to help eggs and sperm mature in a nutrient-rich environment so they can be as healthy as possible, it is important to avoid dietary and environmental stressors that damage cells, and to include all the protein, essential fatty acids and vitamins, minerals and antioxidants that help to build strong eggs and sperm and protect them from accelerated wear and tear.

The Balanced Diet

Theoretically, you should be able to obtain all the nutrients you need from a healthy, balanced diet. However, research shows that only 15 per cent of women and 13 per cent of men manage the recommended five daily portions of fruit and vegetables, not to mention the two portions of fish a week, or wholegrains. Our hectic lifestyles often mean skipping breakfast, grabbing a sandwich and eating it over the computer, keeping going on coffee, tea and cola, eating sugary snacks to keep us going then getting home to pop a ready meal into the microwave and knock back half a bottle of wine.

Even if you do manage to eat healthily, you may not be obtaining the RNIs (Reference Nutrient Intakes) for some of the vitamins and minerals essential for fertility, like folic acid, selenium and vitamin D.

Folic Acid

As soon as the thought of having a baby enters your head, start taking 400 mcg of folic acid a day. This is the one crucial vitamin supplement that you really need to take three months before you conceive, if possible. This is easy enough if you know that you're going to have IVF at a certain time. But if you are just 'thinking' about it, not really trying but not using contraception either, then you must still take it. In fact, many experts recommend that all women of childbearing age routinely take folic acid as a matter of course. Folic acid helps to prevent neural tube defects such as spina bifida, and research has also linked folic acid with the possible prevention of other conditions such as cleft palate and heart defects. It is particularly important in early pregnancy as it is needed to make red blood cells and in the production of DNA, the genetic blueprint of a developing embryo.

Couples tested at the clinic for nutrient deficiencies consistently show low levels of omega 3, magnesium and vitamin D. Food manufacturing and processing and long storage periods all contribute to the depletion in nutrient content of our food, compared to the levels of 50 years ago. This is where a carefully chosen, informed diet and supplement advice can really help.

Now you're ready to start looking at the other areas of your diet and lifestyle that will help you succeed in having a successful pregnancy.

Back to Basics: Protein, Carbs and Fats

Protein, carbohydrates and fats are the backbone of the diet and they all play an essential role in fertility and pregnancy. However, the information can be so confusing as to what constitutes 'good' and 'bad'. How much protein for IVF? What if you are vegetarian or vegan? Is fish safe? Are dairy and soya good or bad for fertility? Are all carbs bad? What about low fat? As you will see, a balanced diet contains a mix of all three.

Protein

Protein is made up of amino acids, which are the building blocks of all cells, our eggs and sperm, hormones and immune cells. Protein is responsible for repairing damage, and the growth of all cells, tissues and organs, including, of course, the developing embryo. It is needed for good ovulatory function and studies with IVF have shown that women who consume very little protein produce fewer follicles and eggs. Conversely women who eat very high-protein diets also damage their fertility because the result of excessive protein consumption is high levels of ammonia, which can adversely affect implantation.

During IVF particularly, protein is very important because the ovaries are working hard to produce many eggs. However, there is no evidence that eating more than the recommended amount of protein produces a more successful outcome.

The RNI for women is 45g/day. To give you an approximate idea, a chicken breast contains about 27g, an egg 6g, 250g yoghurt 13g, ½ cup quinoa 14g, 12 almonds 3g and 50g tofu 11g. All food contains some amino acids, and a good mixed diet will supply everything you need, but animal foods contain all the essential amino acids in one 'package'. But our modern diet often contains too much animal protein, which is not ideal for fertility. Studies have shown that a high consumption of red meat and chicken (every day) led to poorer ovulatory function and lower rates of conception, and a higher consumption of vegetable proteins improved ovulatory function. So we certainly don't believe in encouraging vegetarians to eat meat when nuts, seeds, quinoa and pulses are an excellent source of protein, but they may have to work harder at getting the balance right. Animal sources are meat, chicken, fish, dairy and eggs, and vegetable sources are pulses like lentils, beans and chickpeas, nuts, soya and the grains quinoa and amaranth. How much protein each individual needs is not an exact science so we recommend that you eat a small amount of protein with each meal, and have a good mixture.

We think that a little red meat is fine a couple of times a week as it is an excellent source of iron, zinc, B12 and protein. We want you to eat with your partner too and so it's better to have a good range of foods that you both like. But try and ensure your meat is free range or organic. Avoid processed meats like ham and salami that contain the preservatives potassium and sodium nitrite/nitrate: they are not good to eat in large amounts. Free range, organic chicken is going to be a better option than intensively farmed, with less fat and water and fewer chemicals, so again twice a week is fine. Eggs are an excellent protein, very rich in other nutrients too and versatile. Recent research has debunked the cholesterol myth, that is, they don't raise blood levels of cholesterol, and they also keep you full and so are a very useful food for weight loss.

Can I Eat Fish?

The advice on fish is often quite confusing. Fish is a very good food to eat for fertility; it's low in saturated fat and a good source of protein, iodine and selenium. However, all fish are affected to some degree by the pollutants in rivers, lakes and oceans but oily fish more so because these chemicals – PCBs (polychlorinated biphenyls), dioxins – and heavy metals like mercury concentrate in the fatty parts of fish like tuna, salmon, mackerel, sardines, marlin, swordfish and shark. Some other fish are also affected like sea bream, sea bass, turbot, halibut, rock salmon (aka dogfish) and brown crab. Canned tuna is not counted as a good source of oily fish because the canning process removes most of the omega 3 fats, but it is lower in mercury than fresh tuna so is okay to eat twice a week. Intensively farmed salmon is also low in omega 3 because they are fed diets high in omega 6, not their usual omega 3-rich plankton, and wild salmon is becoming extinct. This is probably an occasion when taking a good sustainable, pharmaceutical grade (this means it's been filtered and purified) fish oil supplement is a better idea than trying to work out what oily fish to eat. It should come from the skin, not the liver, of a fish. There is also the major issue now of fish sustainability and ethical farming, and many of our clients are concerned about this, so the advice is eat fish but choose well. Download the Marine Conservation Society Good Fish Guide (www.fishonline.org) to see exactly what you can eat. Don't eat shark, swordfish or marlin; apart from these, we would advise that one portion from the above list is fine, tuna (one fresh, one tinned or two tinned) a week is fine and otherwise well farmed, sustainable white fish and shellfish two to four times a week.

What About Dairy?

We recommend a moderate intake of dairy foods as long as you have no known intolerances. Many women cut all dairy from their diet, thereby depleting the body of valuable protein, calcium, riboflavin and iodine. Of course, if you are lactose intolerant you need to avoid dairy foods, although many people tolerate goat's milk, buffalo mozzarella and live yoghurt. Low-fat products of any kind are not great for fertility as, to take fat out, something else has to go in its place and full-fat dairy products contain important vitamins like vitamin D that are only absorbed with fat. A lot of the new information on dietary changes has originated from the USA Nurses' Health Study. This is a huge study of 238,000 nurse participants, which investigates factors influencing women's health. The prime focus of the study is cancer prevention, but it has also produced many invaluable insights into diet, physical activity and other lifestyle factors that promote improved health, including reproductive health.

This study has shown that a daily serving or two of whole milk and foods made from whole milk seems to offer some protection against ovulatory infertility. Good sources are full-fat yoghurt, cottage cheese and crème fraiche. Even a scoop of creamy vanilla ice cream now and again is fine. Remember this is whole milk, so you have to weigh up the calorific content. Organic dairy products contain fewer hormone-disrupting pesticides, and higher levels of omega 3 fats and betacarotene.

Some research has suggested that consuming soya is detrimental to fertility. However, in many cultures soya is a staple food and their levels of infertility are no higher than our own. The research was conducted in-vitro, and also on animals who consumed nothing but soya. In a normal mixed diet, including a small amount of soaked or fermented soya like tofu three to four times a week is helpful especially for vegetarians as soya provides protein, calcium and some iron. Ensure it is organic and GM free.

Slow Carbs Not No Carbs

Many women have become nervous about eating carbohydrates, because of concerns about putting on weight. Cutting carbs out of your diet or having too low an intake causes tiredness and low mood – you do need carbohydrates. They provide energy, B vitamins, minerals and fibre, but they do need to be the right kind.

Simple carbohydrates are usually refined so are low in vitamins and minerals. They are very quickly digested and absorbed causing spikes in blood sugar which lead to rapid unwanted changes in hormones. They include 'white' foods like refined bread, pasta, rice, sugary foods, fruit juices and soft drinks and, of course, alcohol. Simple carbohydrates are more likely to be converted to fat.

Complex carbohydrates have all the vitamins and minerals retained and because they are more fibrous, are broken down more slowly by the body and are less likely to be converted to fat. They slowly increase blood sugar levels, giving you more energy and fewer cravings. Complex carbohydrates ('brown') foods include wholegrains such as oats, wholemeal bread and pasta, brown rice, rye and pulses.

Balancing Your Blood Sugar

Maintaining a balanced blood sugar level is very important to fertility because if it is too high or too low it can seriously impact your hormones, your energy levels and your weight. Low levels will make you tired, jittery, irritable, and make headaches and pre-menstrual symptoms worse. You will also crave sugar, probably give in to that craving which will then rocket up your blood sugar levels and your body will produce insulin in a valiant attempt to bring the level down again. This will then lead to low blood sugar levels and the cycle begins again. The more refined, sugary food and drink you have the more you will crave, as levels go up and down. This cycle over the long term can have a devastating effect on your fertility and your health. When levels are low your body will release the hormone adrenaline, your 'flight and fight' hormone, which affects the way your cells use progesterone, the major hormone of the second half of the menstrual cycle. Adrenaline is a stress hormone, not a maintenance hormone, and many experts argue that constant high levels of stress hormones have a negative effect on our reproductive hormones. When blood sugar levels are high, the constant release of insulin eventually leads to an inability of the cells to respond properly to it and a condition called insulin resistance may occur. This cycle of elevated glucose and insulin levels is a major factor in polycystic ovary syndrome (PCOS), contributing to obesity and a vicious hormonal cycle. Many experts believe that because the ovaries contain many receptors for insulin, these unregulated levels may actually damage a woman's eggs.

Understanding the Glycaemic Index and Glycaemic Load

The body's ability to regulate these levels depends on the rate at which glucose is absorbed. This, in turn, depends on what we eat and the type of carbohydrates we consume, back to simple and complex again. A good way to understand how this works is to look at both the Glycaemic Index (GI) and the Glycaemic Load (GL) of foods. The GI is a ranking of how quickly glucose is absorbed from various foods. Foods are scored from 1, very slow release, to 100, very fast release. The lower the number the more slowly you will digest the foods, you will feel satisfied for longer and have more energy and fewer cravings. The GL gives a fuller picture as it is based on the portion size as well as the GI ranking. For example, the GI of cooked carrots is high, so you would automatically think it isn't a good idea to eat them. However, you would have to eat a lot of cooked carrots to raise blood sugar significantly. Moreover, cooked carrots are high in betacarotene which is very good for fertility. Eating carbs with a little protein also helps to slow down the release of glucose, for example fruit with nuts or seeds, wholemeal toast and a boiled egg or vegetable soup with lentils. So, to keep your blood sugar stable:

- never skip breakfast
- eat protein and carbohydrates together
- don't leave long gaps between meals which will encourage cravings
- avoid processed, refined, sugary foods and drinks
- read labels, look for total sugars content; you would be amazed at how much sugar is contained in quite innocent, healthily packaged foods, especially breakfast cereals

Low GI Foods, 40 and Under on the Index

These are slow-release foods. All pulses – beans, including baked beans, lentils, chickpeas; the brassica family of vegetables – cabbage, broccoli, Brussels sprouts and cauliflower, especially the stalks; wholegrains, nuts, rye bread, oats and oat bran, apples, plums, pears, cherries, avocado, leeks.

Medium GI Foods, 41–60 on the Index

These are fine if you eat with a little protein: sweetcorn, mangos, oat cakes, wholegrain pasta, brown basmati rice, figs, steamed potatoes in their skins, beetroot, raw carrots, wholemeal bread.

High GI Foods – Over 60 on the Index

Try and eat these foods in moderation, with a little protein, but avoid the foods in italics which are really just pure refined sugars. Baked potatoes, mashed potatoes, *white bread, white rice and pasta, honey,* cooked carrots, parsnip, swede, squash, *sugar,* ripe bananas, *jam, sweets and chocolate, sugared breakfast cereal,* watermelon, raisins, *biscuits, desserts, ice cream, cakes and pastries, rice cakes,* cous cous.

The American Nurses' Health Study found that it was not the overall amount of carbohydrate eaten that affected fertility and ovulation but the GI ranking of the foods their research participants ate, that is, how quickly they were converted to glucose in the body. Women in the high GI intake group were 92 per cent more likely to have problems ovulating than those in the lower groups, so whether you're trying naturally or going through IVF, blood sugar balance is important.

Sugar Accelerates the Ageing Process

Sugar can affect fertility in other ways too. A high-sugar diet accelerates the ageing process, and particularly if you're a little older preparing for IVF, you want to delay age-related damage as much as possible. The process to blame is called glycation, and is caused by the attachment of sugar to proteins which together form destructive molecules called advanced glycation end products, known rather appropriately as AGEs. AGEs affect the structural tissues that are made of collagen and elastin. They cause wrinkles in the skin, literally making it hard and brittle. And there is collagen in the ovaries, and building the walls of the follicles from which the egg ruptures. AGEs are also related to increased oxidative stress, another side effect of ageing and cellular damage. Moreover, recent studies have shown that accumulation of AGEs may influence IVF success rates by affecting implantation and embryo development. Of course, the odd glass of wine or bar of good chocolate is not going to affect your chances. It's the everyday consistent consumption of those refined carbohydrates that counts. So treat yourself every now and again but otherwise say no.

Fats

The whole subject of dietary fats is very topical at the moment, and with government campaigns urging us to lower our fat consumption it's no wonder that many people are a little confused. Fat is absolutely crucial for every function in the body and low- or no-fat diets are an absolute no for fertility. The body needs fat for energy and growth, fats make the texture and taste of food good, and they help the absorption of fat-soluble vitamins like A, D, E and K which are vital for fertility. However, there is no doubt that some fats are much better than others and the type of fat eaten is crucial to fertility.

'Bad' Fats, 'Good' Fats

Saturated fats are naturally solid at room temperature, and are usually found in animal products, coconut and palm oil. A diet too high in these fats is linked to heart disease, obesity and cancer. High amounts also encourage inflammation which is detrimental to fertility. Many reproductive conditions that may affect fertility are associated with inappropriate inflammatory responses, for example endometriosis and some auto-immune disorders. However, your daily portions of full-fat organic dairy are fine.

Trans-fats are the real villains in fertility. They are formed by adding hydrogen to liquid oils to 'saturate' them and make them solid. They are used in food manufacture and found mostly in baked goods, margarines and snacks and are labelled as 'hydrogenated' or 'partially hydrogenated' fats. These fats are linked with obesity, they interfere with our metabolism of essential fatty acids and they affect both male and female fertility. Research from the Nurses' Health Study (see page 143) shows that just 4 grams a day of trans-fats could impact on ovulation. They also affect sperm. This is the equivalent of only one doughnut or a handful of French fries.

The 'good' fats are the poly- and monounsaturated long chain fatty acids. They are liquid at room temperature and so have the ability to keep our cell membranes fluid, which is crucial for fertilisation. Olive oil and rapeseed oil are monounsaturated and are the most stable of the fats. The polyunsaturated fats in oily fish, nuts, seeds and vegetables are the most beneficial for our health. We cannot manufacture them ourselves so they have to come from the diet and are known as the Essential Fatty Acids (EFAs), omega 6 and omega 3.

The importance of omega 3
In recent years, however, there has been concern that we are eating too many omega 6 fats and not enough omega 3 long chain fatty acids, causing an imbalance in our fatty acid ratio. This is because omega 6 fatty acids are far more prevalent in the modern diet, which contains high amounts of vegetable oils. The EFAs that are most valuable in fertility and pregnancy are the omega 3 fats eicosapentaenoic acid (EPA) and docosahexaenoic acid (DHA) and adult humans find it even more difficult to manufacture them. At the clinic we strongly believe that these fats are critical for fertility and pregnancy. Oily fish are the best source because the complicated process of making them has already been done for us by the fish. However, because generally our levels are so low and our omega 6 levels so high, we would have to eat literally pounds of fish a day to reach the optimal levels of EPA and DHA. We see this in the clinic because we can do a blood test that shows us the ratios.

EPA and DHA omega 3 fats have a profound effect on fertility; they convert into anti-inflammatory messengers called eicosanoids which are hormone-like substances that regulate the maturation of the egg, ovulation and menstruation. These fats also play an important role in labour. There are some thoughts that they may also decrease unwanted natural killer cell activity, although this whole area of reproductive immunology is controversial. These fats have blood-thinning qualities so increase blood flow to the uterus and ovaries, and may be particularly useful in IVF because the hormone therapy used raises the levels of unhealthy fats in the blood, and omega 3 fats reverse this process. Supplementing with omega 3 during pregnancy may prevent premature birth and increase foetal growth by increasing foetal blood flow. Omega 3 may also reduce the risk of pre-eclampsia and post-natal depression. Studies show that DHA plays a vital role in the development of the foetal nervous system and eyes. Finding out exactly what is your ratio of omega 6 to omega 3, and then supplementing with the advised amount three months before you start trying to conceive or have an IVF cycle, will help you to build up those vital stores, because it takes at least three months to build up the stores of omega 3 in the body.

In the meantime try to reduce your intake of omega 6 fats from vegetable oils. Don't use corn oil or sunflower oil in cooking and read labels. Use olive oil or rapeseed instead. Avoid margarines and spreads as they are high in omega 6 fats. Many claim to contain omega 3 also but the majority are not from marine sources, which for fertility are the most useful. Eat wild fish, as many farmed fish eat diets of wheat and soya which are high in omega 6, not their natural diet of EPA-rich plankton. Heating unsaturated oils damages them so it is better to use the minimum of olive or rapeseed oil to cook and then drizzle on some cold after cooking. This way you will

Good Sources of Omega 3 Fats

- Wild oily fish and seafood
- Flaxseeds, flax oil
- Rapeseed oil (Canola)
- Hempseeds, hempseed oil
- Walnuts
- Pumpkin seeds, sesame seeds
- Avocados
- Dark green leafy vegetables

obtain all the goodness without the damaged fats. In fact there is certainly a ring of truth in the claim that lard is the safest fat to cook in. It is saturated and highly stable and resistant to damage when heated and then it is converted in the body to oleic acid, the major constituent of olive oil, so roasting your potatoes in a little lard is probably a good idea; however, remember those calories! Unsaturated fats are also very vulnerable to free radical damage, so include lots of fresh vegetables and fruit in the diet.

Vitamins and Minerals and Their Effects on Fertility

A healthy balanced diet is essential for fertility, and for optimum health generally to prepare you for pregnancy. However, there are certain nutrients that have a special role in fertility. As well as looking at symptoms, blood tests are a useful way of identifying deficiencies.

Vitamin A

Not found in pre-natal multi-vitamins because very high amounts are toxic to the foetus, but it is very important for the absorption of protein, follicular development, embryo growth, thyroid health and immunity. Sources: full-fat dairy, eggs, oily fish (see beta-carotene below).

Betacarotene

The vegetable precursor of vitamin A. High levels in the corpus luteum positively correlate with strong progesterone levels. Sources: yellow, red, orange fruit and vegetables, dark green leafy vegetables.

Vitamin E

A major antioxidant, works with vitamin C and selenium to reduce free radical damage, thins the blood, regulates menstrual flow. Sources: wheat germ, nut and seed oils, green leafy vegetables, nuts.

Vitamin B6

Increases the brain chemicals, serotonin and dopamine, which control FSH and LH. Helps regulate oestrogen and progesterone levels. Sources: wholegrains, bananas, potatoes, chickpeas, lentils, seeds, fish, milk products, oats, avocado.

Folic Acid

Prevents neural tube defects (NTDs). Needs to be taken as a 400 mcg supplement at least one month, but preferably three, before conception. Sources: green leafy vegetables, pulses, oats, wholegrains.

Vitamin B3

Needed for regulation of blood sugar and production of reproductive hormones. Sources: eggs, fish, chicken, peanuts, wholegrains, avocados.

Vitamin B12

For red blood cell formation, works with folic acid to prevent NTDs, helps regulate ovulation. Sources: animal-derived foods – meat, chicken, fish, dairy, eggs. The B12 from seaweed is unusable by humans. Vegans need to test blood levels and supplement accordingly.

Vitamin C

Helps to regulate ovulation. May boost the action of clomiphene. Vitamin C is a major antioxidant, working with vitamin E to help protect your developing and maturing eggs from oxidative stress-related damage.

Vitamin D

Blood tests at the clinic have revealed that many women are deficient in vitamin D, the 'sunshine' vitamin. More and more research is showing just how important vitamin D levels are for fertility and IVF. A small study showed that women deficient in vitamin D had a lower clinical pregnancy rate than those whose vitamin D levels were adequate. Vitamin D deficiency in early pregnancy has been described as an ongoing epidemic. Some scientists recommend that pregnant women – or women thinking of becoming pregnant – have their vitamin D levels checked about every three months. Many women going through IVF are prescribed blood-thinning drugs like Heparin which interferes with vitamin D and calcium metabolism.

Vitamin D can be classified as both a vitamin and a fat-soluble pro-hormone. It is obtained naturally from two sources: sunlight and food. However, it is found in few foods and we get most of our vitamin D from the action of sunlight on our skin. Natural food sources of vitamin D include eggs and oily fish, such as herring, salmon, mackerel, sardines and tuna. Some foods, such as breakfast cereals and bread, are fortified with vitamin D.

- In a study of 67 women with anovulatory infertility, 93 per cent were deficient in vitamin D. Supplementing with vitamin D helps to restore normal ovulatory function. Vitamin D deficiency was highly prevalent among women with PCOS (see pages 176 and 251). Supplementation (alongside calcium) can help to normalise irregular periods.

- Deficiency of vitamin D is common among people with inflammatory and auto-immune disorders ranging from rheumatoid arthritis to multiple sclerosis. This may be relevant for women who have experienced unsuccessful IVF cycles.
- Vitamin D deficiency is linked to miscarriage. It also makes it five times more likely that women will develop pre-eclampsia.
- Supplementing with vitamin D may enhance the immune function of the placenta and protect it from infection.

Iron

Forms oxygen-carrying red blood cells. Deficiency causes anovulation and serious problems in pregnancy. Low iron levels are linked to infertility. Sources: red meat, chicken, fish, eggs, pulses, dark green leafy vegetables, dried apricots and prunes, seeds. Vegans and vegetarians should have a blood test to check their levels before trying to conceive or undergoing IVF at least six weeks before, in order for levels to be adequately repleted if necessary.

Iodine

Essential for the correct functioning of the thyroid gland, which strongly influences fertility. Iodine concentration in the ovaries is high and studies have found a correlation between levels in follicular fluid and follicular development. Crucial in pregnancy for foetal brain development. Sources: fish, shellfish, dairy products, iodised salt.

Magnesium

Research has shown that many women have low magnesium levels. Low levels may be implicated in hormonal irregularities and miscarriage. Sources: green leafy vegetables, nuts especially almonds, seeds.

Selenium

Another powerful antioxidant protecting developing eggs and the embryo from free radical-induced damage. It is a vital trace element for thyroid function whose proper functioning is essential for fertility. It is also linked with the prevention of miscarriage and pre-eclampsia. Sources: Brazil nuts are high in selenium but also in potentially toxic barium and radium so care must be taken not to exclusively rely on them for selenium intake. Other sources are seafood, eggs, garlic, the onion family, broccoli, mushrooms, asparagus.

Zinc

Zinc is particularly important for gene regulatory hormones, and is crucial for the synthesis of DNA and the receptor proteins for oestrogen, progesterone and testosterone, as well as vitamin D and thyroid hormones. Sources: oysters, seafood, meat, sunflower seeds, wheat germ.

Free Radicals and Antioxidants

Free radicals, or reactive oxygen species (ROS), are produced as a natural by-product of our metabolism, playing an important role in cellular repair and signalling, and we have developed our own anti-oxidant system to deal with them, both from within the body (endogenous) and from the diet (exogenous). However, when this system becomes overwhelmed for various reasons, free radicals begin to cause damage to normal healthy cells. Increasingly, free radicals are being linked to egg and sperm damage. Sources include smoking, UV radiation (too much sun exposure), recreational drugs, alcohol, foods high in poor-quality fats, industrial cooking oils and over-heated damaged fats, fried and burnt foods, and pollution.

As we said, a certain amount of free radical damage is normal. This increases with age as our endogenous antioxidant system wears down; it is what ages us and makes our skin wrinkle. However, it also ages eggs and sperm, perhaps prematurely sometimes. Free radicals target the fatty fluid membranes of all our cells leaving the DNA damaged and the cell (in this case the egg and sperm) no longer able to function. Inflammation causes free radical formation that researchers now think may be linked to endometriosis, miscarriage, pre-eclampsia, auto-immune diseases, premature ageing and unsuc-cessful IVF cycles. Couple this with a diet low in antioxidants but high in foods and lifestyle habits that encourage free radical formation and you have a recipe for damage. The oocyte (egg cell) is the largest cell in the body, 500 times bigger than a sperm cell. The mature oocyte has an abundance of cytoplasm, giving it a greater capacity to repair free radical damage, with the right antioxidants. Sperm, on the other hand, are much smaller and their highly fatty membranes make them more vulnerable to damage which affects their shape (morphology) and renders them unable to function.

Eating a diet rich in antioxidants and boosting antioxidant intake with very carefully chosen, well-researched supplements is extremely important. Antioxidants reduce damage and protect cells, playing a vital role in fertility, assisted reproduction and pregnancy. They also protect the oocyte, sperm and embryo, particularly at critical times of reproduction. Some of the most important antioxidants include vitamins C and E, zinc, selenium and betacarotene. Other powerful antioxidants also include nutrients like alpha lipoic acid, N-acetyl cysteine, resveratrol and pine bark extract (pycnogenol). So to maximise your intake of antioxidants it is a good idea to eat a broad range of fruit and vegetables of different colours. Usually the richer the colour and the stronger the taste – earthy, bitter, sulphuric or sweet and delicious – the more powerful the antioxidants. Light cooking retains them, so steam rather than boil. Good sources include broccoli, curly kale, blueberries, pomegranates, red peppers, prunes, kidney beans, cloudy apple juice, tomato puree, nuts and seeds and cold pressed olive oil.

Inflammation

Many disorders related to infertility are now being linked to abnormal inflammation. Allergies, asthma and eczema as well as auto-immune conditions like rheumatoid arthritis, lupus, Crohn's disease and ulcerative colitis are all flammatory conditions. Endometriosis, miscarriage and pre-eclampsia are also linked with high levels of inflammation. One of the reasons obesity is such a factor in infertility is because excess fat releases inflammatory chemicals. At the clinic we look at dietary and lifestyle factors that may influence the inflammatory response. A diet which is high in poor-quality fats and sugar, a poor digestive system, stress and lack of sleep, alcohol and recreational or prescription drugs can weaken the immune system. The omega 3 fats are important as they have strong anti-inflammatory properties.

Alcohol and Nutrition

Alcohol increases the amount of free radicals in the body. It also contains empty calories, is high in sugar and stored as fat. A high alcohol consumption causes the stomach to secrete too much acid and histamine. This causes inflammation and interferes with the body's ability to absorb nutrients, such as thiamine, folic acid and vitamin B6. It makes the body less efficient in utilising vitamin D, and the kidneys will excrete extra magnesium, calcium, potassium and zinc. All of these nutrients are vital to fertility, especially folic acid.

Alcohol and IVF

The latest research suggests that alcohol should be completely avoided the week before and during an IVF cycle. The chances of an unsuccessful cycle increased after consumption of over six units a week (the equivalent of two large glasses) and white wine was especially significant for women. If a woman drank between two and three large glasses of white wine a week, the chance of a successful IVF cycle was reduced by 24 per cent. Researchers think that it may affect the number of eggs produced and reduce implantation, but they do not know why, or why white wine is so significant. Previous research has found that alcohol does delay the time it takes to conceive, and the more you drink the longer it takes to become pregnant. At the clinic we always recommend that women completely avoid alcohol in the weeks leading up to and during an IVF cycle. Apart from that you can enjoy the odd glass of wine (particularly red) now and again but try to keep it under four units a week and no more than two in one evening; you have to carry on with your life.

Caffeine

Some studies have linked more than three cups of coffee a day with miscarriage, and certainly the latest research seems to suggest that we should consume even less caffeine than was previously thought if trying to conceive. Moreover, there is caffeine in many other things we enjoy – tea, green tea, colas, chocolate, and even some medications. Tea seems to be a better bet than coffee for conception. Researchers showed that women who drank half a cup of ordinary black tea a day were twice as likely to conceive as women who didn't. We usually advise that a cup of tea a day is fine, and have a cup of really good coffee at the weekend for a treat. During an IVF cycle avoid coffee altogether. Avoid green tea as it contains a chemical that blocks the action of folic acid, as well as containing caffeine. Herbal teas are fine but just don't drink more than one cup of any one particular type a day. Decaffeinated versions are useful for weaning you off tea and coffee, but we would recommend the water-decaffeinated versions, as otherwise solvents are used to remove the caffeine. However, because they also contain other chemicals that may be detrimental to fertility we would not really recommend them in the long term.

Salt

Although we do need a certain amount of sodium in our diet most of us eat far too much salt. Salt elevates blood pressure, which of course is dangerous in pregnancy, and contributes to weight gain by retaining water. It can also trigger inflammation. Too much salt just upsets the basic biochemical balance of your body. The most common culprits are processed foods such as ready meals, soups, condiments and salty snacks. Learning to read the labels is crucial – you would be amazed at the amount of salt there is in the most innocent-looking foods, often five or six times the recommended daily amount. Don't be misled by 'healthy eating' labels either: products that advertise themselves as low fat often contain hidden sugars and salt to put back the flavour. Even bread can contain a lot of sodium, as well as hidden fats.

The current RNI (Reference Nutrient Intake) is 6g of salt. However, labels usually declare the amount of sodium not salt, so in order to translate this into salt you need to multiply the sodium by 2.5, while also taking into account the portion size: for example, if a product is labelled so much sodium per 100g, you have to work out how much an actual portion size is. Six grams of salt is less than a teaspoon. For example, tomato ketchup contains 0.1g sodium for about 2 teaspoons. If you multiply this by 2.5 you get 0.25gm, ¼ of your daily intake of salt. So you can see how easy it is to have masses of salt without even adding it to your food. Look out for any ingredients that contain the word 'sodium' such as disodium phosphate, monosodium glutamate (MSG), sodium hydroxide, sodium nitrite, sodium proprionate and sodium sulphate.

You can add a pinch of salt to home-cooked food (remember the total daily amount is just less than a teaspoon) but don't have it at the table. Increasing fruit and vegetables that contain potassium will help to balance sodium too. These include bananas, avocados, carrots, celery, pineapple, leafy greens, dried apricots, melon, apples, potatoes.

Organic Food

Ideally all the food that we eat would be relatively free of pesticides and additives. Pesticides are known as 'gender bending' or hormone-disrupting chemicals, as their chemical composition is similar to that of human oestrogen. They accumulate in fatty tissue as they are fat soluble, so the fattier the food, the better it is to buy organic, e.g. butter, cheese and fatty meats. Certain foods contain more pesticide residues than others. The 'Top Ten' list compiled by the Pesticides Action Network are: flour, potatoes, bread, apples, pears, grapes, strawberries, green beans, tomatoes and cucumbers. Moreover, organic foods appear to contain more nutrients, probably due to the farming methods. Because organic cows feed on clover, their milk is higher in omega 3 fats. Many antioxidants in plants are made as a defence mechanism against pests because they are bitter tasting, so using an artificial pesticide lowers these disease-fighting chemicals in plants. But there is a balance to be had here with issues of cost, locally grown and seasonal variations. So try to buy organic as much as possible, particularly for animal-derived foods, wholegrain products and root vegetables. Remember to wash fruit and vegetables before eating. For more information see The Soil Association – www.soilassociation.org, The Organic Research Centre – www.efrc.com and The World Wildlife Fund – www.wwf.org.uk

Your Digestive System

So many of the women we see have digestive disorders such as irritable bowel syndrome, constipation, diarrhoea and bloating. Nowadays many of us eat on the run, grabbing lunch and eating it over the computer, then arriving home late, and if you are trying to eat a good meal with your partner, it may be well after nine o'clock before you eat. Then, of course, no one wants to go straight to bed, so you end up falling asleep on the sofa, dragging yourself off to bed, and before you know it the alarm has gone off, you're still full from the night before and so you miss breakfast. It really doesn't matter how well and healthily you are eating if you end up with a compromised digestive system.

The TCM Way

In Traditional Chinese Medicine (TCM) there are certain laws of nature, and it is believed that if you go outside of these laws your system becomes out of balance and it is harder to stay well. There are certain times of the day when one organ is believed to peak in performance. For example, 7am–9am is the peak time for the stomach, when you should eat a good breakfast, but 7pm–9pm is the 'rest' time for the stomach, so that is when you shouldn't eat. However, in Western countries we tend to eat late because we just have to; long gone are the days when you had the luxury of sitting down at 6pm for a good home-cooked meal.

In the Chinese tradition it is also important to eat food as near to its natural state as possible. However, TCM practitioners hold that warming foods (yang foods) are better for fertility, and that too many raw foods are harder to digest. But a salad on the side of a hot dish

Good Yang Foods for Fertility

- ginger
- chicken
- eggs
- black pepper
- red peppers
- oats
- wheat germ
- kidney beans
- onions and leeks
- root vegetables
- shellfish
- beef
- millet
- sea vegetables
- walnuts
- sesame seeds

should be fine. How you eat, where you eat and the amount of times you chew your food are all very important in TCM. Practitioners believe you should take your time, concentrating on trying to do only one thing at a time. If you are eating, eat; if you are drinking, drink; if you are thinking, think. It is also important not to eat when you are upset or angry as it will affect the digestive process.

Nutritional Planning

If you lead a busy life and come home late then it can seem to be a trial to put the right sort of foods on the table. However, there are some things you can do to help. Firstly make a weekly meal plan so you both know exactly what you are going to eat. Keep it simple and during the week eat more fish, chicken and vegetarian foods which are just lighter and easier to digest than red meat and heavy sauces. Use your freezer for simple things like chicken breasts or thighs, or a fish fillet. A little lemon juice, olive oil and fresh herbs and it can go straight into the oven. Make double the amount of freezable dishes. Steam fresh vegetables lightly; broccoli florets only need about four minutes. Slow cookers are another wonderful investment making a small cheap cut of meat and a few well-chosen vegetables into a fabulous delicious meal. Go lightly on the carbs which are heavy and hard to digest. Think about how much you eat. If you usually feel uncomfortably full after a meal, adjust your portion sizes to give your digestive system a rest. Chewing your food properly will help to increase levels of saliva; when this is mixed with food it helps the breakdown and absorption process. If you don't chew properly and eat too fast, you are preventing your digestive system from working efficiently.

Digestive Problems

Constipation can be a real problem with many women, particularly going through an IVF cycle, as the progesterone prescribed can slow down contractions of the bowel, and we regard good regular bowel movements as essential, particularly for the excretion of old hormones. We don't recommend laxatives as they just irritate the bowel, and lots of wheat bran can interfere with your absorption of important minerals like iron and zinc. Fibrous foods, plenty of water, stress management and taking the time to go are the best remedies.

If you suffer from:

Constipation

- Eat soaked linseeds, especially effective in prune juice.
- Try mixing the juice of half a lime in a little milk and drink first thing in the morning.
- Eat pulses, wholegrains, oats especially oat bran, apples and pears, prunes and figs, cherries and kiwi fruit, all vegetables including stalks.
- Take a good probiotic supplement.
- Magnesium helps to relax the bowel, so eat almonds and green leafy vegetables.
- Take some exercise.
- Good posture really helps, so straighten up.
- Make time to go and don't rush yourself.

Bloating and Flatulence

- Take small mouthfuls and chew your food really well.
- Eat slowly and stop when you are full.
- Eat lightly cooked vegetables rather than raw.
- Eat fruit between meals rather than after.
- Avoid sugar, fizzy drinks and carbonated water.

- Avoid wheat bread and pasta, try rye, millet and buckwheat.
- Eat a plain, live/bio yoghurt a day.
- Drink fennel tea.

Indigestion
- Eat little and often rather than three large meals.
- Eat slowly and chew your food well.
- Avoid red meat, fatty foods, alcohol, tea, coffee and fizzy drinks.
- Try fresh carrot and cabbage juice mixed with apple (you will hardly notice the cabbage).
- Don't drink with meals, drink water between meals.
- Try to eat lightly in the evening.
- Don't bend down or lie flat after eating, keep your trunk upright.
- Drink peppermint tea.

Coeliac Disease

This is an auto-immune condition in which the protein in grains called gluten is not digested and the immune system reacts by destroying the absorptive cells of the intestine. This leads to diarrhoea, bloating, poorly formed and malodorous stools, extreme fatigue and, of course, undernourishment due to malabsorption of nutrients. Research has linked undiagnosed, untreated and even subclinical coeliac disease with infertility and recurrent miscarriage. If you suffer from IBS-type symptoms or any of the above then a quick blood test can identify if gluten is the problem. Interestingly Irish people or people of Irish descent have a high incidence of coeliac disease. Special care must be taken with the diet as nutritional deficiencies are common, especially of the fat-soluble vitamins A, E and D and the carotenes, zinc, selenium and some of the B vitamins.

Gut Bacteria

Looking after your gut bacteria is extremely important. There are about 100 trillion bacteria, together weighing between one and three kilos, that live in the human gut. They are both beneficial and potentially harmful, although in a healthy gut they manage to live side by side with the beneficial bacteria outweighing the harmful. They help digestion, reduce constipation, manufacture B vitamins and vitamin K and help to metabolise oestrogen. These bacteria are also critical to a healthy immune system; they seem to be able to modulate immune cell signalling, and play an essential role in reducing inflammation. Scientists have also discovered that bacteria may be involved in obesity, with a high sugar and saturated fat diet changing the type of bacteria to ones that favour obesity by conserving energy. The type of food you eat can greatly influence how the 'good' bacteria thrive. The key seems to be in the consumption of plant-based foods, especially the fibrous, insoluble, indigestible parts which provide the critical fuel for these bacteria, known as prebiotics. So the diet of your gut bacteria is as important as your own! Avoid high-fat, sugary, stodgy foods and too many animal-based products, and eat plenty of fruit, vegetables (and their stalks like broccoli and cauliflower), seeds and nuts. Especially beneficial foods are believed to be onions, leeks, garlic and chives, artichokes, chicory and bananas, live yoghurt and fermented foods like sauerkrat, kefir, miso and tempeh.

Alkalising Foods

Most of our body fluids like blood, urine, cervical secretions and semen have an alkaline pH. The body employs buffering systems in order to maintain this very exact pH, but if we constantly eat very acid-forming foods, these systems have to work very hard, leaching calcium from the bones and stressing the kidneys. Very high-protein diets are acidic, as are diets that consist of lots of sugar, meat, grains, tea and coffee, alcohol, salt and, of course, the ultimate, fizzy drinks. Alkalising foods are fruit and vegetables, especially green leafy ones like watercress, wheatgrass, carrots, asparagus, pineapple, avocados and mango.

Weight Problems

As has been previously discussed, weight issues, both over and under, can seriously hinder your ability to become pregnant. Being overweight is a risk factor for IVF failure, miscarriage and pregnancy complications, and many IVF clinics will not offer treatment to women who are obese. Abdominal fat in particular releases all sorts of undesirable inflammatory chemicals and excess hormones. Studies show that you may be programming your baby to be overweight also, predisposing it to health problems way into its future. Obesity is also associated with polycystic ovary syndrome and its associated fertility problems.

Being underweight can affect your fertility just as much as being overweight. Studies have shown that even small changes in body weight (loss of 5–10 per cent of ideal body weight) may be associated with alterations in the menstrual cycle and infertility. Reproductive hormones depend on fat for their production and metabolism and there is a risk of producing too little oestrogen, or hormones with a low potency, a bit like comparing full-fat oestrogen with skimmed oestrogen – we want the full-fat version! Insufficient fat can also cause a woman's eggs to develop poorly. Additionally being very underweight significantly reduces the chance of a healthy pregnancy. The risk of miscarriage and premature birth increases, problems with breast-feeding can arise and an underweight baby has a much greater risk of developing chronic disease later in life. And interestingly, poorly nourished mothers give birth to underweight babies who are also then predisposed to obesity and chronic disease. Women following very low-fat diets also increase the chance of being malnourished as many of our most essential nutrients for fertility are actually fat soluble and must be accompanied by fat in the diet.

Over- or underweight is an area that does require some guidance as neither condition, from a fertility point of view, is particularly receptive to the straight 'calories up or calories down' approach. Maximising your fertility is not just about calories, it's about the protein, good fats, wholesome carbohydrates and nutrients that you eat, and many of our clients have put themselves on very restrictive quick-fix diets to lose weight, or on doughnuts and chips to gain weight. These kinds of extreme approaches have side effects: most obviously you will just not feel very well! A three-month plan ahead of trying to conceive naturally, or planning an IVF cycle, will often be quite enough to make that small but highly significant difference. We devise meal plans based around your lifestyle, we show you how to eat less but stay satisfied, and for underweight women we understand that it's completely counterintuitive to be told to put on weight, but there are ways of padding out your diet in a healthy and satisfying way. Just a 5–10 per cent weight gain or loss can make that critical difference to getting, and staying, pregnant.

Many women who struggle with 'comfort eating', or food restriction and other emotional issues with food, benefit from an added psychological intervention. We all know what we should be doing, but patterns of behaviour are often very hard to break, and this is where fertility counselling, hypnotherapy or cognitive behaviour therapy may be of benefit. At the clinic we aim to provide an integrated approach to weight management to ensure that you have a healthier relationship with food and therefore a long-term sustainable change.

Of course many women are naturally slim and many others are naturally curvy and the tool most often used for determining healthy body weight is the Body Mass Index (BMI), which takes into account the variety in size and shape of women, with an ideal reference range for pregnancy of between 20 and 25. So, working towards your ideal body weight will help conception, pregnancy and the health of both you and your baby.

The Importance of the Lean:Fat Ratio

BMI gives a good guideline, but it is also important to consider the lean:fat ratio. For example, some women may be in the normal BMI range but if they are exercising a lot they may have a very high lean body mass (muscle weighs heavier than fat), so may have insufficient fat stores. This fat is often called 'sex fat' as it is vital for oestrogen production and storage to ensure a woman's body has the energy reserves to get her through pregnancy, and deliver a full-term healthy baby at the end of the journey. This 'sex fat' capacity is rather like the fat-storage capacity of a camel's hump ready for a trek across the desert. Dr Rose Frisch explains this link between body fat, fertility and the effects of exercise in her book *Female Fertility and the Body Fat Connection*.

Women who are trying to lose weight can also speed up this process by exercise, and for this reason there may be times when weight reaches a plateau, or even increases as the lean mass increases. For this reason, at the clinic we tend to always check body fat percentage as well as BMI to manage weight issues. Some women may choose to see our fitness expert who can tailor-make a fitness programme and is a key support in our weight-management plans.

Weight Loss Tips

Aim for a slow, steady, sustainable weight loss of between one and two pounds a week. Some weeks you may lose a little more, and some weeks, less. But don't worry; it will average itself out. You may have a few slip-ups along the way. The important thing to realise is that it doesn't matter! You have not slipped off the track in order to then punish yourself by eating everything around you with the promise that you will start 'the diet' again on Monday. Just carry on eating normally and healthily. This is when a diary can be really helpful as you can begin to identify patterns of erratic eating and lapses in your new plan. Remember that this not a faddy diet designed to merely lose weight; eating good healthy food and exercising will not only improve your health, but also your self-esteem, your skin and hair, your energy levels and every other aspect of your health as well, of course, as your fertility. Because of this it is far less likely that you will go back to your old eating habits, thereby keeping that weight off for good.

- Always eat breakfast; this will boost your blood sugar and kick-start your metabolism.
- Eat an afternoon snack. Nuts, seeds and fruit, a rye cracker or oat cake with hummus, cottage cheese, mashed avocado, a small chunk of lower-fat Edam or Gouda and sliced apple or pear will all keep you satisfied until your next meal. Plain, unsalted popcorn is a good alternative to crisps.
- Always have protein with every meal – nuts including nut butters, seeds, eggs, fish, yoghurt, cheese, chicken, lentils, beans, chickpeas (including hummus). This will slow down the digestion of your food, allowing a steady release of glucose into the blood. Eating lean meat is hard work for your digestive system and so uses more energy.

- Eat slowly and chew your food really well. Try and sit down, don't eat on the run or grab things from the fridge or cupboard. Take your time over eating. Make the food on your plate look good and appetising.

- It takes the brain 15 minutes to recognise the feeling of 'fullness', so tell yourself that if you really feel hungry after that time you can have some more. The chances are you will not feel like eating more.

- Your body is not a dustbin! If you have leftovers either store them for lunch or supper the following day or throw them away.

- Plan menus in advance so you know exactly what you are going to shop for and eat.

- Lunches at work can be difficult. Making your own is the ideal solution. Otherwise choose sandwiches with wholegrain bread, protein and some salad or vegetables. Have fruit salad or yoghurt instead of crisps. Avoid bread, pasta, potatoes and white rice in a restaurant or canteen; stick to fish or chicken and lots of vegetables/salad. Have salad as a starter and avoid rich sauces and dressings. Try and go for a walk outside after lunch; this will improve your digestion and your energy levels.

- Before going to a restaurant always have a small snack like some nuts and an apple and this will ensure that you are not ravenous and tempted immediately by the bread basket!

- Avoid diet or slimming foods, or meal replacements or any foods that are marketed as low sugar, low fat, light, lite, diet, fat free or sugar free. These are more than likely going to be laced with a cocktail of artificial sweeteners and other additives. Removing fat also removes much of the good taste from food, and sugars are then added to make the foods more palatable. Artificial sweeteners may also intensify cravings and slow down your metabolism. Learn to read labels.

- Eat foods high in fibre. These will also fill you up, creating a feeling of fullness, and stabilise blood sugar levels as they slowly digest. Vegetables, fruit, oats, barley, beans and pulses all contain high amounts of fibre.

- Be careful about portion control. If you have big plates, start using smaller ones, sized in between the dinner plate and the side plate. Fill your plate with a variety of vegetables, the more colours the better.

- Keep foods containing high levels of saturated or processed fats to a minimum, such as pork (ham, sausages, bacon), lots of full-fat dairy produce, fast foods (burgers, battered fish, fries, crisps and roasted nuts). Remove the skin from chicken and the fat from red meat. Organic and free-range meat contains less saturated fat and more lean muscle.

- Oven bake and roast foods: adding a little olive oil and herbs will make most food taste delicious, including vegetables. Otherwise lightly steam vegetables or have raw in a salad.

- Reduce starchy carbohydrates for your evening meal. Have small portions of 'good' carbs like brown basmati rice, wholegrain pasta, steamed or boiled potatoes in their skins, sweet potato, butternut squash or a slice of wholemeal bread.

- Eat foods rich in calcium, which appears to be helpful in weight loss: dairy products, green leafy vegetables, nuts and seeds.

- Try and wean yourself off the 'need' for something sweet after dinner. This is not a need – it's a 'want' and a habit! Try substituting a little dried fruit, or slices of fresh fruit; a slice of fresh pineapple can also help digestion. Smelling real vanilla essence may help to reduce chocolate cravings.

- Keep cool. The body uses more energy to warm you up.

- Try and keep sugary or junk foods to a minimum but allow yourself regular treats. This may be eating what you like in a restaurant once a week, ice cream at the cinema, a croissant on Saturday or chocolate on Sunday. Look forward to it and enjoy it. If the basic framework of your diet is good then it's fine to have the odd treat.

- Keep a diary of the times when you feel that you're coming off track, i.e. when you feel like giving up and tucking in. This may be after a row, watching a certain TV programme or just feeling low.

Weight Gain Tips

Although research tends to concentrate on why people are overweight rather than underweight, it appears that, just as overweight people eat more than they think they do, underweight people eat less than they think. They also consume fewer calories, particularly in the form of fats, and do more exercise. Stress plays a part too with overweight people 'comfort eating' and underweight people being too busy to eat, or 'in a state'. The key to healthy weight gain to prepare for pregnancy is to eat both calorie- and nutrient-rich foods, not to suddenly start eating junk foods.

- Eat three meals a day with a mid-morning snack, an afternoon snack and a snack before bed. Eating breakfast will stimulate your appetite. Never skip meals.
- Stop drinking fizzy drinks, fruit juices, tea and coffee, which fill you up. Even water before or with a meal can blunt your appetite so drink between meals only.
- Make eating easy. Make a list of your favourite foods and make sure that you have thought about what you are eating. Make time to shop and stock up with good nutritious food.
- Avoid artificial sweeteners. These have many unhealthy side effects including increasing sugar cravings. Avoid 'diet' foods in

which the fat content has been reduced only to be replaced by a cocktail of artificial additives.

- Be aware of hunger, tune in to your body and recognise the signs that you need to eat.

Nutritious Food for Gaining Weight

- Olive oil – buy cold pressed, organic unrefined, and have it with vegetables and bread and use plenty in cooking. Mix with walnut oil for salads, and sesame oil for stir fries, and use lots
- Avocados
- All plain nuts
- Nut butters
- Seeds
- Coconut milk; in Indian and Thai curries. It is also delicious in smoothies
- Dried fruit. Good snacks and delicious soaked, and poached and pureed
- Oily fish like salmon (organic or wild), mackerel, herrings, sardines
- Mayonnaise, add garlic and fresh herbs and dip in home-made potato chips roasted in olive oil
- Hummus (not low fat)
- Sundried tomatoes and pesto
- Full-fat natural organic yoghurt and crème fraiche
- Bananas
- Mangos
- Home-made carrot, banana or date and walnut cake or flap-jacks
- Wholemeal bread and pasta
- Brown basmati rice
- Sweet potatoes, butternut squash, pumpkin

- Eat good-quality protein but don't avoid carbohydrates. You need them for energy, fibre, vitamins and minerals.
- Start adding fats into your diet. They are the best and easiest way of increasing your calorie intake and fats are absolutely essential for good hormone production. Use more plant fats and less animal fats. Avoid things in breadcrumbs and batter and don't fry foods.

Restricted Diets

There are many couples who, for various religious, ethical and health reasons, restrict certain food groups and may just need a little guidance towards other foods that can fulfil their nutritional requirements. Also just being aware of what goes well with what to ensure maximum nutrient absorption can be helpful.

A good vegetarian diet can be one of the healthiest in the world, but a bad one that relies heavily on carbohydrates and dairy is not going to help your fertility. Ensuring a wide variety of plant-based proteins, eggs, a little dairy, nuts and seeds and, of course, vegetables and fruit will maximise your fertility. South Asian and Middle Eastern diets are often low in iron and zinc because flat, unleavened breads interfere with their absorption.

Vegans need to be especially conscientious because animal-derived foods contain many easily absorbed nutrients. The most common deficiencies are protein, the omega 3 fats EPA and DHA, calcium, iron, zinc, selenium, vitamin A, vitamin D, riboflavin and vitamin B12. We would always advise blood tests to ascertain levels and then probably advise a mixture of specific foods and supplementation.

Polycystic Ovarian Syndrome (PCOS), Endometriosis and Fibroids

These are all conditions that are implicated in fertility problems. They cannot be 'cured' as such, but certainly diet and lifestyle changes can help manage and reduce the symptoms and increase the chances of conception.

PCOS

We see many women at the clinic suffering from PCOS-related fertility problems. One of the defining features, and often the most distressing, is the presence of high levels of circulating testosterone, which can cause acne, male pattern baldness and excess facial and body hair. PCOS is strongly associated with being overweight; in fact just losing between 5–10 per cent weight can help to restore fertility. Abdominal fat is the key, the 'apple shape', because this fat has a life of its own. It is highly active metabolically releasing inflammatory chemicals called cytokines and prostaglandins which affect hormones, egg development and implantation. If you are unsure if you carry your fat around your middle calculate your waist:hip ratio. Divide the measurement of the narrowest part of your waist by the measurement of the largest part of your hips. This should be less than 0.8. If it is greater than 0.8 then try to take steps to lower it.

Insulin and Insulin-resistance

At the very root of the abdominal fat issue is the way the body uses the hormone insulin. Insulin is the hormone that regulates blood glucose and high levels of blood glucose cause correspondingly high spikes of insulin. Instead of taking glucose back to the liver to be stored, insulin takes it to the abdominal fat cells where it is stored as fat. PCOS sufferers have a high number of insulin receptors in their abdominal fat. Insulin also causes the ovaries to produce testosterone. PCOS also has an impact on SHBG (sex hormone binding globulin). The role of SHBG is to package up excess hormones making them unavailable for use. PCOS causes lower levels of SHBG which allows the testosterone to circulate freely causing the acne, hirsutism and alopecia.

PCOS and Diet

Diet is critical for women with PCOS. This involves weight management (where appropriate), blood sugar management, antioxidant nutrients and the right supplement advice. We may advise using a combination of chromium for blood sugar balance and omega 3, inositol and magnesium for improving insulin sensitivity, as well as probiotics and antioxidants. Try and reduce animal-derived products and substitute these with vegetarian sources like quinoa and especially beans, lentils and chickpeas. Cut out sugar and reduce alcohol consumption. The best diet for PCOS is a low-refined carbohydrate diet with plenty of fibre, plant protein and good fats. Some herbs can also help with reducing the symptoms of PCOS. These include black cohosh, saw palmetto and milk thistle although do seek advice from a registered herbalist, especially if you are actively trying to conceive. Agnus castus is commonly used but it is not always appropriate as it can raise LH levels (which may already be too high), and lower FSH levels (which may already be too low), so a blood test is always necessary to ascertain exactly which herbs are suitable for you. Do not take herbs with fertility drugs, or if you are planning an IVF cycle, as they may interfere with hormone test results.

Exercise

Exercise is extremely beneficial for PCOS sufferers. It helps with weight loss, reduces stress hormones, improves insulin sensitivity and improves oestrogen metabolism. Rebounding on a mini trampoline is excellent as it is cheap, quick – just 15 minutes a day will give you an excellent work out – and the pumping action helps lymphatic drainage which is the body's way of processing toxins. Make a promise to yourself to never use lifts or escalators, and perhaps get off the bus or tube a stop earlier. PCOS cannot be 'cured' but, in our opinion, it certainly can be managed to help you regain your fertility.

Endometriosis

Endometriosis is another complex condition of varying degrees, often with the addition of debilitating, painful, heavy periods (see page 254). Women with endometriosis may also have high levels of immune cells and inflammatory chemicals in the peritoneal fluid which can affect both tubal contractility and the sperm's ability to fertilise an egg. Endometriosis is a multi-factorial condition which includes sensitivity to high levels of oestrogen and involvement of the immune system with a high level of inflammatory mediators being released.

Diet and Lifestyle Factors
Women who suffer from endometriosis may benefit from a diet low in animal products and high in anti-inflammatory nutrients. We may advise supplements including probiotics to help modulate the immune system, omega 3 to reduce inflammation and pain, magnesium to help relax the smooth muscle of the uterus and antioxidants to combat the free radical damage that accompanies inflammation. The herb agnus castus can also be very helpful with correcting the hormonal imbalances involved. Consult a herbalist for advice. Some studies have suggested that tampons bleached in chlorine may worsen symptoms so try using unbleached ones, or better still use pads as tampon use

may also increase pain. It makes sense to allow your menstrual bleed the most obvious exit route to try and reduce the chance of the wayward endometrial cells migrating backwards along the tubes. Sex and exercise during menstruation may exacerbate symptoms of endometriosis. Similarly a high caffeine and alcohol intake may also worsen symptoms.

Fibroids

Fibroids can also be associated with heavy, painful periods and fertility problems depending on their size and position. Like endometriosis they are associated with a sensitivity to high oestrogen levels. As with PCOS fibroids are often associated with overweight and obesity, so weight loss and an organic diet low in animal products may be recommended. Agnus castus may be useful for women with fibroids and research has also suggested that iodine deficiency may be implicated. Iodine-rich foods include dairy products, sea vegetables and shellfish. Because of the heavy bleeding that is often a feature of fibroids, iron deficiency anaemia can occur so this would need to be addressed as anaemia can also affect fertility.

Male Factor

Sperm quality is crucial for fertility. Sperm need to survive the long and difficult journey through the woman's reproductive tract to reach the egg, transporting the male DNA and perpetuating the species. Yet, in spite of this critical function, human sperm quality is given less attention than the sperm of a bull or a rabbit! Farmers and vets are well aware of the value of ensuring good nutrient status in their animals because good breeding stock means money.

Sometimes Life Is Unfair

Many couples express frustration at what they see as incredible unfairness – we all know the fat bloke down the pub who drinks 10 pints a night and smokes 20 cigarettes a day and has four kids; the mate who has a big cocaine habit and had to do it just once before his wife was pregnant; and what about drug addicts and alcoholics who seem to be able to just look at a girl to get them pregnant? For every one of them, though, there is another who has problems getting his partner pregnant. It's also important to consider whether those babies with unhealthy fathers are as healthy as they can be. Probably not. For example, we know now that the children of smoking fathers suffer a higher incidence of leukaemia and this is due to genetic mutation caused by the toxic chemicals in cigarettes. The ancient Greeks and the Romans also believed that excessive alcohol consumption by men caused them not only to perform less well in bed but to have less-healthy children. Plato wrote that a man 'steeped in wine ... is clumsy and bad at sowing seed, and is thus likely to beget unstable and untrusty offspring, crooked in form and character ...'

What About Age?

We now also know that sperm quality deteriorates with a man's age too. Yes, there are men well into their seventies and even eighties who father children but they really are the exception. Moreover, studies show that the incidence of autism is increased with older fathers. As in women this may be due to an increase in oxidative stress and free radical damage, which increases with age.

Minimising Genetic Damage to Sperm

Your sperm makes up half your baby's genetic blueprint. Fortunately, we are now beginning to learn more and more about human sperm, and the impact of certain toxins and nutrients. If you are spending what might turn out to be a small mortgage on assisted conception (or even if you aren't) then it's certainly worth preparing your sperm. This will not only help fertilisation, but will also help your partner minimise her risk of miscarriage (chromosomally abnormal sperm can still fertilise an egg but eventually the woman's body will reject a developing embryo with faulty DNA).

If a woman is older then it is even more important for a man to have the best sperm possible. Older eggs are just tougher to fertilise. With natural conception, and even with IVF, the strongest sperm is the winner, but with ICSI this process of natural selection is lost. It is therefore essential that the DNA of all the sperm is as good as it can possibly be.

Sperm is particularly vulnerable to free radical damage, which often results in abnormally formed sperm, and a poor motility and morphology result, or fragmentation of the DNA. Eating a diet rich in antioxidants that protect against free radical damage is vital, but supplementing the most important antioxidants may also be recommended. Some causes of oxidative stress are poor nutrition, pollutants such as smoking and excessive drinking, obesity and poor detoxification processes by the body. Free radicals can also cause sperm to become hyperactive while still in the reproductive tract, which affects their motility and forward progression. Semen normally contains antioxidants to protect sperm against free radicals. If this natural defence system is impaired in some way, the effect on sperm can be extremely damaging.

Sources of Free Radicals

- Smoking
- Recreational drugs
- Alcohol
- Processed foods, particularly foods high in artificial additives
- Fast foods
- Foods that contain high amounts of poor-quality fats and oils, particularly processed meats, margarines, biscuits and pastries, and takeaways
- Fried, barbecued and burnt foods
- Exposure to environmental pollution such as traffic fumes. Keep car windows closed in traffic jams and wear a mask if you regularly cycle in heavy traffic

Alcohol

Even moderate alcohol consumption can affect male semen quality, and higher consumption may lead to serious problems with sperm morphology, leading to an increase in malformed sperm. Alcohol also affects motility – imagine trying to swim the Channel and then head-butting your way through a wall after a few pints! Daily drinkers may have an increased susceptibility to poor sperm morphology. Alcohol can deliver a double blow to sperm, as it is also a major source of free radical damage and depletes the body of valuable vitamins and minerals like folic acid.

Caffeine

Caffeine may cause sperm to become hyperactive in the seminiferous tubules, which affects motility on ejaculation. It may also be associated with chromosomal damage and the effect on sperm appears to be dose related, so keeping to a moderate total caffeine intake is important. Caffeine is contained in tea, green tea, chocolate, colas and some medications, as well as coffee.

Weight

Excess weight can affect male reproduction because a process carried out in fat cells called aromatisation can cause the conversion of testosterone to oestrogen, which can affect sperm count. Moreover, obesity can lead to the development of an apron of fat around the genital area which can lead to overheating of the testicles, potentially reducing sperm numbers. A sedentary lifestyle may also be a factor in poor semen parameters so walking as much as possible, using stairs instead of lifts and incorporating some form of regular exercise may be beneficial.

Dietary and Environmental Oestrogens

The dozens of synthetic chemicals found in everyday life, from shampoos, cosmetics and household cleaning products to pesticides, plastics, food wrappings, tin can linings and heavy metals like lead and arsenic, are known as hormone disruptors because their molecular shape is very similar to that of oestrogen. The delicate balance between the hormones oestrogen and testosterone in men is disrupted and may well be a cause of much male infertility. To limit your exposure to hormone-disrupting chemicals eat organic as much as possible and avoid contact with strong chemicals.

Antioxidants

These are the most potent antioxidants for improving male fertility.

Vitamin E
A fat-soluble vitamin and the main antioxidant in sperm membranes. It works with selenium in its antioxidative capacity. If you are taking prescribed medicines for blood pressure or blood-thinning medications such as aspirin, heparin or warfarin, please seek medical advice before taking vitamin E.

Selenium
This antioxidant mineral is vital for healthy sperm formation, particularly motility. It also protects against toxic metal contamination. The amount of selenium in food depends on the amount in the soil; as it is believed that the soil is often highly depleted of this mineral, supervised supplementation is recommended.

Vitamin C (ascorbic acid)
A water-soluble vitamin. Its most important role in male fertility is the prevention of agglutination, when sperm clump together. This often happens when antibodies bind to sperm and can result from present or past genito-urinary infection. Vitamin C is also a powerful antioxidant and present in high levels in seminal fluid. Overheating and smoking easily destroy it.

Zinc
A trace mineral, and perhaps one of the most important nutrients in male fertility. Zinc deficiency decreases both testosterone and sperm counts. It is highly concentrated in the seminal fluid and seminal plasma, and the head of sperm contains high amounts. Zinc concentration is significantly correlated with sperm density, motility and

viability. However, zinc supplementation needs to be carefully monitored because immune function can be impaired if doses are too high.

Additional antioxidants that have also been shown to improve sperm are N-Acetyl Cysteine and pycnogenol (pine bark extract).

Other Important Nutrients

L-Arginine

An amino acid that may affect sperm count and motility. The heads of sperm contain large amounts, and abnormal sperm counts often indicate a deficiency of arginine in the semen. Arginine also improves blood flow and can be very helpful for erectile dysfunction, alongside pycnogenol. (Note: people who suffer from the herpes virus should avoid foods rich in arginine as it stimulates replication of the virus.)

L-Carnitine

This amino acid plays a crucial role in the metabolic processes of energy production that fuel sperm motility, and high levels are normally found in sperm cells. Vegans should be aware that there is virtually no carnitine in plant foods, and supplementation may be necessary.

Co-enzyme Q10

A vital catalyst in the conversion of food to energy within cells. In sperm cells it is concentrated in the mid-piece where it is an energy promoter and antioxidant. Research is showing that it may be effective in improving fertilisation rates following ICSI.

Folic acid

Some research has shown that this may reduce abnormalities in the sperm.

Supplements For Men

Men hate taking pills, that's for sure! However, this is one occasion when some nutrients just have to be taken in supplemental form if there are problems. Much of the research has been carried out using specific doses of nutrients and it is just too difficult to ensure the correct amount in foods. That is why we do suggest carefully researched supplements, but we try to be very careful and exact with our recommendations. There is a specialised test for ROS (reactive oxygen species) or free radical damage, and also folic acid and vitamin D. We suggest a general multi-vitamin that covers all the basic nutrients we have covered here for every man trying to conceive but if there are problems we recommend 'topping up' specific nutrients. But because sperm is produced on a three-month cycle, we do stress the importance of just thinking of this as a three-month project. This may be either the three months prior to an IVF cycle, or, if trying naturally, we would advise a retest of the sperm after three months. If there is an improvement then it is worth carrying on. If not, then stop – simple as that.

If you are planning on conceiving naturally or, indeed, having an IVF cycle, then you can really help to improve your sperm and therefore your chances of success by giving yourself three months to make that sperm the very best it can possibly be. At the clinic we do consultations for men that last half an hour (not too long!), often on the phone (not too much time away from work!), which involve a simple, non-judgemental information-giving, of the dos and don'ts for healthy sperm based on the latest research. Part of our ethos at the clinic is that everyone has different dietary needs, likes and dislikes, lifestyles, eating habits and relationships and so our job is to make our advice as easy, attractive and functional as possible for each individual man. Try to think of it as a three-month project, ticking the boxes and just doing your best.

Foods Containing Vital Nutrients for Male Fertility

SELENIUM	VITAMIN E	VITAMIN C	ZINC	ARGININE	CARNITINE	VITAMIN B12	FOLIC ACID
Brazil nuts (max 3/day)	Nut and seed oils	Citrus fruits	Meat	Nuts especially:	Beef	Meat	Green leafy vegetables
Wheat germ	Nuts and seeds	Kiwi fruit	Fish	Walnuts	Pork	Fish especially:	Beans
Oats	Wheat germ and wheat germ oil	Strawberries	Chicken	Almonds	Lamb	Trout	Lentils
Garlic and onions	Wholegrains	Blackcurrant	Eggs	Brazil nuts	Dairy products	Salmon	Asparagus
Barley	Eggs	Red pepper	Pumpkin / Sunflower seeds	Beans		Sardines	Oatmeal
Butter	Green leafy vegetables	Broccoli	Wholegrains	Lentils		Eggs	Dried figs
Smoked herring		Cabbage	Beans and pulses			Cheese especially:	Avocado
Brown rice		Brussels sprouts	Ginger root			Edam	
Wholegrains		Melon	Rye				
Red Swiss chard		Mango	Oats				
		Watercress					
		Spinach					
		Papaya					
		Parsley					

Acupunctu
Complementary
Therapies

When I opened my clinic in 2003 it was one of the first fertility clinics in the UK to integrate complementary therapies with conventional medicine. Since then, I have seen a big increase in the number of clinics using complementary therapies for women trying for a baby or undergoing fertility treatment, including IVF. I believe that complementary therapies have a huge amount to offer in this field of medicine when used correctly. Finding the right therapy or mix of therapies for each individual's needs is a vital part of the work we do. This chapter focuses on acupuncture, which is one of my preferred approaches, although other therapies are used at the Zita West Clinic, including nutritional therapy (see Chapter 7), hypnotherapy (see Chapter 5), qigong, manual lymphatic draining and massage.

I believe that a combined approach to fertility, encompassing mainstream medicine and a holistic approach using complementary therapies, ensures every aspect of the body is looked at. I take a

dical history first, and then look at areas such as nutri-
lifestyle and emotional and psychological wellbeing.

When you are choosing a therapy, spend a little time researching
what is available and thinking about your needs. I have found that
everyone has some area of their life that is out of balance, be it physical, emotional or spiritual, in their lifestyle, work or relationships.
You will need to find a therapist you can work with. The beauty of
working with a team like mine is that we are able to pool our resources
to find the right treatment for the client. An overall plan might start
with a nutritional consultation, then following with acupuncture,
hypnotherapy or cognitive behaviour therapy, depending on the needs
of the individual. In this way we look at the whole picture.

Complementary therapy can offer a lot of support to women both
trying to conceive naturally and going through assisted fertility treatment. It makes them feel they are being proactive in increasing their
chances of pregnancy and, very importantly, helps to reduce their
stress levels. It gives the individual time and space to be listened to by
someone who is not emotionally involved. In recent years some
complementary practice has benefited from increased education and
regulation about treating people with fertility issues. Although there
is limited hard evidence showing the effects of complementary therapies, in our experience, many women feel that they do benefit from
having these treatments. Generally, provided a treatment is safe and
makes you feel better, then you are likely to benefit from it.

In recent years the medical profession has become more open and
accepting of complementary therapies in the light of increasing
research and evidence. Some doctors, however, are still dismissive of
complementary therapies and some hold a healthy scepticism. This
can be difficult for women who wish to combine complementary and
conventional approaches.

Therapy Dos and Don'ts

- Therapists sometimes use language that can make you nervous. Always ask the therapist if you don't understand; don't go home thinking that something is wrong.

- Therapy costs can spiral out of control. Remember that you are very vulnerable while you are going through fertility treatment. Don't feel obliged to go for therapy, and don't worry that the magic won't happen if you stop. Always work within a time-frame. Review what you are doing after three months. Don't waste more time than that.

- Always keep in mind your age and how long you have been trying for a baby. Valuable fertility time can be wasted if you are moving from one therapist to another without keeping an eye on time passing.

- Don't lie there with needles in you if you hate needles. You should get some pleasure or relaxation from the treatment.

- Don't let the therapist control what you are doing in terms of your fertility treatment. I feel very uncomfortable when a client tells me her therapist says she shouldn't take fertility drugs or go through another IVF cycle for six months because she needs that time to get back into balance. Be guided by your IVF doctors.

- If the therapist is spending most of the session discussing him- or herself and not you, move on – they are not focusing on you enough.

I am always disturbed when I hear claims made by complementary therapists of high success rates for women with fertility problems such as unexplained infertility. Some therapists put a figure on what they claim as their success rate. These claims really need to be questioned

and seen in the light of all the other things (including the passage of time) that contribute towards pregnancy.

I would not in any way want to diminish the role of the complementary therapist in supporting women with fertility problems. However, while I believe there is a place for complementary therapies in the treatment of fertility problems, they should be used in conjunction with mainstream medicine. I am pleased to say that this is happening more and more.

What is Acupuncture and How Does it Work?

Acupuncture originated in China more than 3,000 years ago. It is important to appreciate that as Chinese medicine was developing, practitioners did not have access to the methods of research and examination available to modern medicine, and they became highly skilled in using detailed observation of the patient to understand body functions and make their diagnoses. This approach remains central to the practice of acupuncture today. It also leaves a rich legacy of terminology and language to describe the complex interconnection of physical, mental and emotional factors in our health that reflect what early practitioners saw, and this can sound a little strange to modern ears if taken absolutely literally.

Acupuncture involves the insertion of fine needles through the skin at specific points on the body, called acupuncture points. The Chinese observed that the body can be mapped with energy channels, called meridians, associated with the various body systems in which energy, or qi (chi), flows. Acupuncture points lie at precise locations on the meridians. An obstruction to the flow of energy may result in physical, mental and emotional imbalance which eventually can lead

to disease. By stimulating the acupuncture points the free flow of energy can be restored and this allows the body to re-establish its natural balance.

What Affects Our Qi?

Many things can affect qi. Exercise can help keep it circulating freely. The Chinese do various exercises, such as t'ai chi and qigong. The aim of these exercises is to promote the circulation of qi within the body, the belief being that vitality of the person is enhanced. Our thoughts and emotions also affect the state of qi. Some people are more emotional than others. Having negative emotions, such as anger, sadness or grief, can deplete or block the flow of energy.

Qi is also influenced by what we eat. Chinese dietary therapy is based on the concept that foods have healing qualities. Foods are classified according to their actions based on their energetic qualities such as hot, cold or neutral. Eating, for example, too much energetically cold foods, such as raw vegetables, salads and uncooked foods, can weaken the spleen's function of transforming food properly for nutrition. In traditional Chinese medicine the spleen is responsible for the digestion of food. If the spleen's function becomes weak and cannot extract energy from food then that person's vitality or qi will be compromised. Cold food can further cool the body down especially if you are constitutionally sensitive to cold.

When it comes to fertility the Chinese advise women to avoid the excessive consumption of cold foods and drinks as they believe this might lead to the phenomenon called 'cold in the uterus'. The uterus has to provide a hospitable environment for the developing embryo, therefore you need to keep it warm by eating warm foods and dressing up properly. I am often surprised to see how little women wear sometimes on a cold day. Because it is often cold and damp in the UK, it is even more important that you wear proper shoes and don't expose the lower back. These are just some examples of things that can affect your qi and how you should look after it, but your practitioner will be able to advise you further to suit your personal needs.

What Happens on Your First Visit?

The first acupuncture session normally lasts an hour. During that time the acupuncturist will ask questions about different aspects of your health and lifestyle. There will be questions, for example, about sleeping patterns, eating habits, digestion, urination, your medical and fertility history, just to mention a few. You might think these questions are not related to your presenting conditions; however, this information can be crucial for your practitioner to identify where the imbalances in your body are. When we treat fertility we always treat you as a whole person rather than your chief complaint in isolation. If you are a woman there will be thorough questioning about your periods, the regularity of your cycles, blood flow and the colour of the bleeding. We would like to know about your ovulation as well, whether you are aware when you think you ovulate and the physical signs of it if you have any.

The therapist will then palpate your pulse on both wrists. In Chinese medicine there are 28 pulse classifications, which describe the way the pulse feels under the fingertips. Your tongue will be examined for its size, shape, colour and coating. Your tongue and pulse readings will provide your practitioner with a great deal of information about how your body is working and how to tailor your treatment. Finally, your acupuncturist will ask you to lie on the treatment couch and will insert a few very fine needles through the skin.

In my experience, I find that women (and men) are often slightly anxious on their first visit, especially if they have never had acupuncture before. Very often they ask whether it is going to be painful or not. I tell them that the sensation they experience is quite personal, and the arrival of qi on the needle brings about a specific sensation. This can be experienced as dullness or soreness around the insertion site but very often it is a pleasant pain. Once the sensation settles down, your body can feel heavy and this will put you into a very relaxed state, making the session very relaxing and enjoyable. Whether you are comfortable with the thought of being needled or not, at the clinic we aim to put you at ease.

From the traditional Chinese medicine (TCM) standpoint, fertility is not treated in isolation from the rest of the body. Women often ask to be treated for a specific condition when they come to the clinic, for example for polycystic ovarian syndrome (PCOS) or lowering high FSH. When I start asking about the different aspects of their health, be it physical, mental or emotional, clients can get irritated as they don't understand what it has to do with the treatment of their presenting condition. Your presenting signs and symptoms are the result of the physiological problems of one or more systems in your body, which in turn is the result of your fertility problem. The acupuncturist will therefore try to identify and rectify those problems so that your body can regain optimal balance and function. Treatments will therefore always focus on resolving the cause of the problem rather than treating only the presenting condition or its signs and symptoms.

To do that, your practitioner first needs to collect information based on the signs and symptoms of your general, mental, emotional health and lifestyle. Chinese diagnosis also draws a lot of information from observing the appearance of your tongue and the quality of your pulse. The collected information can then be differentiated into specific groups described as 'patterns', and this method is one of the most important diagnostic principles in TCM.

The selection of acupuncture points to be used will be based on your Chinese diagnosis; so your treatment can be very different from another person's, even if that person has the same presenting medical condition as you.

When acupuncturists explain their diagnosis, they sometimes use terminology that seems unfamiliar or ambiguous. For example, your acupuncturist may give a diagnosis of 'kidney deficiency', which in TCM terms is almost always associated with infertility, or blood deficiency. This doesn't mean that you have problems literally with your kidney organ itself or problems with your blood, that you need to run to your GP to have assessed. These are only TCM terms used by your acupuncturist and do not refer to the kidney function in a biomedical sense. If you don't understand what your acupuncturist is describing then ask for help and explanation. Do not go home feeling anxious and worried that something is wrong with you.

If you are trying for a baby naturally, the treatment will be influenced by where you are exactly in your menstrual cycle. If you are around ovulation time, for example, there would be some additional points to help with ovulation.

Individual Approach

Each acupuncturist brings his or her own uniqueness into the treatment room: no two acupuncturists will give exactly the same treatment. One of the most important parts of the treatment is the rapport you have with the acupuncturist. Certainly for me, while treating, that relationship has to exist to be able to meet my client's emotional needs. It is an intriguing insight into the way acupuncture works that, having done this work for some years now, I would describe many women trying for a baby as tending to hold their emotions in the abdomen. I think this reflects the way acupuncture focuses on a mind–body connection. In Chinese medicine the two are not separated. TCM identifies a connection through a meridian called the 'bao mai' that links the heart to the uterus and the kidneys: these are all important for reproduction. The organs have physical as well as emotional connections. For example, the kidney association is fear, and the heart is joy and is the seat of the emotions. We can relate to this instinctively in the West, using such terms as 'broken-hearted' or 'heavy-hearted'.

Strong emotions such as worry, fear or anger can upset the heart and affect the flow of qi to the uterus. Using acupuncture points along this meridian helps a woman to reconnect to her lower abdomen. We also use visualisation techniques – I will ask a woman to describe and talk about her uterus, or I'll ask her to tell me how she feels emotion-

Case Study

Eleanor, 35, had tried to get pregnant for three years. She'd had a termination when she was much younger and had really beaten herself up about this. She got pregnant with IVF and miscarried. She felt that her termination was coming back to haunt her. Like a physical scar she kept picking at this emotional wound. She had irregular cycles and also terrible stress and tension in her abdomen. Every day she woke feeling as though there was a hand-like vice gripping her the whole time, as she described it, and there was a heavy, sinking feeling in the lower part of her abdomen. She didn't want to think about or connect to her lower abdomen as she felt it was all probably a mess due to the termination. We used acupuncture and visualisation to help her to connect to her lower abdomen again, and abdominal massage to release tension. This was followed by hypnotherapy to help her subconscious mind let go. Eleanor was due to do an IVF cycle and was fearful it wasn't going to work. It did work and she is now pregnant with twins.

ally. Some say 'empty', 'aching', 'heartbroken', 'flat'. In asking women questions about this area some will say they can make a connection but many will say they can't. It may often be that they are unable to connect to this whole area or visualise it for powerful reasons such as past traumas (a termination, for example), low self-esteem and, in some cases, abuse. Many women have had disappointment after disappointment, so they have cut themselves off on some psychological level. Women who have had many operations in the past, or gynaecological problems such as fibroids, may protect themselves by cutting these connections from their minds.

Techniques Used During Treatment

A variety of techniques and equipment may be used with acupuncture. Different acupuncturists will use different needling techniques largely influenced by their training. There are different sizes and types of needles and different depths of insertion. Women often feel anxious about the needles especially if they don't like blood tests. Acupuncture needles are very fine, individually packaged and completely sterile. Some acupuncturists may use other equipment including moxibustion and electro-acupuncture.

Moxibustion

Acupuncture points can be stimulated by burning a herb called mugwort, commonly known as moxa, over the point. The name 'moxibustion' is derived from its Japanese name Mogusa (which means burning herb). Moxa is used in several ways, such as directly on the skin or indirectly through a needle. Direct moxibustion is carried out with a smouldering moxa stick, which is held about a centimetre away from the skin to warm the acupuncture point. Other kinds of moxibustion involve the burning of a moxa cone or a ball of moxa wool on the head of the needle. Rolled moxa balls can also be placed on a slice of ginger or garlic over the acupuncture point, and then moxa is lit. Moxa disperses cold and warms the meridians, which leads to a smoother flow of blood and qi. Moxibustion has a therapeutic effect and can be used for many conditions. The person being treated will experience a pleasant warm sensation that penetrates deep into the skin and feels very relaxing.

Electro-acupuncture

Electro-acupuncture is the stimulation of acupuncture points by an electrical current. Tiny clips or electrodes are attached to the needles which provide continuous stimulation. The duration of a standard treatment is up to 30 minutes. Patients may experience a mild 'tapping' sensation, or numbness or heaviness. These sensations can decline during the treatment so that the frequency or intensity may need to be adjusted to increase the sensation. Electro-acupuncture is effectively used to reduce chronic pain and muscle spasms. It stimulates the release of endorphins, the body's natural pain reliever. The use of electro-acupuncture has been found to be beneficial for triggering ovulation, especially in women with anovulatory menstrual cycles, and to increase blood circulation to the pelvic organs. We use electro-acupuncture to stimulate blood flow when a woman is going through an IVF cycle.

Lifestyle and Chinese Medicine

The ancient Chinese believed that if you stay within the laws of nature your body stays in balance and you remain well. Simple laws look after your mind, body and spirit: many women do not think about their reproductive health until trying for a baby. Here I am going to list just some general dos and don'ts from the Chinese medical perspective, regardless of whether you are just contemplating trying for a baby or already in the process of trying.

- Get plenty of sleep.
- Cut down on your working hours and reduce stress in your life as much as possible.
- Avoid stimulants, such as coffee, smoking and cigarettes.
- Eat good-quality food with lots of vegetables and fruits.
- Eat cooked and warm food at least once a day.
- Do regular exercise but don't overdo it.
- Dress up warm in cold, rainy weather.
- Wear proper warm, dry footwear. Wear slippers indoors. An important kidney point is on the base of the foot. The Chinese believe that if a lot of cold enters the body it affects the flow of qi.
- Don't expose your midriff or lower back by wearing low-cut trousers in cold weather.
- Don't go out with your hair wet.

Nurture Yourself

There is a good analogy of the plant and the seed. The seed grows to a plan; it has a direction. It determines exactly what flower it is going to turn into – what colour, how high and so on. It is going to grow, but it also needs nourishment – good soil and enough water, warmth and sunlight – in order to be able to grow. If you put a seed in poor soil, with no nourishment and no water, its roots don't go deep enough, and therefore it cannot grow. Nourishing yourself on every level – the food you eat, building your reserves through adequate rest and sleep, practising breathing exercises and using acupuncture – helps establish or correct that delicate balance that makes the conditions right for conception.

Acupuncture and Fertility

I am most grateful to Eva Stecz, one of our acupuncture specialists at the clinic, for contributing to this section of the chapter.

In recent years there has been a lot of comment in the press about the benefit of acupuncture for fertility concerns. Although there is not always hard evidence showing the effects of acupuncture, the results of some studies are very promising. Acupuncture has been shown to be effective in the following ways:

- Acupuncture restores the communication along the HPO axis, helping to regulate the menstrual cycle (see page 203).
- Acupuncture reduces stress by decreasing the activity of the sympathetic nervous system (see page 75). High stress levels are associated with reduced chance of conceiving.
- Acupuncture improves blood circulation to the pelvic organs including the ovaries and uterus, allowing the reproductive organs to work to their full potential.
- Improved blood circulation to the uterus ensures optimal endometrial thickness, creating a hospitable environment for the embryo to implant.
- Acupuncture is shown to be successful in helping to trigger ovulation in some women with ovulatory dysfunction (see page 229).
- Acupuncture may improve sperm parameters (see page 207).

From the Western medical perspective the cause of infertility may be explained by physiological aspects such as ovulatory problems, blocked tubes, implantation failure, or poor sperm parameters; or other factors which may contribute including age, body weight and so on.

Acupuncture and Assisted Fertility

In recent years acupuncture has gained more and more credibility for its use alongside fertility treatments and IVF. It is believed that acupuncture can enhance the outcome of assisted fertility in various ways.

Some things in fertility are clearly genetically pre-programmed and cannot be changed. For example, the quality of a woman's egg is already predetermined, so the issue is more about the environment that the egg is developing in (see the seed analogy on page 200).

Improving Blood Flow to the Pelvic Organs

The pelvic organs, and in particular the ovaries and uterine lining (endometrium), rely on a good blood supply. Boosting the blood flow to this area maximises the supply of oxygen and nutrients. This in turn helps the ovaries and the uterus to function optimally.

Blood flow can be compromised by age and stress. As already discussed (see page 75), reproduction is a non-essential system, so is the first system to be compromised under any stress. As we age, the blood flow to the pelvic organs is reduced. If you suffer from long-term (chronic) stress it is very likely that your nervous system is overloaded and will release hormones (adrenaline and cortisol) which contract the uterine artery and inhibit blood flow to the uterus.

An acupuncture study by Stener-Victorin has shown that the use of electro-acupuncture significantly improves the blood flow along the uterine artery. Several other studies demonstrate that acupuncture initiates the release of endorphins, which, in turn, alleviates stress levels in general.

There is strong data suggesting that a thicker endometrial lining is associated with improved pregnancy rates in women going through assisted fertility. For successful implantation to occur, the uterus has to create an optimal environment in which the uterine lining is thick enough for the embryo to implant. However, this might not be the case, and one cause can be decreased blood flow to the uterus which may affect endometrial receptivity. One study looked at the effect of acupuncture on uterine blood flow by measuring the amount of blood flow to the area before and after acupuncture treatment. The study concluded that there was a significant increase in the uterine arterial blood flow after the acupuncture treatment – a factor which may improve the chances for successful implantation.

Regulating Hormones Prior to IVF

Effective communication along the hypothalamic-pituitary-ovarian (HPO) axis (the hormonal pathway between the brain and the ovaries) is vital if the ovaries are to respond appropriately to stimulation by the follicle stimulating hormone (FSH). If there is a breakdown in communication, the ovaries cease to pay attention to the signals coming from the pituitary gland and hypothalamus. The pituitary gland responds by, in effect, shouting louder and louder to get a reaction – resulting in the FSH level rising.

Many clinics will check your FSH and oestradiol levels around Day 2 at the start of an IVF cycle. It has been shown that, if these two hormones are in balance at their optimal levels, you will respond better to the stimulating drugs, which then can boost your chances of a successful cycle.

Acupuncture can help to correct hormonal imbalances prior to the start of your IVF cycle, helping to restore communication along the HPO axis and also increasing blood circulation to the ovaries. In some cases it may take only a few weeks of weekly treatments to restore the balance.

Balancing the Immune System

Women who have had previous IVF cycles, creating good-quality embryos but repeatedly failing at implantation stage, may be found to have immune problems (see page 419), although this is a very controversial area in medicine. Several studies have demonstrated acupuncture's ability to regulate certain immune cells, such as cytokine production in people suffering from headaches, allergic rhinitis, asthma and rheumatoid arthritis. In view of this, it is possible that there may be a role for acupuncture in normalising placental immune cells which would benefit women with implantation failure, but to date there has not been any research in this area.

Reducing the Side Effects of IVF Medication

Some women may experience side effects with the use of different fertility drugs as they progress through their cycle – these may include headaches, hot flushes, abdominal pain or bloating, breast soreness and mood changes.

Usually, these side effects are short-lived and once you stop the medication your symptoms will gradually subside and disappear. Many of these symptoms can be effectively relieved by regulating the circulation of qi (energy), using specific acupuncture points on the body.

How Many Acupuncture Treatments Are Needed?

At the clinic we have created an acupuncture programme for women going through IVF. I am very often asked about the optimal number of treatments women should have when doing IVF. Work done by Dianne Cridennda in the US concluded that women who received around nine treatments of acupuncture appeared to have the maximum benefit for IVF outcome. Treatments were performed in the lead-up to IVF, during down-regulation, ovarian stimulation and twice on the day of embryo transfer. I therefore encourage women to have a minimum of four sessions prior to the start of their IVF cycles if this is manageable and then ideally five sessions specifically targeted through the cycle.

Some women can feel very emotional and vulnerable during an IVF cycle so, if for nothing else, I always encourage them to have acupuncture to reduce their stress levels.

At the clinic we have made an informal survey of women's experiences of complementary therapies with us and how they enhanced their experience of IVF, and the majority of women thought it helped them to relax and focus on their goal. They found it an escape from the clinical side of IVF and felt calmer, more positive and supported. It helped them to feel they were being proactive in doing absolutely everything they could, and that the practitioners were an invaluable source of support and advice.

Acupuncture During an IVF Cycle

The use of acupuncture alongside IVF treatment is a large part of the work we do at the clinic. Over the last few years there have been many contradictory reports about the effectiveness of acupuncture. One week you will read in the popular press about how acupuncture

Acupuncture Before and After Embryo Transfer

A 'Meta-Analysis (Systemic Review)' published in 2008 looked at seven trials involving 1,366 women undergoing IVF. The randomised controlled trials, that used acupuncture treatment within one day of embryo transfer – mostly 25 minutes before or after – showed that acupuncture increased the chances of pregnancy by 65 per cent compared with the control groups. The conclusion in this particular review was that acupuncture given with embryo transfer improves the pregnancy and live birth rate among women going through IVF.

As always with science, further research can change the way of thinking and when this data was reviewed again a year later (2009), with the inclusion of another study, the conclusion was that acupuncture did not make any difference to IVF success. So – this remains in the balance.

The medical profession is divided on the use of acupuncture treatment in the days following embryo transfer. Some IVF units will encourage you not to have any acupuncture at all after your post-transfer treatment. At the Zita West Clinic, we give acupuncture at specific times prior to the IVF cycle starting; during the down-regulation phase; through the stimulation phase; and on the day of transfer. Transfer day can be stressful for women. We encourage them to have acupuncture before and after the transfer if the timing permits. If this is not possible, aim to have a treatment either before or after transfer. Do not put additional stress on yourself by travelling huge distances to have acupuncture or trying to fit it in both before and after. We also offer women a very gentle treatment for stress and relaxation between Days 7 and 10 because this is when high anxiety kicks in for many of them. You should not have acupuncture on the abdomen or use any form of heat in this area at any time after the embryos have been put back.

boosts ovulation; how it helps with IVF success rates before and after embryo transfer; and then there will be another report saying that it doesn't make any difference at all. As an acupuncturist, I feel the reports don't reflect our clinical practice because they don't compare like for like. Every person who comes in to see me or another therapist has a different diagnosis. You never treat two people in the same way. In the practice of acupuncture it doesn't make sense to give a single treatment in isolation, such as before or after IVF, and I find that women who come regularly to the clinic for acupuncture in the lead-up to their IVF are a lot more relaxed than those who just come on the day of the embryo transfer, many never having had acupuncture before.

Improving Sperm Parameters

Acupuncture may help to improve sperm quality including low sperm count, poor motility and structural abnormalities. Several studies have shown a positive effect on these sperm parameters. In one study, 28 men who were diagnosed with idiopathic (unexplained) infertility received acupuncture twice a week over a period of five weeks. Sperm samples were analysed at the beginning and end of the study and the researchers found significant improvements in sperm quality in the acupuncture group compared with the control group. Acupuncture treatment was associated with fewer structural defects in the sperm and an increase in the number of normal sperm and in motility. In view of the fact that it takes up to three months for sperm development, there is a case for suggesting that a three-month course of acupuncture may be optimal, but this is yet to be tested.

Acupuncture and IUI

There is currently no research on the use of acupuncture with IUI. Acupuncture has a clear role in improving sperm parameters so would be of benefit for men helping to improve sperm quality prior to IUI. Women going through IUI may benefit from improved pelvic blood flow, boosting ovarian function and endometrial thickness, balancing hormones and reducing stress. At the clinic we offer acupuncture treatment prior to IUI and acupuncture treatment a week after insemination. The efficacy is yet to be tested by appropriate randomised controlled trials.

It is clear from this that more well-designed large prospective studies are needed into the use of acupuncture and complementary medicine in the field of natural fertility and alongside IVF treatments. However, evidence or no evidence, the feedback from the majority of women up and down the country who have had acupuncture and other complementary therapies is that they have benefited enormously and felt proactive and relaxed, listened to, supported and nurtured though what is a very stressful time for a lot for women.

Part 3

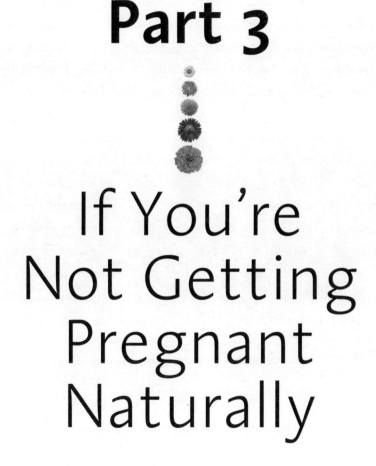

If You're Not Getting Pregnant Naturally

Chapter 9

Investigations for Women and Treatment Options Before IVF

It is quite normal to take six months to a year to conceive. For older women, it could take considerably longer. This is why your GP may not seem too interested in doing any tests or investigations until you have been trying for a baby for at least a year – really trying! If you are under 35, the general recommendation is to wait for a year before you start investigations, but if you are over 35, you should start to be investigated after six months. In some ways this is quite illogical, because it tends to take older women longer to conceive than younger women, but the whole process of fertility tests and investigations takes time, and older women do not have that luxury. Also, if a more assisted route is needed, then success rates decline with age. In-vitro fertilisation (IVF) cannot compensate for lost years. This chapter looks at the normal course of tests and investigations and common gynaecological conditions. Some couples may need to move directly to IVF (page 287), but other couples will benefit from less invasive forms of treatment such as ovulation stimulation or intrauterine insemination (IUI) (page 243).

Causes of Infertility

The main causes of female fertility problems are: problems with ovulation; tubal problems; problems with the womb or cervix; and sexual difficulties. Investigations need to determine why the sperm are not getting to the egg, and why a fertilised egg is not implanting. This involves checking:

- Ovulation and the hormonal control of the cycle
- Egg pick-up, transport and potential for fertilisation in a healthy tube
- The womb, the cervix, the womb cavity and lining
- Lifestyle factors that could negatively impact conception
- Emotional and psychological factors
- Production of healthy sperm

If you think of the female reproductive system, there could be problems anywhere along the way for you. These could be abnormalities you may have been born with; hormonal problems; damage related to previous abdominal or pelvic surgery; or damage from sexually transmitted infections. There is the added concern that with increasing age, there is a decline in both the number and quality of eggs, and more time to develop gynaecological conditions, such as fibroids (see page 258).

Sexual difficulties are a frequent, but often overlooked, cause of fertility delays. If you are having any sexual difficulties – whether these are temporary difficulties related to the pressures of trying to conceive or longer-term problems – don't be embarrassed. Your GP will be used to dealing with such common problems. He or she may want to examine you or your partner to check there are no physical problems, and possibly do a blood test to exclude any medical causes. You may be referred to a psychosexual counsellor to work through your difficulties. Or it may be considered more appropriate for you to go straight to a more assisted route such as IUI or IVF and then to resolve any sexual difficulties at a later date. Self-insemination may be appropriate in some circumstances (see page 38).

Many couples are keen to find a medical problem, hoping that it can then be fixed, but often there are no obvious physical causes to explain the delay in conceiving, and a couple will be diagnosed with 'unexplained' infertility. In at least a third of couples, both partners will be found to have factors that may be contributing to their delay in conception. So, before going straight down an assisted fertility route, there is a series of tests, usually starting with the least invasive investigations, to try and identify a possible problem. These tests are generally shared between your GP and a specialist fertility unit.

Investigating Fertility Problems

Visiting Your GP and Starting Basic Fertility Tests

As a general rule, the first port of call is an appointment with your GP, who will look at your medical history and order some first-line tests. This involves blood tests to check whether the woman is ovulating, and a semen analysis (sperm test) to check the man's sperm quality.

All too often the male side is neglected, so it is really important that the man is investigated at the same time, even if the woman suspects she may have a problem or he has fathered a child before (for more details on sperm analysis, see Chapter 10).

'Day 21' Progesterone Test to Confirm Ovulation

The first blood test is usually a progesterone test to confirm ovulation (release of the egg). After ovulation the collapsed follicle produces the hormone progesterone, so a significant rise in this hormone confirms that ovulation occurred in that cycle. This test needs to be timed very specifically for midway through the luteal phase (second half) of your cycle. It is often referred to as the 'Day 21' progesterone test but it should only be done on Day 21 if you have a 28-day cycle. The timing of this test can create difficulties if you have irregular cycles. If you are aware of your wetter secretions, then try and time this test for about a week after your peak day (the last day you notice the wetness) or about a week after you get an LH surge with an ovulation predictor test. You will only know that the test has been well timed if you have a period about a week after the progesterone test was taken. (For problems with ovulation and understanding progesterone results, see page 230.)

At the same time as initiating your progesterone test (and the semen analysis on your partner), your GP will usually want to make sure you are immune to rubella (German measles) (see page 10). You are also likely to be offered a chlamydia test if you have not had a full sexual health screen recently.

Day 1–3 Blood Tests

Your GP will usually arrange a blood test to be done between Days 1 and 3 of your cycle to check the interplay of the hormones:

- Follicle stimulating hormone (FSH)
- Luteinising hormone (LH)
- Oestradiol

If your cycles are irregular or you have any other symptoms, your GP may also check:

- Testosterone
- Prolactin
- Thyroid function
- A full blood count which includes haemoglobin to check for anaemia

The results of these tests will reveal whether you may need medication to help you ovulate or to get your hormones back into balance (see page 228).

Age and Extra Investigations

If you are in your mid- to late-30s and have been trying to conceive for six months, and making the changes suggested in this book, there are two tests that can help you make a swift decision about whether you need to move on to a more assisted route:

- an AMH blood test to check your ovarian (egg) reserve
- an antral follicle count (special ultrasound scan which counts the number of small resting follicles)

The findings from these tests can help you decide if you should consider going straight down the IVF route, rather than through lengthy investigations (see page 48, Fertility MOT, and page 300, for AMH and IVF). AMH tests may not be available on the NHS.

Your GP may refer you to your local fertility unit at this stage, so that by the time you get to your appointment with the fertility specialist, you will have the results of your blood tests, a semen analysis (from your partner) and possibly a pelvic scan. This information will allow your fertility specialist to consider your next steps and a clear treatment plan.

Your Initial Consultation at a Specialist Fertility Unit

You are likely to have mixed emotions about going to a fertility clinic. It can feel very exciting to be getting professional help at last, but it can also be frightening. You are likely to worry about what is wrong with you, and it's so easy to imagine the worst. Even just walking into the clinic or sitting in the waiting room can make many couples feel uncomfortable, and anxious that someone might recognise them.

Often you will find that your mind races ahead as you wonder who could be at fault. You might be thinking to yourself, 'Is it me or is it my partner?' You look back on how many sexual partners you have had; whether you could have an infection you didn't realise you had. You imagine what your friends will think of you; whether you should tell your family; how you will manage financially if you need treatments such as IVF; how you will manage work-wise. Will you need surgery, medical treatment, drugs? Will the treatment be painful? What if it doesn't work? If you've had a pregnancy terminated in the past you will wonder if that could have any bearing on what's happening now. You will ask yourself why you got pregnant so easily before. Then you will wonder about your partner – how many partners has he or she had in the past? Have they got some unknown infection? Will the past rear its ugly head?

It is easy to see how anxieties can grow by the second in this rather alien clinical environment. When you finally meet up with your gynaecologist, your head buzzing, he or she will take a more detailed history, look at the results of any tests you have already done with your GP and decide what (if any) further investigations need to be done, or what treatment may be appropriate.

Pelvic Ultrasound Scan

If you have not already had a pelvic scan, this will usually be recommended at this stage. The internal ultrasound scan uses high-frequency sound waves (not x-rays) to visualise your ovaries and womb and identify problems such as polycystic ovaries, fibroids or polyps. It can also detect problems such as congenital abnormalities (birth defects) in the womb. An ordinary pelvic scan (sometimes known as a trans-vaginal scan or TVS) cannot detect problems with your tubes. As the insides of your tubes are only about a hair's breadth wide, the only way to check whether they are patent (open) is to put a dye through them (see below).

If your blood tests and scan are normal and your partner has a normal semen analysis result, then you may be advised to continue trying for a while. However, if there is a problem on the scan, or there is reason to suspect there may be a problem with your tubes, then you may progress fairly quickly to a more detailed look at your pelvis and the patency of your tubes. You need to have the results of your ovulation assessment and the sperm test before you proceed to the more invasive dye tests. In some circumstances (such as significant problems with the sperm), you may need to proceed directly to IVF or intra-cytoplasmic sperm injection (ICSI). (For more on the role of ultrasound scans and monitored cycle – see page 260).

Tests to Check Tubal Patency

There are several tests to check tubal patency and look in more detail at the other reproductive organs. They may identify anatomical problems such as a uterine septum (dividing wall in the womb), which may be delaying pregnancy. Tests are usually done in the first 10 days of your cycle to avoid the possibility of dislodging a pregnancy that may already have started. You will normally be given antibiotics to reduce the risk of infection. These tests can all take time and so the whole process of investigation can become very frustrating and, at times, highly stressful for couples.

- **HSG** The simplest test to check the woman's tubes is with an x-ray and dye test called a hystero-salpingogram or HSG (hyster = uterus; salpinges = tubes). The radio-opaque dye is inserted through the cervical opening, so this is similar to having a smear test. The x-ray pictures give an outline of the womb and tubes. The HSG can identify areas of adhesions (scarring), polyps and fibroids, as well as congenital abnormalities. The dye may show up blockages anywhere along the tube. At times the tube can go into spasm, possibly as a reaction to the dye, making it hard to be sure about the patency of the tube. For most women the test will be painless, but it can cause varying levels of discomfort or pain, particularly if there are any difficulties getting the dye through the tubes. The dye itself may clear very minor blockages and some women will conceive purely as a result of this procedure.

- **HyCoSy** A similar, slightly more sophisticated test known as a HyCoSy is increasingly used. This stands for hystero-salpingo-contrast sonography – a test that uses an ultrasound scan and contrast medium to get a more detailed image of the womb, ovaries and tubes. This test is used to check for polycystic ovaries, fibroids, polyps and other problems in the pelvis, alongside checking that the tubes are patent.

- **Laparoscopy** Some women will require a laparoscopy and dye test. This is a more invasive investigation, but is often considered the 'gold standard' test. It is usually performed if a woman has a history of pelvic surgery (such as appendicectomy), pelvic pain or other symptoms, or if an HSG highlights a possible problem. A laparoscopy requires a general anaesthetic and two or three very small incisions – one around your bellybutton and one or two lower down on either side of your pelvis (lower abdomen). A small instrument known as a laparoscope is used to take very detailed photographs. Laparoscopy has the advantage of being able to look all around at the outside of the tubes and womb and to check for adhesions (scarring) and endometriosis. In order to get a good view of your insides, the gynaecologist first uses carbon dioxide gas to inflate your abdomen. A dye is usually passed through the inside of the tubes to check they are open (patent). An exploratory laparoscopy also gives your gynaecologist an opportunity to treat conditions such endometriosis or adhesions (scarring) at the same time. A hysteroscopy (see below) may be performed at the same time as laparoscopy.

- **Hysteroscopy** This involves inserting a very narrow endoscope through the cervix to view the uterine cavity. It is not normally done in the first round of investigations, but may be suggested to provide a more detailed view of the size and shape of the inside of the womb and to get a particularly detailed view of the endometrium (lining). This may be suggested prior to IVF and is usually done under a general anaesthetic. Hysteroscopy also allows a gynaecologist to diagnose or treat conditions such as polyps, fibroids, adhesions or a congenital septum.

Investigation of Fertility Problems

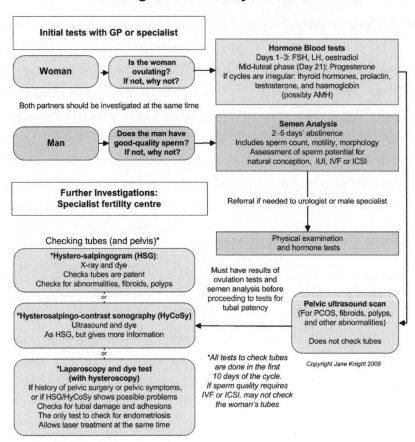

The chart above summarises the normal investigation pathway. The precise nature and the time-frame over which this takes place will depend on many factors including the woman's age, time trying to conceive, medical conditions and whether you are doing tests on the NHS or privately.

Treatment Options

Depending on the outcome of the fertility investigations, whether a possible cause has been diagnosed or whether you have 'unexplained' infertility, a decision has to be made as to whether you need some extra help with conception. If so, the most suitable treatment options will be discussed. If the delay is possibly due to mis-timed intercourse, or irregular cycles, then some women may benefit from having their menstrual cycles monitored by ultrasound scan to identify ovulation and then optimising the timing of natural sex or 'timed intercourse' (see page 260). The main fertility treatment options range from ovarian stimulation through to IVF and beyond.

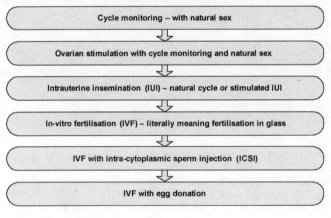

Fertility Treatment Options

Cycle monitoring – with natural sex

Ovarian stimulation with cycle monitoring and natural sex

Intrauterine insemination (IUI) – natural cycle or stimulated IUI

In-vitro fertilisation (IVF) – literally meaning fertilisation in glass

IVF with intra-cytoplasmic sperm injection (ICSI)

IVF with egg donation

Copyright Jane Knight 2009

Although there is a logical progression starting with the least invasive treatment option, each couple's situation is considered on its own merit and some options may be inappropriate.

1. Boost Ovulation with a Fertility Drug
If you are having problems with ovulation or erratic cycles, then your doctor may consider you a suitable candidate for an ovulation

stimulation or boosting drug such as clomiphene (Clomid) or sometimes another drug known as Tamoxifen. This is only appropriate if your partner has good-quality sperm and your tubes are clear (patent). You can take clomiphene for up to six cycles, during which time you will be monitored to check that the drug is having the desired effect. You will have scans and a blood test for progesterone to confirm that ovulation is occurring and have optimally timed natural sex (for more on clomiphene, see page 239). There may be situations where it is more appropriate to miss out this step and move directly to stimulated IUI.

2. Intrauterine Insemination (IUI)

If you are not pregnant after three to six cycles of ovulation stimulation, your gynaecologist may suggest intrauterine insemination (IUI). There are a number of clear indications for the use of IUI (see page 244). With IUI you may or may not have additional ovarian stimulation. Perhaps unsurprisingly IUI with ovarian stimulation tends to be more successful than natural cycle IUI. Your IUI cycles will be monitored and, around the time of ovulation, the gynaecologist or specialist nurse inserts specially prepared sperm through the cervix into the womb. It is very important that you have had appropriate tests to check your tubes are clear before IUI is attempted. (For more on IUI, see page 243.)

3. In-vitro Fertilisation (IVF), With or Without ICSI

Women who have blocked tubes inevitably go straight to in-vitro (literally 'in-glass') fertilisation (IVF). This may also be an option for women with patent (open) tubes with unexplained infertility or who have tried IUI for three to six cycles without success. With IVF, the ovaries are stimulated to produce a large number of eggs so that they can be collected, usually under general anaesthetic, and fertilised by the sperm in a laboratory. A safe number of embryos (usually one or two) will then be transferred into the woman's womb between two and five days after the eggs have been collected. During an IVF cycle a woman has to give herself injections of ovulation-stimulation drugs and other drugs to support a pregnancy, while being monitored carefully with ultrasound scans and blood tests.

There are two different ways that the egg can be fertilised in the laboratory: either straight IVF, where prepared sperm are placed next to the egg in a Petri dish; or ICSI (intracytoplasmic sperm injection), where the embryologist injects a single sperm directly into the egg. So, with ICSI, the woman goes through an IVF cycle in exactly the same way; the only difference is that a more complex technique is used in the laboratory to achieve fertilisation (see page 337).

Choosing between the Treatment Options

Most clinics will understandably use a step-wise approach, starting with the least invasive treatment. For example, at first they may try ovulation stimulation only, then move on if necessary to IUI and possibly IVF. This makes sense in that for some couples, depending on the nature of their problem, a boost with a fertility drug may be all that is needed. With this approach it can take about a year to 18 months to get to the IVF stage. If you are in your late 30s or older, there is a good case for doing IVF sooner rather than later.

There seems to be a clear role for IUI in the right circumstances (see page 244). IUI can achieve around 15 per cent success per cycle when combined with ovarian stimulation. However, there are currently debates among the medical profession about the value of IUI for couples with unexplained infertility as the success rates for this group are so low (see page 226).

IVF is not an easy decision. For some couples there may be religious or ethical considerations or different beliefs around IVF, while for others one partner may want to do IVF while the other doesn't feel ready. I can honestly say from my experience that once a woman has made up her mind to do IVF, she is very driven in the process, and while it may take her partner longer to catch up, she will generally want to move forward as quickly as possible. There are exceptions, of course, and some women have real concerns about the IVF drugs and will not want to consider an assisted route.

Finding Out There is a Problem

If either you or your partner is found to have a problem, this can feel devastating. It can be made more difficult if the news is not delivered as sensitively as one would wish. So many couples I see are still reeling from hearing bad news or have had a rushed explanation about their results and are unclear of the way forward. It is never easy in a short consultation with a doctor to really grasp what is being said. When we are already feeling anxious and then hear bad news we often find that somehow our brain switches off and it is very hard to make sense of the conversation or to think of any appropriate questions at the time. So, even if a doctor or nurse spends considerable time explaining things, we may not be able to grasp the full implications but need to go away and have time to digest things.

Many women report that the only discussion they have had with a specialist has been at an 'inappropriate' time, such as when they were coming round from the anaesthetic following a laparoscopy. It is very difficult to take in new information at the best of times, but when you are still feeling groggy you are certainly not at your most receptive. Ideally, make sure your partner is with you at a time when you are likely to be receiving results. Two heads are usually better than one, and you have a better chance of asking questions and remembering what has been said, or finding someone else who can explain the results at a later time.

Many men and women find they need more time to come to terms with negative test results, and this is where a session with a fertility counsellor can help you to get things back into perspective (see page 115). This may be especially helpful for men who have had bad news about their sperm, which may then mean that their partner will need to go through some form of assisted conception. Men can find this very difficult as they are in this rather bizarre situation where they seem to be the one with the problem, but the way to fix it is for the woman to get the treatment – that is to go through an IVF cycle, possibly with ICSI. It is probably the only medical scenario where this role reversal occurs. In more extreme situations where no suitable sperm can be found, sperm donation may be needed (see page 460). This is, of course, a very big step and couples require appropriate support and professional counselling to consider the implications of using a donor (see page 463).

Women who find out they have a problem may be relieved on one level, feeling that something can be done, but there may also be other anxieties about whether lifestyle or past behaviour may be a contributing factor. Women who have had eating problems or been fanatical exercisers may start to wonder whether past abuse of their body may have had any influence on their present situation. Women with pelvic problems may be anxious about whether this could be related in some way to past sexual health issues or to an earlier termination. Again, it may be valuable to spend time talking through your anxieties with a fertility counsellor, to help you let go of the past and to move forward positively. (Gynaecological problems are discussed on page 228.)

The outcome of fertility investigations usually means that there are decisions to be made. For example, if the woman's tubes are blocked or the sperm are of poor quality, then IVF may be the next step. I often find, when talking to couples, that if they discover they both have a problem there is a huge sense of relief from both parties

– somehow the burden is shared. Even if it seems that the problem is one-sided, it is very common that other factors are discovered during assisted conception which may have been compounding the problem.

Finding Out There 'Isn't a Problem' – 'Unexplained' Infertility

Of the couples we see, at least one-third have been told that the standard investigations show there is 'nothing wrong' – there is no explanation for why they are not conceiving. This can be reassuring in one way, as it can give hope for conceiving naturally, but it can also be very difficult to cope with – there is nothing obvious to 'fix'. Even after three years of 'unexplained' infertility, many couples will still conceive naturally – it simply takes longer. This is why the national clinical guidelines recommend that for couples with 'unexplained' infertility, doctors consider 'expectant management' – in other words, a 'wait and see' approach – for up to three years of trying, provided a woman's age and previous history allow this. The problem here, of course, is that for so many women time is at a premium, and even for younger women, the uncertainty can seem intolerable.

The diagnosis of 'unexplained' infertility implies that the man's semen analysis is normal, the woman is ovulating and her tubes are open. So, why no conception? Some couples may have been investigated more thoroughly than others before the diagnosis is given and it is possible that a more subtle problem may be identified on further investigation. For example, a laparoscopy might show fine adhesions, even though an HSG showed the tubes to be open; a woman may be ovulating regularly, but her egg quality could be poor making fertilisation less likely. It may therefore be appropriate to consider more comprehensive investigations. The big difficulty doctors have when faced with a couple with 'unexplained' infertility is what – if anything – further investigations would add, when in the longer term the solution is likely to be IVF anyway. Also the whole procedure of IVF can be considered an investigative process as it allows the doctor to examine more closely each stage of the reproductive process and to observe the sperm and egg in the laboratory.

Couples with 'unexplained' infertility should reconsider whether their sexual health is optimal. Many people have infections they may be unaware of, such as ureaplasma or mycoplasma. There is some controversy about the role these bacteria may play in fertility as they are naturally present at low levels in most sexually active couples, but there is some evidence that these infections may be linked to delays in conception or miscarriage. The presence of these bacteria does not indicate that you or your partner has been unfaithful in any way. They can become troublesome if you become unwell or 'run down' in the same way that candida or 'thrush' can become a problem. Tests may not always be offered routinely as part of an NHS sexual health screen, but can be organised privately. (See page 280, interview with Sam Dawkins, sexual health doctor.)

Some couples with 'unexplained' infertility may want to do more detailed investigations of the sperm, including tests for sperm DNA fragmentation. Although this has a role, it is important to consider what will be learnt from such testing and whether the information gained would alter the course of treatment (see Chapter 10). It is increasingly recognised that even though a routine semen analysis may be normal, men who smoke or drink to excess are likely to have a high level of sperm DNA fragmentation which may delay conception.

It is possible that some women with 'unexplained' infertility may have problems with implantation – the egg and sperm may be fusing but the embryo fails to implant for some reason. A few of these women may have immune problems. This is where tests and treatments start to become highly contentious as we move into the area of reproductive immunology (see page 419).

The treatment will vary. Some research has shown that for couples with 'unexplained' infertility, the use of clomiphene (see page 239) or IUI (see page 243) does not significantly increase a woman's chances of pregnancy compared with continuing to try naturally, so there are two options here: 'do nothing' or be fast-tracked to IVF. This is why some units may suggest IVF rather than clomiphene or IUI for 'unexplained' infertility. The option of 'doing nothing' is, unsurprisingly, not a popular one, but it is even more important for couples with 'unexplained' infertility to be aware of the woman's fertility time and to have frequent sex. Some women have a shorter fertile window (around three days instead of the usual six days) and may notice fewer days of fertile secretions (to identify the fertile time, see page 27).

If there is no obvious medical cause for the fertility delay, then it is reasonable to start to question whether there could be a psychological component. A lot of the work we do in the clinic with couples with 'unexplained' infertility falls into the mind/body area – looking at stress, tensions in relationships and reasons why couples may be struggling to conceive due to psychological or emotional blocks. This is explored more fully in Chapter 6.

Gynaecological Problems and Hormone Imbalances

As you progress through the often lengthy process of fertility tests and investigations, you will inevitably come across more and more medical terminology. It is very likely that you will have already convinced yourself (often from a few vague symptoms) that you have a hormone imbalance or gynaecological problem. The following information provides a brief overview of different gynaecological conditions. If, after the appropriate investigations, you are found to have a problem you will inevitably want to research it more thoroughly. There is so much information on the internet that it is hard to know where to find reliable 'evidence-based' information. Each condition is potentially a book in itself, but see Resources (page 487) for further useful information and support groups. The best source of advice will still be your GP or fertility specialist who will be able to help you consider how the condition may or may not impact on your chances of achieving a successful pregnancy.

Problems with Ovulation

Problems with ovulation are possibly the single most common cause of fertility delays, accounting for up to 20 per cent of fertility problems. This is why the first test a doctor will do is usually a blood test to confirm the presence or absence of ovulation (see page 213). It is important to remember that although the release of the egg is crucial, it is only a momentary part of a complex sequence of hormonal events. Things can go wrong at every step of the way: from the hypothalamus at the highest level in the brain right through the whole chain of events leading to the production of hormones by the ovaries to sustain a pregnancy. So, problems with ovulation or 'ovulation disorders' can have a range of causes – some of which can be 'fixed' more easily than others, depending on the level and the severity. The spectrum of problems can also range from being just the occasional stress-induced irregular cycle right through to the complete absence of ovulation and periods (amenorrhoea).

As a general rule, the more regular and consistent your menstrual cycles are, the more likely it is that you are ovulating normally. If your cycles are irregular (varying by more than seven days in length) you may still be ovulating normally (that is, releasing an egg about 14 days before the next period is due), but it is more likely that you have a problem with ovulation. A positive LH (luteinising hormone) or ovulation predictor test is not proof that ovulation is occurring. The predictor test is doing just that – predicting that it will happen (and it usually follows) – but it does not guarantee that the egg has been released. Ovulation still needs to be confirmed with a progesterone test halfway through the luteal phase (second half) of your cycle.

Try and remember the fact that causes most confusion about ovulation:

- *If you release an egg*, only two things can possibly happen. Either:
  1. you conceive – and get a positive pregnancy test about two weeks later

  or:

  2. you don't conceive – and have a period about two weeks later
- *If you don't release an egg*, you will still get a 'period' at some stage as the womb lining will eventually break down. The 'period' (which is strictly speaking an anovulatory bleed) may occur earlier than expected; on time; delayed; or so delayed that a bleed has to be medically induced.

So, getting a 'period' does not prove ovulation.

Interpreting the Test Results

The timing of your progesterone test is crucial. Your test results are normally interpreted after the date of your next period is known, to ensure that the test has been appropriately timed. If your period starts about a week after the test was performed, it is likely to have been a well-timed test. The most common reason for a poor test result is a mis-timed test. As a general rule:

- A progesterone level above 30nmol/l is considered proof of ovulation (in that cycle).
- A level between 16 and 30nmol/l indicates a strong possibility of ovulation, but most likely a mis-timed test. Repeat the test in another cycle.
- Less than 16nmol/l indicates absence of ovulation. Repeat the test.
- A consistently low result usually indicates the need for referral to a specialist.

If your progesterone result is low, then you will have further blood tests to find out why you are not ovulating and determine any underlying problem.

Many women feel anxious that they may not be ovulating. Remember, it is quite normal not to ovulate in absolutely every cycle – even in perfectly healthy fertile women – but if you have two or more consecutive cycles where you suspect you may not be ovulating, or you feel that your cycles have changed in length or in the nature of the bleeding, then do discuss this with your doctor. Rest assured that with today's drugs there is much help at hand to help restore your hormone balance and stimulate ovulation. Most women with ovulation problems will conceive with the appropriate medication, without needing more invasive procedures such as IVF.

Causes of Ovulation Problems

Cycles tend to become irregular and often shorter, with ovulation occurring less frequently, as a woman gets older and her egg reserve diminishes, so this is always of potential concern. Additionally, when stressed, cortisol (an adrenal stress hormone) can cause irregular cycles and problems with ovulation. Bear in mind that although fertility may be all-important to you at present, in terms of personal survival, reproduction is considered a 'non-essential' system, so when the physiological demands on the body are great, reproductive processes are often the first system to be temporarily suppressed until the 'stressful' situation is resolved and the body recovers its natural balance.

Women are very fortunate in having a visual warning sign that may indicate problems with ovulation. If periods become irregular (more than a week's variation in cycle length) or stop altogether, it is a cause for concern. This can occur due to conditions such as thyroid problems (see page 247); anaemia (see page 250); endocrine disorders; PCOS (see pages 176 and 251); and premature ovarian failure (see page 412). Ovulation disorders can also be caused by chronic illnesses unrelated to reproduction, and occasionally no obvious cause can be found. Problems with ovulation should always be investigated to exclude any serious causes. Women who are on the contraceptive pill will not get a warning sign of irregular periods, so underlying problems can go undetected for longer.

- **Hypothalamic amenorrhoea** Ovulation is under the overall control of the hypothalamus which is located in the centre of the brain. The hypothalamus also controls the body's response to internal and external influences, and controls the thyroid hormones, body temperature, sleep, thirst, appetite and fluid balance. So, altogether the hypothalamus has a really significant role. In its reproductive capacity, the hypothalamus releases gonadotrophin-releasing hormone (GnRH) to regulate the nearby pituitary gland and its output of follicle stimulating hormone (FSH) and luteinising hormone (LH) which in turn act on the ovaries to control ovulation and the menstrual cycle. This sequence of hormonal events is known as the Hypothalamic-Pituitary-Ovarian Axis (HPOA). Men have a parallel communication system operating between the hypothalamus, the pituitary gland and the testicles, so men may have similar communication difficulties anywhere along the way from deep within the brain to the production of sperm in the testicles right through to ejaculation.

At times, such as if you are highly stressed or seriously underweight, the hypothalamus fails to send GnRH messages to the pituitary gland, which in turn affects the production of FSH and LH. The follicles fail to grow, there will be no ovulation and no period. This is known as hypothalamic amenorrhoea ('amenorrhoea' means absence of periods). If periods stop at any time, the first thing is to check for pregnancy with the hCG (human chorionic gonadotrophin) test. If this is negative, then the next thing is to try and find out the cause of the problem. A series of hormone blood tests will be needed to exclude other causes (such as a raised prolactin level). If the level of FSH, LH and oestrogen is very low, then this may indicate hypothalamic amenorrhoea. The treatment may be a fairly simple lifestyle change, such as gaining weight or reducing exercise, as a way of kick-starting the whole hormonal process; but if this does not work, hormone treatment may be needed. This is often given in the form of a series of injections, or sometimes a continuous hormone-releasing intravenous pump.

- **Weight-related amenorrhoea (absence of periods due to low body weight)** Oestrogen is stored in body fat, so the percentage of body fat is critical to maintain ovulation and normal menstrual cycles. A woman needs to have at least 22 per cent body fat to ovulate effectively. If the weight and body fat percentage falls too low ovulation and periods will cease (amenorrhoea). Women whose weight and body fat is borderline low may be ovulating but having short luteal phases, with insufficient time for implantation (see page 30). Increasing weight and body fat percentage may be all that is needed for normal fertility to return.

- **Exercise-related amenorrhoea** Women who exercise to excess and competitive sportswomen – such as dancers, gymnasts, cyclists, runners and swimmers – are likely to have problems with ovulation, irregular periods or no periods at all while competing. Amenorrhoea resulting from exercise also increases the risk of osteoporosis due to low oestrogen levels. Reducing the exercise intensity, or in some cases stopping all exercise, will generally restore hormone balance.

- **Raised prolactin levels (hyperprolactinaemia)** Prolactin is a hormone normally produced by the pituitary gland during pregnancy and breast-feeding to stimulate the production of breast milk, but it also suppresses ovulation and menstruation, which is why it is known as nature's contraceptive. A raised prolactin level at other times can be caused by stress, exercise (especially running), PCOS (see pages 176 and 251) or hypothyroid (see page 247). It can also be caused by certain drugs used for the treatment of anxiety, depression and high blood pressure. If your prolactin levels are very high, your doctor may refer you for a brain scan to exclude a pituitary tumour. Some women with high prolactin levels will notice some breast leakage, even if they have never had a baby. Breast leakage should normally cease completely within a couple of months of stopping breast-feeding. If you have any abnormal breast leakage, discuss this with your doctor. Drugs such as cabergoline or bromocriptine are used to reduce prolactin levels and restore natural hormone balance and subsequent fertility.

- **Abnormal LH levels** Luteinising hormone (LH) is involved in the maturation of the egg, triggering ovulation and the development of the corpus luteum (see Chapter 2). Women with PCOS (see pages 176 and 251) may have abnormally high levels of LH, which can be damaging to the egg, reduce the chances of conception and increase the risk of miscarriage. Women with abnormally high LH levels may be offered ovulation stimulation drugs (see page 238). Abnormally low LH levels will not trigger ovulation and result in amenorrhoea (see hypothalamic amenorrhoea, page 232).

- **Raised testosterone** Testosterone, an androgen or male hormone, is produced in small amounts in a woman's ovaries. Abnormally high testosterone levels may be present in women with PCOS (see pages 176 and 251), resulting in acne, hirsutism (excessive facial or body hair) and sometimes thinning of hair on the scalp. Your doctor may want to do more detailed testing of your androgens to rule out any other unusual hormonal conditions.

- **Stress** Everyone's degree of stress is different, but if your adrenal glands are busy producing the stress hormone cortisol to fight crises and emergencies, they will divert blood flow away from your reproductive organs to prepare the large muscles for action – the so-called 'fight or flight' response. The 'domino effect' of the GnRH, FSH and LH will be interrupted, resulting in insufficient oestrogen and a failure to ovulate. Remember, ovulation and reproduction are the most dispensable of all bodily systems. Some systems (such as breathing) are essential; the functioning of other systems (such as the gut) can be reduced without affecting personal survival in the short term, but reproduction can easily be shut down completely until the stressful situation is over. This is where long-term stress can become a problem, as many women (and men) fail to recognise the adverse consequences of long hours and a challenging job on top of all of the other stresses of life. This is why I strongly believe that stress management helps with ovulation problems by getting the autonomic nervous system back into balance.

- **Problems with ovulation after stopping the Pill** I consistently see women who have come off the Pill and are concerned about their cycles not getting back to normal. For most women, fertility returns immediately after the Pill (or even with missed pills), but other women may experience a delay.

Post-Pill Facts

- There is no reason to delay conceiving after you have stopped taking the Pill, unless you are specifically told to do so by your doctor.
- Although some women conceive immediately after stopping the Pill, it is not unusual to have some cycle disturbance for up to nine months (sometimes longer).
- Women over 30 who are trying for a first baby are more likely to experience fertility delays after coming off the Pill.
- There is no evidence to suggest that the Pill causes long-term fertility problems.
- One study found that at 12 months only 32 per cent of women who had stopped the combined Pill to get pregnant had conceived, compared with 54 per cent of condom users – but by 18 months there was no difference in conception rates.
- If you have had contraceptive injections it may take even longer to conceive.

Case study

Sophie, 32, came to see me because her cycles were all over the place since she had stopped taking the Pill over nine months earlier. She had had only four periods since then and was feeling very depressed. I found out that she had been on the Pill since she was 16, with just two short breaks. She was now desperate to get pregnant and had become obsessed with taking her temperature, monitoring her secretions and trying to make her body more alkaline. She had cut out wheat, dairy and red meat but had not managed to give up alcohol. She was keen to get pregnant naturally rather than going down the medical route, and she was taking her folic acid conscientiously.

I reassured her that she was still young and it was early days. I explained that it was not at all unusual to take up to a year, or even longer, to conceive after stopping the Pill, particularly in women over 30 trying for their first baby. I suggested some lifestyle changes she could make over a time-frame of three months. We agreed that if this approach didn't work we would start to look at a more medical approach, doing hormone tests and a scan, and testing her partner's sperm. Being so organised, she had had a blood test for rubella while she was still on the Pill to ensure she was immune when she started to try for a baby.

Sophie agreed to attend a session on fertility awareness, to get a better understanding of her cycles. As she was very slim, I asked her how important her figure was to her. She told me that it was very important as she worked in the fashion industry, and she was happy with her weight. I encouraged her to try and put on some weight because the hormone oestrogen is produced and stored in body fat. I also explained that a woman who is too thin when she conceives has a higher chance of miscarrying or having a very small or pre-term baby with more risk of complications at birth. Her body needed enough energy reserves to carry a pregnancy to full term and to be able to breast-feed the baby. Sophie was also doing too much exercise: nearly nine hours a week. When I explained that physical activity is linked with problems with ovulation and infertility, she agreed to cut down, and to try and relax through yoga and sleeping well instead.

Her food diary was very erratic. I was concerned that she had cut so much out of her diet – no wheat or dairy, virtually no carbs and little protein. Her body was in starvation mode. She wasn't eating breakfast, which is essential for balancing hormones, and her alcohol consumption was high: 20–30 units a week. I encouraged her to eat breakfast, a mid-morning snack, lunch, a mid-afternoon snack and an evening meal, mixing protein with carbs. She agreed to cut down on her drinking, having three to four evenings a week when she didn't drink and keeping to under six units a week. Within three months with a combination of improving her nutrition and decreasing her exercise, her lean:fat ratio improved and she resumed regular cycles.

Treatment Options Before IVF

Treatments for Ovulation Problems

Many couples can be helped by minimal medical assistance, without requiring IVF. Provided time is on your side, you may be offered a range of options, including:

- A fertility drug such as clomiphene to boost ovulation

- Clomiphene plus intrauterine insemination (IUI)
- Injectable FSH- and LH-based drugs combined with IUI

The first-choice drug for inducing or boosting ovulation is usually clomiphene. If clomiphene doesn't work, another drug, Tamoxifen, may be tried. At times, particularly for women with PCOS (see pages 176 and 251) and insulin-resistance, metformin may be offered. Sometimes other FSH-based drugs are given by injection (see IUI section, page 243). Most women will ovulate with the use of these drugs and many will conceive. However, there are situations where ovulation may not occur despite the use of ovulation-boosting drugs. Some women – particularly those with PCOS – may benefit from ovarian 'drilling', a surgical procedure designed to make the ovaries more responsive to drug treatment. This is performed by laparoscopy during which the ovary is punctured several times by a surgical needle and diathermy (heat). This procedure tends to lower testosterone levels, and some women may respond better to fertility drugs afterwards. As with any surgical procedure, it is really important to have a full discussion with your gynaecologist and to really understand the pros and cons of the operation in your particular circumstances.

Clomiphene
Clomiphene may be used for the treatment of the following:

- Absence of ovulation, for example in women who have come off the Pill
- Irregular cycles
- PCOS (see pages 176 and 251)
- Unexplained infertility

Clomiphene acts on the hypothalamus and pituitary gland to stimulate FSH and LH production and therefore stimulate the growth of follicles in the ovary. It is given in tablet form. Doctors believe that the earlier clomiphene is administered, the more effective it is in promoting the growth of follicles; therefore it tends to be given over five days at the beginning of the cycle, usually on Days 2–6. The dose is typically 50mg, but this will be increased if there is no response after three cycles, although regimes will vary slightly. Ovulation will occur 80 per cent of the time.

While you are taking clomiphene it is very important that you are monitored to see how your ovaries are responding. This is usually done by ultrasound scan around Days 10–12 of your cycle. The scan is to make sure that one or, at most, two follicles are growing, and to check that the womb lining is developing well. If one or two follicles are developing then a Day 21 blood test will usually be done to check progesterone levels and see if ovulation has occurred (see page 214). If it has, then the same dose will be given in subsequent cycles; if it hasn't, the doctor may increase the dose. The maximum that will be given is 150mg.

There is a risk that more than two follicles will grow and reach maturity. If this is the case the cycle will be abandoned as there is then an increased risk of a multiple pregnancy. If you are told to avoid sex because you have too many follicles, it is really important to do so, however difficult it may seem, because a multiple pregnancy can have devastating consequences.

- **Who should take clomiphene?** If you are having regular periods and it is confirmed by a progesterone blood test or an ultrasound scan that you are ovulating then you are not usually a candidate for clomiphene. I am amazed, however, at how often it is given under these circumstances. Sometimes this is because women almost demand it, or so that there is a feeling of 'doing something'.

If your cycles are irregular, clomiphene helps you to have more regular ovulatory cycles – producing more mature eggs and therefore a better opportunity for fertilisation.

The success of clomiphene is dependent on the particular condition you have. Generally speaking, of the women who receive clomiphene, 80 per cent will ovulate and 30–50 per cent will become pregnant – but there are many factors involved in its success. Age, for example, is a big factor, and clomiphene is not as successful in older women. Another factor is the length of time you take it. Taking it for too long without a break can cause problems including thinning of the womb lining. Many women report reduced amounts of cervical secretions while on clomiphene, making it more difficult to identify the fertile time.

- **Side effects of clomiphene** Clomiphene can have many side effects. Some women are absolutely fine on it, but others have side effects including:
  - hot flushes
  - cysts
  - abdominal pain and discomfort
  - dizziness
  - visual disturbances
  - nausea
  - vomiting
  - insomnia
  - breast tenderness
  - headaches
  - depression
  - blood spotting between periods
  - heavy periods
  - weight gain

○ rashes

○ hair loss (in some cases)

Many women will feel very fragile emotionally and can experience mood swings.

Clomiphene Treatment for Unexplained Infertility

Clomiphene is often used for women with unexplained infertility, but its use in such circumstances is debatable. A study reported in the *BMJ* in 2008 challenged the common practice and the current NICE guidelines of recommending clomiphene or unstimulated intrauterine insemination (IUI) as a first-line treatment for couples with unexplained infertility. The Scottish research found there was no higher pregnancy rate using clomiphene or unstimulated (natural cycle) IUI compared with 'expectant management' or a 'wait and see' policy. Our hunch is that the 'wait and see' group may benefit significantly from education in fertility awareness and psychological support, but this has not been studied. Some NHS clinics are taking the Scottish research on board and offer couples with unexplained infertility the full choice of treatment, including going straight to IVF. Although this might seem like a giant leap, the interim steps can be a waste of valuable fertility time and may not be cost-effective. The whole process of IVF also acts as a way to determine other factors which may be causing a problem; in effect, it acts as another investigation to find an 'explanation' for the 'unexplained'. This may be in a woman's best interests, particularly if she is older.

Daily FSH Injections

If you have gone on to take the higher doses of clomiphene and you are not pregnant or have not ovulated, then your doctor may suggest you have injections of follicle stimulating hormone (FSH). You will start with a low dose and build up until one or two dominant follicles can be seen on an ultrasound scan. You may also be given a human chorionic-gonadotrophin (hCG)-based drug to trigger ovulation. This helps to mature the follicle and stimulate the release of the egg 36 hours later. You will usually be monitored prior to ovulation while having this course of treatment. Again, if you produce more than two follicles the cycle will be abandoned as it is unsafe to continue.

HMG Injections

Another drug that might be given is HMG (human menopausal gonadotrophin). This is a mixture of luteinising hormone (LH) and follicle stimulating hormone (FSH). Given as a course of injections, usually for seven to ten days on alternate days, it stimulates your ovaries to develop and mature the follicles. You are closely monitored with an ultrasound scan and blood tests. The scan gives a good indication of when the egg follicles are of sufficient size for the injection of hCG to be given to mature the egg(s) and trigger ovulation. Ovulation usually occurs 24–36 hours thereafter, and you are encouraged to have sex every day, or sometimes HMG is given in conjunction with intrauterine insemination (IUI).

Intrauterine Insemination (IUI)

Intrauterine insemination involves injecting specially prepared sperm through a soft catheter via the woman's cervix into the uterine cavity around the time of ovulation. IUI may be performed as part of a natural menstrual cycle (unstimulated) or combined with ovarian stimulation (stimulated). IUI is a fairly straightforward procedure which only takes a few minutes – rather like having a smear test. The treatment can be repeated on successive cycles – usually for three to four cycles so chances of success increase over time.

Main Indications for IUI

- PCOS and other ovulation problems
- if there are anatomical problems
- for women with mild endometriosis
- for men who suffer from premature ejaculation or erectile difficulties
- for couples who are unable to have intercourse due to psychological distress
- for men with immunological infertility (not recommended in severe cases, i.e. 80 per cent binding or more in the MAR test)
- for women who have cervical secretions that are hostile to sperm
- for women who have had treatment for problem smears, for example if a cone biopsy has reduced the number of glands producing cervical secretions
- for men whose semen parameters are slightly outside of the normal range
- for couples who are geographically apart from each other for extended periods of time

Monitoring the Cycle

Some clinics use ultrasound scans to determine the timing of the insemination, while others rely on the woman using ovulation predictor kits at home. The aim is to be producing two or three follicles. If there are more than three follicles, the cycle may either be abandoned or possibly converted to IVF to avoid the risk of multiple pregnancy.

Timing Insemination for Natural Cycle IUI

With unstimulated or natural cycle IUI, a woman observes her normal menstrual cycle and checks for the LH surge with an ovulation predictor kit. The insemination is then generally performed within 24 hours of detecting the LH surge.

Timing Insemination for Stimulated IUI

The ovaries are stimulated (superovulation) usually by clomiphene tablets or sometimes FSH-based injections. When two to three follicles reach a certain size (usually around 18mm), an injection of hCG is normally given to mature the follicles and trigger ovulation. Insemination is then carried out between 12 and 30 hours after the hCG. Most women are given some form of ovarian stimulation as this more than doubles the success rate. Each clinic will vary in how they are set up to do techniques such as IUI and they know what works best within their particular clinic setting.

Sperm Preparation

The man is normally asked to abstain from sex (ejaculation) for two to three days before the insemination to optimise the sperm sample. This is especially important if there is a low sperm count. On the day of the insemination, the man produces his sperm sample by masturbation. The sample is then 'washed' to separate out the motile and non-motile sperm from the seminal fluid. Sperm washing can also remove some antibodies. Frozen-thawed sperm or donor sperm can be used if needed. There must be a minimum sperm count for IUI, but this will vary between clinics. Sperm preparation takes about one to two hours.

After the Treatment

IUI is a relatively painless procedure. The woman normally lies down and has a short rest before leaving the clinic. I encourage women to lie down for around 20 minutes if possible. Avoid strenuous exercise on the day of treatment, but most people carry on with life straight afterwards. You can resume lovemaking as soon as you wish after the procedure. A pregnancy test can be done about 14 days after the insemination.

Can the Sperm Fall Out Again?

Many women are concerned that the sperm might fall out. You may lose a little fluid afterwards, but most of the swimmers will be well on their way to the fallopian tubes. They have already been given a head-start, so you can carry on life pretty normally.

Complications of IUI

There are minimal complications with IUI. Some women will experience mild cramping during the insemination. As with any procedure, it is possible to introduce infection, but this is rare. The main risk associated with stimulated IUI is multiple births with the risk of twins around 10 per cent.

Success Rates

Success rates with stimulated IUI are around 10–15 per cent, per cycle, but vary widely between clinics. Some studies show that IUI is more likely to succeed if two treatments are given, spaced 12 hours apart. Other studies show that a single well-timed insemination is just as successful. The lowest statistics for IUI success are where there is only one follicle. The other factor is the quality of the sperm. Higher sperm counts increase the odds of success.

Women who are going through IUI treatment often say that they don't feel as if they are part of the 'real buzz' of their fertility clinic, because they have not signed up for the full works of IVF. They often complain of feeling marginalised and express anxiety about the lack of monitoring and what they perceive as sub-optimal timing of their inseminations. Remember, the egg is viable for up to 24 hours, and sperm live for a few days so try not to get too anxious about the timing of the technique. However, I firmly believe that couples are not always given the full attention they deserve when going through IUI and that in the right setting, and with optimal timing, higher success rates could possibly be achieved.

Common Gynaecological Conditions

Some readers will be aware of existing medical or gynaecological conditions which may impact on fertility; other women may find that some of these conditions are detected during the process of fertility tests and investigations. It is important that you stay in close contact with a specialist if you have a known or pre-existing condition and that your fertility specialist and medical specialist are working in collaboration to monitor your health and wellbeing.

Thyroid Function

The thyroid gland (in the neck) controls metabolism and energy balance. It is under the overall control of the hypothalamus and pituitary gland and is stimulated by thyroid stimulating hormone (TSH). The thyroid uses iodine from food sources to produce two thyroid hormones: thyroxine (T4) in large quantities and triiodothyronine (T3) in much smaller amounts. T4 is converted into the much more potent T3 when it reaches its target tissues. Thyroid levels are kept constant by drawing on supplies of stored iodine, much in the same way that the body maintains blood sugar balance. If your thyroid gland is not making enough thyroid hormone your body slows right down, whereas if your thyroid gland is producing too much thyroid hormone you feel as if you are on fast forward all the time.

General Symptoms of Hypothyroid (Underactive Thyroid)
- Weight gain and inability to lose weight
- Feeling cold
- Tiredness
- Dry skin, hair and nails
- Low libido

- Irregular or heavy periods
- Anovulatory cycles (no ovulation)
- Constipation
- Slowing down mentally, depression

General Symptoms of Hyperthyroid (Overactive Thyroid)
- Weight loss despite increased appetite
- Sweating, dislike of heat, thirst
- Rapid heartbeat, palpitations
- Changes in periods, often light and infrequent
- Anovulatory cycles (no ovulation)
- Diarrhoea
- Anxiety, restlessness, irritability, poor sleep

So, thyroid symptoms can be wide and varied. I don't want you to read this and think: 'Goodness, I have a thyroid problem,' because all of these symptoms can be caused by other conditions, including stress. Symptoms usually develop quite gradually, and many people notice only the occasional symptom. If there are thyroid problems in your family, it increases the chance of you having thyroid problems. There is also a chance that you may have thyroid antibodies (Hashimoto's disease), where your body starts to attack the thyroid gland eventually destroying the thyroid cells so that they cannot produce thyroid hormones. Thyroid function tests are available on the NHS, although the test is not too expensive if you opt to have it done privately. A full assessment of your thyroid function requires a blood test to check levels of TSH, T4 and T3 and sometimes for thyroid antibodies. Although thyroid testing is not routine NHS practice when investigating fertility delays, one fertility clinic found that 5 per cent of women attending their clinic had thyroid problems, often without symptoms.

Case Study

Dawn, 36, had one child and was trying for a second. She suffered from anxiety and had been on antidepressants. Dawn was convinced that the stress and anxiety were stopping her from getting pregnant. During the consultation I asked her about her anxiety and discovered that many of her symptoms were mimicking or very similar to those of thyroid problems. Tests revealed that she had an underactive thyroid. She went to see her doctor and was put on thyroxine; her anxiety lifted, which goes to show how sensitive the thyroid is and how easy it is to miss. We also looked at when she was having sex as her cycles were irregular (another reason why the thyroid needs to be checked). Dawn and her partner were having sex just once a week, so I explained that this was not often enough. The more often they had sex, the more likely pregnancy was to happen, no matter how anxious she was.

Normal thyroid function can be affected by nutritional deficiencies, infections and stress. If you are very stressed you will have raised levels of cortisol, which can inhibit the conversion of T4 to T3, so stress management is important. When the thyroid hormones are back in balance, ovulation and fertility are usually restored quite quickly. If you have thyroid problems it is very important that your thyroid function is stabilised before you conceive to protect your future health and that of an unborn baby. Even if you don't have any thyroid symptoms, make sure that you get your thyroid checked if:

- you have not conceived despite having regular sex for more than six months
- you have suffered two or more miscarriages
- your cycle is irregular

- you have had one child and are struggling to conceive a second
- there are any thyroid problems in your family

Anaemia

Anaemia is a reduction in the amount of haemoglobin, the oxygen-carrying pigment, in the blood. Many women are anaemic without knowing it, and women with heavy periods are particularly susceptible. Anaemia can have a big impact on fertility, because if the blood is busy going to all the vital organs to keep them going, it may be diverted away from the non-essential reproductive organs.

The symptoms of anaemia are related to the lack of oxygen in the blood:

- Tiredness
- Lethargy
- Feeling faint
- Breathlessness on exertion
- Sometimes looking pale
- Irregular periods

A simple blood test is done to measure the amount of haemoglobin (iron) in your blood and count up the red blood cells and other constituents. This test may confirm you are anaemic and you may be advised to take extra iron in your diet. If there is no obvious cause for your anaemia (such as heavy periods), you may need further tests to establish the cause as there are many different forms of anaemia, some of which can be more serious.

Polycystic Ovaries (PCO) and Polycystic Ovarian Syndrome (PCOS)

It is really important to understand the difference between PCO and PCOS. The term polycystic ovaries (PCO) simply describes a very common finding on ultrasound scans: multiple small cysts containing immature eggs beneath the surface of the ovaries. The woman has a normal hormone balance and normal menstrual cycles. This does not have an impact on fertility. PCO affects about one in three women.

Women sometimes find out they have polycystic ovaries years before trying for a baby. This can happen when a woman has a pelvic scan for another issue. Sometimes, a woman is told that she will have difficulty conceiving due to the PCO. She is made to feel that she has failed before she has even tried, and those negative messages can go very deep into the subconscious mind. PCO is such a common finding on ultrasound that it is a shame that it is even mentioned; more likely than not, it won't have any impact on future fertility.

The term polycystic ovarian syndrome (PCOS), on the other hand, describes a syndrome, which is a combination of signs and symptoms. PCOS is an endocrine (hormone) disorder in which polycystic ovaries are found in conjunction with symptoms such as irregular cycles, acne, increased facial and bodily hair and sometimes weight gain. The exact cause of PCOS is unknown, but it tends to run in families and can lead to additional health problems, such as diabetes, later in life if not properly managed. PCOS affects 5–10 per cent of women of reproductive age and is the most common cause of anovulatory infertility in the western world.

With PCOS, it is generally accepted that the underlying problem is an inability of the ovaries to produce hormones in the right proportions. Moreover, some women are unable to regulate the levels of ovarian hormones circulating in the blood at any one time. Added to this are other contributing factors such as hormonal issues related to excess weight, and blood sugar abnormalities. Levels of luteinising hormone (LH) are often raised, which can damage the egg and affect fertilisation and implantation. For women having IVF treatment, doctors will take this into account when deciding upon the drug regime (see page 322). It is harder for women with raised LH to use ovulation predictor kits reliably because they will continually get positive results. This gives the impression that they are about to ovulate when the real issue is that the LH level is consistently raised above the threshold for the test.

Some women with PCOS have cycles that are longer than 35 days (oligomenorrhoea) and some will have no periods at all (amenorrhoea) for four to six months. The length of the cycle generally relates to the degree of insulin imbalance, so the more normal the length of the cycle, the better the blood sugar control.

Typical Signs and Symptoms of PCOS

- Irregular periods and sporadic ovulation
- No ovulation and amenorrhoea (no periods)
- Excessive facial or body hair (hirsutism)
- Blood tests showing high LH and testosterone
- Acne
- Tendency to be overweight
- Fertility problems

Women with PCOS have a higher miscarriage rate – up to five times higher than normal – due to the raised levels of LH. If a woman with PCOS manages to conceive naturally, she may benefit from additional progesterone supplementation to maintain the pregnancy to full term. I try to help women with PCOS to conceive naturally before going down an IVF route. We start by managing any weight issues, then if necessary she may need to go on to ovarian-stimulation drugs such as clomiphene (see page 239) or metformin (see below). Clomiphene is the first-choice drug for women with PCOS. Ovulation will occur in 90 per cent of cases, with a 60 per cent pregnancy rate, depending on age. However, in women who haven't got pregnant after nine cycles, very few pregnancies occur. Clomiphene is not usually used for more than three to six cycles as it causes thinning of the womb lining.

PCOS and Insulin Resistance

Many women with PCOS have insulin resistance. The hormone insulin is produced in the pancreas in response to increased levels of glucose in the blood. Insulin acts to regulate the metabolism of blood sugar. With insulin resistance, the body cannot use the insulin properly and the pancreas produces more insulin to keep up with demand. Eventually the pancreas struggles to keep up and there is a build-up of excess glucose. This is why some women with PCOS go on to develop type 2 diabetes. The key areas that need to be targeted for these women are diet and nutrition. I cannot stress enough how important it is to stabilise your blood sugar levels and insulin resistance with a specialised diet and exercise programme. It's essential that you enjoy your diet and exercise routine and that it fits easily into your daily life. (For further advice on nutrition, see Chapter 7.)

Metformin

The drug metformin has been used by many women with PCOS. A hypoglycaemic agent, it brings down blood sugar levels and helps to improve the action of insulin in many ways. For example, it helps to increase the metabolism of glucose in the muscles, and it increases the intestinal absorption of glucose. Published data shows that it improves insulin resistance in women with PCOS. Metformin is often prescribed for women with PCOS to help them lose weight. The side effects can be pretty nasty, however, and include nausea, vomiting, bloating, diarrhoea and other gastrointestinal-tract disturbances.

Endometriosis

Endometriosis is a condition where cells that are normally found in the endometrium (womb lining) are found elsewhere in the pelvis – ovaries or tubes – or in other parts of the body, such as the bowel. These endometrial cells that have escaped the womb respond to the reproductive hormones in the same way as other endometrial cells – they grow then break down and bleed in a cyclic pattern. As these small internal bleeds do not have a direct way out of the body they can result in areas of inflammation and pain and the development of adhesions (scar tissue). Endometriosis is graded mild, moderate or severe.

The cause is unknown although it tends to run in families. One theory, known as retrograde menstruation, is that the endometrial tissue migrates backwards instead of being shed in the usual way through the vagina. It goes out through the tubes and into the pelvis where it can implant on pelvic organs. Another possibility is that there is a link with the immune system, and some women cannot fight off the wayward endometrial cells. Although the exact cause is not clear, a combination of factors is probably involved. Endometriosis is not an infection, so is not transmissible, and it is not cancer.

The symptoms depend on the location of the endometriosis and include:

- Painful, heavy or irregular periods – sometimes dark (old) blood
- Spotting or bleeding between periods
- Deep pain during or after intercourse
- Pelvic pain, particularly during a period or around ovulation

- Abdominal bloating, constipation or diarrhoea, especially during a period
- Pain when passing urine
- Problems or pain on opening bowels or bleeding from the bowel
- Back or leg pain
- Fatigue, lack of energy, depression
- Fertility problems

Symptoms can vary in intensity, and the intensity of the symptoms does not always reflect the degree of endometriosis. Some women with endometriosis are symptom-free. The above symptoms can all have other causes – some serious – so it is important to get medical advice. It can be difficult to diagnose endometriosis as the symptoms can vary. The only way to get a clear diagnosis is by laparoscopy (see page 219).

The link between endometriosis and fertility problems is not clearly understood, but there may be problems including ovarian cysts (endometrioma or chocolate cyst – see page 258); twisted tube(s); ovulatory problems including anovulation, luteal phase defect or unruptured follicles (see page 259); or immunological changes affecting implantation.

As the endometrial tissue grows in response to oestrogen, women who do not wish to conceive will often be advised to take the Pill or other longer-acting contraceptives. This reduces the production of oestrogen and cuts off the fuel supply, thereby suppressing the endometriosis and improving symptoms. At times, surgery may be advisable – laparoscopic surgery aims to clear any areas of endometriosis and remove any adhesions to free up the pelvic organs. The endometrial patches may recur over time, and this is why a woman may be advised to conceive as soon as possible after surgery. Sometimes other hormonal therapies may be used to suppress endometriosis prior to IUI or IVF (see page 178).

Self-care is very important for symptom control. Good nutrition is vital. Some women find acupuncture helpful. Women who find their symptoms distressing or are having difficulties conceiving may find fertility counselling helpful.

Tubal Problems

Healthy tubes should be patent (open) and quite mobile. The fringed (fimbriated) end of the tube (with the finger-like projections) is designed to catch the egg and sweep it along the tube with the help of delicate hair-like cilia that line the tube. If a woman loses a tube for some reason (such as an ectopic pregnancy) then the tube from the opposite side may be able to compensate by sweeping across to collect an egg from the opposite ovary.

One or both tubes can be blocked anywhere along their length. If the woman's tubes are blocked or damaged in any way, it may be suggested she has IVF. This can, of course, be devastating news for women. However, IVF was initially designed to by-pass the tubes, and the chances of IVF working are very high in women with tubal disorders as long as everything else is okay. If there are adhesions (scarring) or the tube has become stuck down, the gynaecologist will try and free it and it may be possible to try and conceive naturally, provided a woman is aware of the potential increased risk of an ectopic (tubal) pregnancy.

Hydrosalpinx

If there are blockages at the fimbriated end of the tube, fluid sometimes collects in the tube. This is because the normal tubal fluid cannot drain out in the usual way into the peritoneal cavity. This is known as a hydrosalpinx. Sometimes the gynaecologist will monitor this to see if the fluid increases or goes away. If there is no improvement, the tube may have to be surgically clipped or possibly removed. Sealing off the tube prevents the build-up of fluid draining back into the womb, creating a hostile environment for implantation during IVF.

Adhesions

These are bands of fibrous scar tissue that bind together two membranous surfaces which should normally be separated from each other. They may be the result of endometriosis (see pages 178 and 254), infection or previous surgery (such as appendicectomy). Adhesions can form anywhere within the pelvis. If they are quite flimsy, they will cause little problem. More rigid adhesions can prevent movement of the tubes or bind the ovaries to the back of the womb or to the bowel. Adhesions can also form in the cavity of the womb, affecting implantation. A severe form of this is known as Asherman's syndrome, where much of the cavity is obliterated. The impact on fertility will therefore depend largely on the position of the adhesions.

A gynaecologist will generally operate only if adhesions are causing pain or preventing a pregnancy. This is because the surgery to divide or remove adhesions can cause the development of further adhesions, defeating its purpose. Any surgery for pelvic problems will normally be done using laparoscopy or keyhole surgery to minimise the risk of adhesions (see page 219).

Uterine Abnormalities

Uterine abnormalities can include polyps, fibroids and malformations of the womb, such as a septum in the cavity or other congenital malformations. Uterine abnormalities occur in 5 per cent of women, and the most common abnormalities are fibroids and uterine polyps. Many women go on to get pregnant once these have been removed, depending on their size and where they are in the uterine cavity.

Fibroids

Fibroids, sometimes referred to as myoma, are found on the uterine muscle. This common gynaecological condition occurs more frequently in women over 30. Interestingly, black women of African origin seem to be at a higher risk of having fibroids than Caucasian women. The position of the fibroid can affect fertility by 25–40 per cent, depending on where the fibroid is located and its size. If fibroids are on the outside of the womb they won't impact on fertility. Small fibroids in the muscle wall are unlikely to cause problems, but if they become enlarged, they could distort the uterine cavity, affecting implantation and causing miscarriage. If fibroids project into the cavity of the uterus they are more likely to cause heavy or irregular bleeding and may prevent implantation.

The management of fibroids is really important to women planning conception naturally as well as women who plan to undergo IVF. Definitive diagnosis is made by ultrasound scan – 3-D imaging can now clearly define the location of a fibroid. A decision needs to be made with your gynaecologist as to whether the fibroid(s) are likely to prevent you from getting pregnant or carrying a pregnancy to term. It is not always necessary to remove a fibroid to conceive, and recovery time will be needed after surgery. As fibroids are fuelled by oestrogen, they can enlarge during pregnancy; this is another factor the doctor will consider when discussing the pros and cons of surgery. You might wish to get a second opinion before opting for fibroid surgery (myomectomy).

Ovarian Cysts

An ovarian cyst is a collection of fluid surrounded by a very thin wall within the ovary. The ovary is, of course, producing small fluid-filled 'cysts' or follicles much of the time, but if a follicle grows larger than about 20mm, it is termed a cyst. Most ovarian cysts are known as simple or functional cysts and are quite harmless – they secrete oestrogen and progesterone and tend to disappear of their own accord. These are a very common finding during an ultrasound scan.

If a cyst forms in the first half of the cycle (follicular cyst), the follicle does not rupture at the usual time but continues to grow to more than 20mm before it ruptures, sometimes with accompanying pain. If a cyst forms in the second half of the cycle (corpus luteum cyst), instead of the corpus luteum degenerating in the usual way, it continues to grow, filling with fluid or blood and expanding into a cyst. These cysts may not produce any symptoms but they can grow to quite a size. They may bleed into themselves or twist the ovary, causing pain. If a cyst ruptures it can cause internal bleeding and sudden sharp pain. A third type of functional cyst is known as a haemorrhagic cyst and results from a small blood vessel breaking in the cyst wall. These cysts can rupture and cause intense pain. Another type of cyst is as an endometrioma, or chocolate cyst, which is caused by a patch of endometriosis forming a cyst in the ovary (see pages 178 and 254). The majority of cysts will disappear with time, but if a cyst persists it may be aspirated and the fluid from the cyst sent off to check for any abnormalities.

If you have a cyst your ovary will generally continue to function and produce eggs, but large cysts can affect hormone balance. There are some concerns that the presence of ovarian cysts reduces the chances of successful IVF, which is why a scan is usually done prior to starting an IVF cycle (see page 217 and below).

Ultrasound Scanning in Fertility Investigations

Scanning techniques are improving all the time. In the early days, scans were performed abdominally (with gel on the tummy), scanning through all the layers of muscle and fat, so the vaginal route was a big step forward in improving the images (see pelvic ultrasound, page 217). In another step forward, 3-D scans are often used antenatally to get remarkable pictures of the unborn baby. Some centres are now starting to use saline infusion sonohysterography, or 'fluid ultrasound', as an improved version of a standard trans-vaginal scan. This provides a view of the uterine cavity and a more detailed image of the endometrium, but cannot give conclusive evidence of tubal patency.

Monitored Cycles

I see many women who need reassurance that their bodies are functioning normally. Essentially, they want to find out if there are any obvious problems. I sometimes refer a woman for a monitored cycle – a series of ultrasound scans through the cycle to monitor the development of the follicle, the timing of ovulation, the development of the corpus luteum and the ovarian blood flow. A monitored cycle is not a standard investigation but many women find these scans very reassuring, and the benefits of having a positive experience of a scan can be empowering. It is important for a woman to be able to visualise her pelvic area positively. As much as I believe in IVF I feel that a more natural approach is appropriate for some couples, provided there is time.

Interview with Mr Bill Smith, Ultrasound Specialist and Technical Director of Clinical Diagnostic Services

How is ultrasound technology used to assess fertility?
Modern ultrasound scanning enables us to monitor a woman's ovulation cycles and fertility status. This can be particularly useful for couples who have had other causes of infertility ruled out, such as tubal problems or low sperm count. Ultrasound can also identify many pelvic and gynaecological disorders which can often be treated, removing the need for assisted conception techniques.

High-resolution trans-vaginal scanning (TVS) is a safe way to gain a tremendous amount of information. It can recognise the characteristic changes that take place during a natural cycle within the womb and ovaries. Colour Doppler Imaging (CDI) is able to demonstrate blood flow through very fine capillary vessels and highlight subtle vascular changes within the ovary associated with ovulation. 3-D ultrasound gives even more anatomical detail, providing a greatly improved assessment of the womb.

What are monitored cycles?

As ultrasound is generally convenient and non-invasive, women tend to find it helpful. Monitoring a woman's cycle can provide tremendous reassurance to patients about their fertility status. In addition, serial scanning offers a good opportunity to communicate with patients. It can give them a valuable insight into ovulation patterns and aspects of reproductive physiology.

A woman's cycle is monitored using vaginal ultrasound, generally on a weekly basis throughout the menstrual cycle. It can reassure some women about ovulation and their womb lining, and give them more information about when they are ovulating. Cycles can be monitored while a woman is taking Clomid or having injections (see Chapter 11). If women are going through IUI, I often use ultrasound monitoring to reassure them that their cycles are working normally, and this gives them the confidence to carry on.

Carrying out between three and five scans during a woman's cycle can provide a wealth of information. For example, it can detect fibroids, endometrial polyps, endometriosis and polycystic ovaries, as well as anatomical malformations that might affect fertility or increase the risk of very early miscarriage. Scans can gauge the number and distribution of follicles, giving an idea of a woman's 'ovarian reserve'. They help us to predict accurately the timing of ovulation and the 'fertile phase' of the cycle. They also provide an effective general screening of the womb and ovaries for female patients. For men, testicular/prostate scans can be helpful when semen analysis reveals relevant issues. Advanced ultrasound imaging has been shown to reduce the need for blood tests to assess fertility status.

What outcome is likely for patients?
A significant number of patients conceive during a monitored cycle. A number will become pregnant during the six months following the initial monitored cycle, whether further cycle monitoring is carried out or not. Experience shows that patients who do not conceive within about six months of the initial monitored cycle might well require ART/IVF treatment.

❋

So, ultrasound is used both to investigate fertility problems and to provide an 'inside view' during different techniques and treatments. Some women will have a monitored cycle prior to starting IVF and certainly all women going through most forms of assisted fertility will be resigned to frequent scans to monitor progress – regularly joining an early morning queue!

Chapter 10

Testing Sperm Health

Introduction by Zita West

My thanks, again, to Dr Sheryl Homa for writing this chapter. Sheryl is a clinical embryologist and scientist who heads up the male fertility programme at the Zita West Clinic. Fertility clinics are usually run by gynaecologists and tend to focus on women; as a result, the man's side is often under-investigated. Here, Sheryl explains the importance of male investigations and the value of a comprehensive semen analysis.

When a couple is having difficulty conceiving, it is a good idea to organise a few general fertility tests, just to check that their reproductive systems are functioning properly. An early diagnosis of a male problem is essential. I see far too many couples spending months or even years investigating female infertility while their biological clock ticks away, only to find that the problem lies with their partner.

Men are advised to have a semen analysis as a first port of call to check their fertility. As male infertility accounts for approximately

50 per cent of all infertility problems, and because a semen analysis is such a simple test to carry out, it makes sense to have this test as soon as you are aware that it is taking some time for your partner to conceive.

The test can be arranged through your GP, but all too often the test may be quite basic and the results given to you without much explanation. It is very important that you have a test that looks at a whole variety of things in the semen, not just the count, motility (movement) and morphology (shape) of the sperm. By focusing just on these parameters, you may be missing some very important clues about your true fertility status, and you may not get a realistic picture of your situation.

The terminology used in the semen analysis can often be very confusing. It really helps to have a thorough explanation of the results given by a sympathetic clinician in an environment where you feel free to ask about aspects of the test that concern you. An abnormal result may be very difficult to reconcile, especially for men who confuse their virility (masculinity) with their fertility (ability to father

Home Testing Kits for Men

Just as there are home tests for women (see page 43), sperm tests can now be done at home. The newest male home test works by allowing the sperm to swim through a barrier that mimics the female cervix. The device then measures the concentration of active sperm able to swim beyond that point. If the level is high enough, then a red line indicates a positive test. While this test may be a good starting point, it does not look at all of the other sperm parameters that contribute to your fertility. As part of a general fertility check, you need to consider the value of a full, comprehensive semen analysis at the relevant time.

a child genetically). You should also be able to discuss the implications of your test result, and your doctor may recommend further testing for you if necessary.

Semen Analysis

Semen analysis varies enormously up and down the country, depending upon the guidelines used to perform the test and how the results are interpreted. Some laboratories look at only a handful of parameters, while others give a much more detailed analysis for a more accurate picture of your fertility.

What Affects Semen Analysis?

A good laboratory will expect you to comply with their guidelines for producing a semen sample so that your results can be reliably compared with the standardised reference range. If you are not compliant, your results may indicate that you are infertile, when in fact you may not be.

Length of Sexual Abstinence

One of the principal things affecting the semen analysis results is the length of time since the last ejaculation – whether through intercourse or masturbation. It is important to have two to three days' sexual abstinence before a semen analysis. If you have fewer than two days' abstinence, the sperm count may seem artificially low for the test, whereas more than five days may start to affect the motility of the sperm. Sperm live for only a few days and will start to die off with time, so although a longer abstinence will allow sperm numbers to increase, the quality will be affected. I recently saw a couple where the man lived overseas. He would return to England occasionally and consequently had an extended length of abstinence. His semen analysis showed very poor results. Once we discussed the importance of regular ejaculation, his repeat sample showed great improvement.

Method of Sample Production

A semen sample should always be produced by masturbation, and the entire sample must be collected. While it is true that men produce a far better quality semen sample when they are making love, remember that the reference values for sperm parameters have been determined only from samples produced by masturbation, and we can only compare like with like in order to get a reliable diagnosis. The main reason why you should produce a semen sample in this way is that vaginal secretions and saliva can actually harm the sperm and give an unreliable result.

Some men may experience difficulties producing a sample for a variety of reasons. This is not uncommon, and discussing the problem with an experienced fertility counsellor may help. As a last resort, sperm can be extracted surgically as part of more advanced fertility treatments.

Time from Semen Production to Testing

A delay in testing may result in the sperm quality deteriorating so you may not get a valid result. I recommend that you try to produce a sample at the place where you are having the test, as the sample should be assessed when it is fresh. However, some men find producing a sample in this way very stressful. If you cannot produce a sample in this way, call the laboratory and they should be able to provide you with a special condom and container to produce it at home as long as you can get it to the lab within 60 minutes. Do not buy a condom from a chemist as most condoms are actually toxic to sperm.

Problems that May Occur

- You miss the pot and lose part of the sample. Don't be embarrassed. Tell the staff as it may affect your result. You may have to return another day to repeat the test.
- You cannot produce a sample. Discuss this with the staff who may suggest you produce a sample at home. If you have concerns about producing a sample on the day your partner's eggs are being collected, this needs to be discussed with your IVF team in advance. It may be possible to produce a sample when you are not stressed and freeze it so that it is there as a backup if needed on the day.

Understanding the Results

To get a complete picture of the semen quality, the test should include information about the following:

- Appearance
- pH (acidity/alkalinity)
- Volume
- Consistency (liquefaction and viscosity)
- Agglutination (sperm stickiness)
- Concentration (sperm count)
- Motility (how the sperm move)
- Morphology (sperm shape)
- MAR test (antibodies)
- Other cells

Results should be analysed according to current World Health Organization (WHO) guidelines, 2009.

Appearance

The colour of the semen sample is important. A normal sample has a greyish appearance and is opalescent. A yellow colour may indicate the presence of leucocytes (white cells), a sign of infection. Other causes of yellow semen are increased length of abstinence or taking too many B vitamins. A brownish tinge is unusual and indicates blood in the sperm, another indicator of infection. This could also be a sign of a more serious problem so you should be referred to a urologist right away. It is important that any infections are dealt with as they can impair sperm function and lead to further fertility problems (see below).

pH

The normal pH of semen is alkaline at 7.2–8.0 and is determined by the balance of fluids coming from the male accessory glands such as the prostate and seminal vesicles. A high or low pH can indicate problems in these glands.

Volume

After two to three days of abstinence from sex, a man should produce 1.5ml or more of semen. Because most of the fluid is produced from the male accessory glands, a low volume may suggest a problem in these areas.

Consistency

The consistency of the sample is important as if it is too thick it can affect the motility of the sperm. A very thick sample would be analogous to the sperm having to swim through treacle. The consistency is determined in terms of liquefaction and viscosity:

- **Liquefaction** When semen is ejaculated it coagulates as it is designed to stick to the woman's cervix, but over the next 10–20 minutes it will begin to liquefy. Liquefaction should be complete at the time of testing, and certainly within one hour of ejaculation.

- **Viscosity** This is a measure of the fluid nature of the sample. Semen should have a fairly watery consistency at the time of testing.

Agglutination

This refers to the presence of motile sperm 'stuck' together and may indicate antibodies in the semen. If the sperm are agglutinated, there are fewer free sperm available to move up towards the egg.

Concentration (Sperm Count)

The count is given in millions per millilitre (ml) of ejaculate and should be equal to or more than 15 million per ml (WHO, 2009) though 60 million per ml is about average. The total sperm count should be a minimum of 39 million in the whole ejaculate. The higher the number the better. Causes of low sperm count include:

- Hormone imbalances
- Infections
- Varicocoele (see Chapter 3)
- Genetic reasons
- Surgery to the testicles or lower abdomen
- Chemotherapy/radiotherapy
- Other conditions such as diabetes or kidney failure
- Age
- Obesity
- Lifestyle
- Heat exposure
- Excessive exercise
- Anabolic steroids
- Drugs
- Stress

- Environmental toxins
- Occupational hazards

Evidence suggests that changes to your lifestyle and a healthy diet may help to improve sperm count in some situations.

Motility

This measures the percentage of sperm that are moving. It is also important to have a breakdown of sperm motility as sperm can move in different ways. It is no good having a large number of moving sperm if they are only jiggling on the spot. At least 40 per cent of sperm need to be moving in some fashion, and 32 per cent should be progressing forward (WHO, 2009).

Causes of poor motility in sperm include:

- Increased length of sexual abstinence
- Defects in the sperm tails
- Anti-sperm antibodies (see The MAR Test, below)
- Infection
- Oxidative stress (see page 282)
- Age
- Weight
- Lifestyle
- Zinc deficiency
- Drugs
- Varicocoele (see Chapter 3)
- Heat damage
- Excessive exercise
- Anabolic steroids
- Environmental toxins
- Occupational hazards

There is considerable evidence in the scientific literature that dietary supplements can help improve sperm motility, so apart from other changes to your lifestyle, it is a good idea to see a nutritionist if you have problems in this area.

Morphology

Morphology describes the shape of the sperm and assesses what percentage is apparently normal. Opinion is divided about the value of morphology tests, mainly because the methods used to assess morphology differ between labs. Furthermore, not all labs use the same reference ranges to report the results, which makes interpretation very difficult. Current best practice guidelines (WHO, 2009) show that the majority of sperm in a healthy fertile man are in fact abnormally shaped. Indeed, up to 96 per cent may be abnormally shaped. The important question to ask is what does having abnormal sperm mean. Abnormal sperm may be less able to move properly and are less likely to be able to bind to the egg. However, the effect of sperm morphology must be interpreted in the light of the other parameters. If you have a very low number of normal sperm but a high count and high

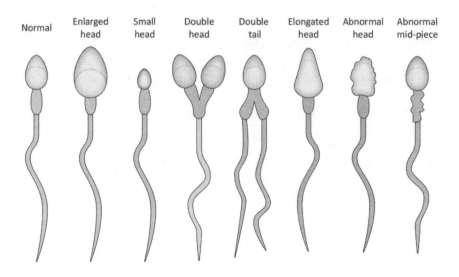

| Normal | Enlarged head | Small head | Double head | Double tail | Elongated head | Abnormal head | Abnormal mid-piece |

motility, there is a good chance that a reasonable number of normal sperm will reach the egg. Alternatively, if the count and motility are low, it is likely to take a lot longer to get pregnant. In these cases, you may be advised to have ICSI treatment (see page 336).

Poor morphology can be caused by:

- Oxidative stress (see page 282)
- Lifestyle
- Genetic predisposition
- Varicocoele (see Chapter 3)
- Heat damage
- Excessive exercise
- Anabolic steroids
- Drugs
- Stress
- Environmental toxins
- Occupational hazards

Although it is not easy to improve morphology by making changes to your lifestyle, I believe it is worth a try (see Chapter 4).

The MAR Test

The MAR (mixed agglutination reaction) test measures the level of antibodies in the semen that attack the sperm. The treatment available depends on how high the levels of antibodies are, so it is important to have this test to determine the most suitable treatment for your partner. If between 50 and 80 per cent of sperm are coated in antibodies, intrauterine insemination (IUI) (see page 243) can be used. ICSI (see page 336) would be recommended if more than 80 per cent of sperm have antibodies on them. Some doctors may prescribe steroids, but these may only be effective if the antibodies are also present in the blood. Furthermore, steroids have some rather nasty side effects and can only be used for a few months, so you should discuss this in depth with your doctor before choosing this option.

Other Cells

Semen samples often contain debris and cells other than sperm in small numbers. These cells may come from the prostate, or they may be immature sperm cells. Alternatively, they may be white blood cells (inflammatory or pus cells) which are usually produced in response to an infection. White cell numbers should be less than 1 million/ml in semen. If the numbers are higher, it would be a good idea to have a full sexual health screen, as infections can contribute to poor fertility (see page 279).

Interview with Dr Allan Pacey, Senior Lecturer in Andrology, University of Sheffield

What can a man do to make sure his sperm is as good as it can be?
The thing about the testicles is that you've got what you are born with. There aren't many things you can do to improve the sperm quality, but there is a lot that can damage the sperm:

- Don't smoke, because smoking damages sperm DNA.
- Get checked out for sexually transmitted infections, such as chlamydia and ureaplasma, which damage the DNA and the genetic quality of the sperm.
- Eat a healthy diet with plenty of fruit and vegetables: this protects sperm from free radical damage.
- Avoid heat. The scrotum is positioned where it is to keep the sperm cool so wear baggy pants and avoid hot baths and jacuzzis. Some women might want to put ice on your balls – don't go as far as this!

- Bear in mind that driving a lot, cycling and hardcore sport such as marathon running push the body to physical extremes.
- Be sensible with alcohol. If it helps you get upstairs to the bedroom then have a drink.
- Don't save up sperm; ejaculate regularly (two to three times per week).
- Have sex two to three times a week but be careful with lubricants and saliva. Arousal is important as it affects the amount of sperm you will release: you are not helping yourself by having mechanical, unpassionate sex.
- If you work with chemicals, especially paints and glues, protect yourself with a mask and make sure there is plenty of ventilation.

Definitions of Low Sperm Parameters

- Oligozoospermia – the sperm concentration is low, fewer than 15 million per ml.
- Asthenozoospermia – less than 32 per cent of the sperm are actively moving forward.
- Teratozoospermia – more than 96 per cent of the sperm are abnormally shaped.
- Azoospermia – the man produces no sperm in his semen. The causes of this can be testicular failure, hormone disorders, damage to testicles through surgery or treatment for cancer, or obstruction caused by infection/inflammation or medical conditions. There may have been a congenital abnormality where the testicles were not descended and had to be brought down by surgery. Up to 15 per cent of men with azoospermia may carry abnormal genes so genetic testing may be carried out.

Procedures to Take Sperm from the Testicles in Men With Azoospermia

The fact that sperm is not present in the ejaculate does not necessarily mean there is no hope. Sperm may be retrieved directly from the testicles by surgical means. If the reason for the azoospermia is an obstruction, there is a good chance of finding sperm this way. Even in azoospermic men with no obstruction in the testicles, sperm can be retrieved in as many as 60 per cent of cases, depending on the cause of azoospermia.

- PESA (percutaneous epididymal sperm aspiration). This is where a small amount of sperm can be obtained directly from the epididymis, and is generally used when there is a blockage.

- TESE (testicular sperm extraction). If PESA is unsuccessful then the sperm may be taken directly from the testes (testicles). This is generally recommended in cases of azoospermia where there is no known obstruction. This procedure can be done on the day of your partner's egg collection. Alternatively, you may wish to have this procedure carried out in advance. The testicular sperm can then be frozen to use for ICSI treatment at a later stage. Although this procedure can be done under local anaesthetic, it can be quite painful because the testicles are very delicate, and you might need heavy sedation or a general anaesthetic. There can be some bruising afterwards.

How important is morphology? The way results are interpreted it is hard to find a man with a normal result.

Many men worry about having high abnormal forms and having a baby with abnormalities. There is such huge variability in a normal sperm sample. The World Health Organization has changed the rules for morphology: a man can have as few as 4 per cent normal shaped sperm and still be fertile (that is, have a good chance of conceiving within one year). Similarly, sperm concentration can fall to 15 million sperm per ml, and motility as low as 32 per cent, and a man can still be considered 'normal'.

The Male Fertility Consultation

Many couples tell us that they feel the whole emphasis has been on the woman's fertility; male fertility has been largely neglected and they are being 'fast-tracked' towards IVF. Undoubtedly, the whole area of male fertility has been revolutionised by ICSI, but there are many situations where, provided the woman's age allows it, intermediate steps may be appropriate to improve sperm health. Very few couples would actively choose IVF in preference to natural conception, so our aim is to identify if any improvement in sperm health is possible to optimise chances of natural conception.

At the Zita West Clinic, I see all of the men who choose to have a comprehensive semen analysis so that we can look at the semen parameters step by step, and discuss the implications of the results. With male problems contributing up to 50 per cent of all cases of infertility, it makes sense to focus on the man at the same time as his partner. We always ask you to fill out a questionnaire before you come in so that we can interpret your results in the light of your medical history as well as your lifestyle. We recommend you attend on your own for a one-to-one discussion to give you the opportunity to talk through any issues that you think might be affecting your fertility. There may be issues you find awkward to talk about in front of your partner that could be crucial to understanding where the problems lie. Depending on your situation, we may suggest further testing to determine the causes of any fertility problems you may have (see below).

If the count, motility and sperm shape are all looking good, I remind men that they should not fall into a false sense of security that there is nothing wrong with them. For these men, I point out that the most important part about a sperm is its genetic integrity, and you cannot tell this just by looking at them down a microscope. It does not matter how many rapidly moving, normal-shaped sperm make it to the egg; if they are genetically abnormal, they will not produce a healthy baby. That is why it is essential to look after your general health and lead as healthy a lifestyle as possible. Remember that many lifestyle factors have been shown to have a significant impact on sperm genetic health.

If your semen sample shows problems, you will usually be asked to repeat the test to confirm the results. Semen parameters can fluctuate depending on your circumstances, and we need to know whether this is a true reflection of your sperm quality or just a transient problem. Poor semen quality is often a result of several contributing factors. You will be asked about any previous or current medical conditions you may have; any surgery to the lower abdomen or injuries to your testicles; any medication you may be taking; and whether you have any history of sexually transmitted infection or urological symptoms. All of these factors are known to affect fertility.

If you have a medical reason for poor sperm quality, don't make a bad situation worse by having a poor lifestyle. I believe there are always things men can do to improve their sperm quality. While new evidence comes to light every day about male fertility, we do not yet have all the answers as to why your semen parameters may be poor. Generally, it makes sense to try to remove any lifestyle issues that may be contributing to the problem, and screen for infections if appropriate. A sperm test should be repeated three months later. It is understandable that you will think about all your friends or work colleagues who have led the most unhealthy lifestyles but still initiated pregnancies and had bouncing offspring. However, the reality is that each individual has a different

Some Frequently Asked Questions

If I have very poor morphology, does this mean I am more at risk of having an abnormal baby?

This has to be one of the most frequent questions I am asked and men are rightly concerned. The most important message to get across is that morphology is not directly linked to the genetic quality of the sperm, except in rare cases where there may be particular types of sperm defects such as double or enlarged heads, round-headed sperm or sperm with irregular shaped (amorphous) heads. Sperm with cytoplasmic droplets may also have a higher risk of DNA damage.

Is there anything I can do to improve the quality of my sperm?

We know that sperm quality is affected by a multitude of factors, some of which are within your control. Because we know that alcohol, drugs, caffeine, cigarettes and heat exposure can all affect the quality of the sperm, it makes sense to try to address these issues if you have poor sperm quality.

What are sperm antibodies and why do they affect my fertility?

Antibodies are produced by white blood cells as part of the body's natural defence system. Antibodies to sperm may be produced as a result of infection, injury or surgery to the testicles or lower abdomen. Only a small number of men are affected. Antibodies coat the sperm surface and become trapped in the cervix, bringing the sperm with them. If the antibodies coat the sperm head, this may also affect the ability of the sperm to bind to the egg. Having antibodies to sperm is not normal, but their presence does not necessarily interfere with fertility until at least 50 per cent of sperm are coated with them.

tolerance level, and if you and your partner are having problems conceiving, then the studies show that your lifestyle may just be affecting you. Furthermore, there is evidence that some men's lifestyles may lead to subsequent health problems in their children.

A referral to a urologist (doctor specialising in urogenital health) or andrologist (doctor specialising in male reproductive health) for medical investigation should always be made for serious problems with male fertility. You will be given a thorough physical examination, and perhaps an ultrasound scan to look for any obstructions. The doctor may check for hormone imbalances, chromosomal abnormalities or genetic defects. They may also take a closer look at the accessory glands (the seminal vesicles and prostate gland) to see if there is any inflammation that might be affecting your fertility.

Sexual Health Screen

If you have had unprotected sex in the past outside of your current relationship, there is always the possibility that you may be harbouring a sexually transmitted infection, which may or may not have symptoms. Infections are associated with infertility and miscarriage, so the next step is to organise a full sexual health screen through your local genitourinary (GU) clinic. This is a very good start and covers the key infections which can cause fertility delays, although they may not test for all likely infections. Other important tests are for ureaplasma, mycoplasma and gardnerella, microorganisms that can be present in the male and female genital tract. We carried out a small audit at the Zita West Clinic, testing 69 men for these two infections: 20 per cent tested positive for ureaplasma and 27 per cent tested positive for gardnerella. These infections may be symptom-free so you will only know you have one if you are tested for them. They are usually treated with a simple course of antibiotics.

Interview with Dr Sam Dawkins who offers sexual health screening at the Zita West Clinic

Which infections do you test for?

For most people, our testing focuses on the 'silent' infections – those they might have without symptoms. These include chlamydia, ureaplasma, mycoplasma, gardnerella and trichomonas. If the patient is having any urinary symptoms, such as burning or stinging, or any discharge, I would also test for others such as gonorrhoea and herpes. These can all be done with a single urine test. We also test for HIV and hepatitis B/C at the patient's request. It's important to be aware that sexual health screening is cheap and easy – and an untreated infection is likely to have a negative impact on fertility.

Where is the best place to be tested?

NHS sexual health clinics don't focus on fertility. Most of their patients either have a symptom they are worried about or are starting a new relationship and want a sexual health check-up. These clinics tend not to test for ureaplasma or mycoplasma – an important omission as there is evidence that they can both have an impact on fertility and miscarriage rate. Most IVF clinics test for just HIV, hepatitis B and C – they are required by law to do this when storing sperm. At the Zita West Clinic we offer a broad range of testing for our clients in a pleasant setting, using the latest screening techniques. I phone or email the results, depending on the patient's preference.

What happens when a result is positive?

Around 40 per cent of the clients I see have a positive result, usually ureaplasma or gardnerella. Most infections can be treated with a short course of antibiotics, and both partners receive treatment.

Other Tests for Male Fertility

Additional testing may be recommended, depending on your circumstances. If your count is very low, a hormone profile and genetic testing may be suggested.

Male Hormone Profile

Hormonal imbalances are quite rare. If a man's reproductive hormones are too high or too low, it may indicate testicular failure resulting in very low sperm counts. Blood tests may be carried out to look at the levels of follicle stimulating hormone (FSH), luteinising hormone (LH), testosterone and prolactin. Treatment options depend on many factors, such as whether the man is able to produce sperm or not, and, if so, its quantity and quality. A reproductive endocrinologist or urologist will decide what needs to be done. Men with hormone imbalances may be given clomiphene (the same drug that is given to women to stimulate the ovaries) as this can kick-start the testicles to produce testosterone. In more serious cases, other drugs might be used. If the man has severe problems, direct access to the testicles to aspirate sperm may be a solution, such as PESA or TESE (see page 275). If this is unsuccessful, then the man may not be able to father his own genetic child and some couples may consider moving on to sperm donation (see page 460).

Genetic Testing

Inherited chromosome abnormalities may contribute to low or no sperm counts. In these circumstances, genetic screening from a blood sample (karyotype, Y-deletion or cystic fibrosis screening) may be offered. Genetic damage to sperm is not always inherited and can occur at any time during a man's life. To screen for non-inherited genetic defects, the sperm sample needs to be analysed directly for abnormal chromosome numbers (aneuploidy) or for damage to the DNA (DNA fragmentation). Genetic defects are not always associated with poor semen parameters. Because genetically abnormal sperm result in abnormal embryos, genetic testing may also be recommended for couples with recurrent miscarriage or years of unexplained infertility. Unfortunately, inherited abnormalities are untreatable, but depending on your situation, pre-implantation genetic screening may be offered as a fertility treatment option. Recent studies show that antioxidants can be very beneficial in improving levels of DNA fragmentation, but more studies are needed.

Some of the causes for non-inherited genetic damage include:

- Caffeine
- Alcohol
- Smoking
- Age
- Environmental toxins
- Occupational hazards
- Chemotherapy/radiotherapy
- Varicocoele (see Chapter 3)
- Exposure to heat

Tests for Oxidative Stress

This test is available at the Zita West Clinic. Reactive oxygen species (ROS) are free radicals produced by sperm and are very important for sperm function at low levels. ROS are maintained at low levels by effective antioxidant pathways, both within the sperm and in the seminal fluid. However, if the production of ROS overwhelms the capacity of these antioxidant pathways to maintain low ROS levels, then oxidative stress occurs, resulting in sperm membrane damage and DNA fragmentation (see above). The largest source of ROS is white blood cells, produced as a result of infection. ROS damage to the sperm can also be caused by exposure to heat, chemicals, varicocoeles, smoking, alcohol and radiation.

A healthy diet and plenty of antioxidants will help to mop up these free radicals (see Chapter 7).

Coping with Poor Test Results

Receiving a poor sperm test result can be devastating for a man. Many men feel inadequate and at a loss as to how to move forward. When men have problems with their fertility, they often describe feelings such as these:

- 'I feel like such a failure.'
- 'I feel guilty and ashamed.'
- 'I have no one to talk to.'
- 'I don't know how to comfort my partner.'
- 'It's all my fault.'
- 'I can't believe she will have to go through this (IVF) because of me.'

A woman can help by supporting her partner as he comes to terms with his test results. Always remember that you are on the same side, and never nag or use the blame game. This can start to affect your relationship and your ability to have sex. Do not give up on having sex as I have seen men with really poor results still manage to achieve a pregnancy with their partner.

What a Man Can Do

- Communicate as best you can with your partner about how you are feeling and ask for support.
- Take time to think about your relationship and what you feel you need from your partner to help you through these next crucial months.
- Consider discussing things with your GP, a fertility counsellor or a trusted friend.
- Look at your lifestyle and the changes you can make (see Chapter 4).

For more on dealing with the emotional side of fertility problems, see page 224.

On a Positive Note...

For decades, determining a man's fertility relied solely on the results of a sperm count, motility and morphology. Unfortunately, too much emphasis continues to be placed on these parameters, and men have sometimes been told erroneously that they will never father their own biological child if these parameters are very poor. The bottom line is that while many men may be infertile (unable to father a child within two years), very few men are actually sterile. With the advent of ICSI treatment with IVF, as long as there are occasional viable sperm present either in the ejaculate or in the testicles, the majority of these men have a good chance of fathering their own biological child.

Part 4

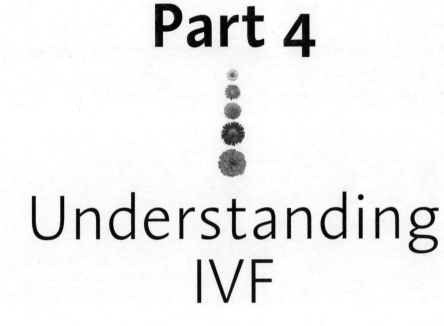

Understanding IVF

Chapter 11

Starting IVF Treatment

One of the questions I am frequently asked is when to start IVF treatment. This is really difficult to answer as it depends on so many factors – age being the main one. Many couples will have spent several years going through investigations and possibly trying other assisted fertility treatments such as ovarian stimulation or IUI (see page 243). Other couples will be 'fast-tracked' to IVF. I would never ever hold anyone back from their plans to do IVF, but sadly this does sometimes happen in the world of complementary medicine, where a therapist may say they want more time and that your body is not ready for IVF. Some women may have time to wait until their body is better balanced, but some women really do not have time to wait and the key thing which determines IVF success is the woman's age. Try and be guided by your clinic doctors.

Once you have decided to begin IVF treatment, there are many practical considerations, but also the emotional ups and downs to deal with. This chapter will help you with the practical decisions, such as how to find a good clinic; questions to ask yourself; and NHS versus private treatment. It provides advice on preparing yourself mentally and physically for the challenging process ahead.

Meeting the Criteria for
IVF Treatment on the NHS

Funding for IVF treatment on the National Health Service varies from region to region across the UK. In 2004, the National Institute for Health and Clinical Excellence (NICE) published guidelines recommending that suitable couples receive up to three cycles of IVF treatment on the NHS. NHS Trusts across England and Wales are now working to provide the same levels of service. As the situation is so varied, your best source of local information will be your own GP or check the NHS or HFEA websites (see Resources).

If you wish to be considered for NHS funding, you need to have a referral from your GP. In some areas, couples have to wait only 18 weeks before free treatment starts, and some NHS clinics have no waiting lists at all. While this is a positive move in so many ways, my concerns are that some couples will proceed to IVF too quickly without giving natural pregnancy a chance or implementing appropriate lifestyle changes (see Chapter 4).

Current guidelines suggest that couples may be eligible for IVF treatment on the NHS if:

- the woman is 23–39 years old at the time of treatment;
- a cause for their fertility treatment has been identified; or
- they have had infertility problems for at least three years.

However, the decision regarding eligibility is made locally, by primary care trusts (PCTs) and priority is given to couples who do not already have children.

Infertility Network UK (INUK), the UK's leading infertility support network, is working with the Department of Health to develop a set of standardised access criteria to help PCTs work towards services which are fair and consistent across the UK. The INUK guidance document is available from their website with explanatory notes. The access criteria endorsed by Department of Health (but not yet applied nationwide) include:

- Failure to conceive after two years of regular unprotected sex
- Woman aged 23–39 years at the time of treatment
- Women should have a BMI of 19–30 (if outside those limits, should be offered advice on diet, exercise and psychosocial support)
- Both partners non-smokers (smokers advised of reduced IVF success and offered help to quit)
- There is uncertainty about the effectiveness of IVF beyond the third cycle, so previous IVF, whether self- or NHS-funded, should be taken into account
- Issues where one partner already has a child
- No NHS funding if either partner previously sterilised

The 'IVF post-code lottery' has been on the political agenda for a long time, and although there has been some really positive progress, and in some areas NHS provision is very good, there is still a long way to go to achieve equitable service provision. The whole issue of funding for IVF can put a huge strain on a couple at a time when they are already struggling with the physical and emotional demands of their fertility problems. Many couples are unable to afford to pay for private treatment. A young woman (26) came to see me in tears because her tubes were blocked and she was desperate to start a family early – it was all she had ever wanted to do. However, she still had to wait until she was 30 to be able to access IVF on the NHS in her part of the country.

I asked Clare Lewis-Jones, Chief Executive of INUK, for her comments on the progress of this initiative to standardise access to NHS funding for IVF:

'It is totally unacceptable and unethical that it still depends on where you live as to whether you can access NHS funding for the treatment you need in order to have a family. Infertility is an illness, a disease, for which there are many treatments available. Our work with PCTs has proved valuable to them and it is no coincidence that funding has improved significantly over the last couple of years. However, we are not there yet and will not cease our campaigning nor our collaborative work with PCTs until we have a fully NHS funded service for fertility treatment. It is vital that PCTs move quickly to implementing the full NICE fertility guideline, before time runs out for many couples.'

Many fertility clinics see both NHS and private clients. Couples may choose to have private treatment for a variety of reasons. Many couples do this to avoid having to wait, especially if they are in their 30s. Others might choose to go to a more specialist centre if they have complicated histories or have already had unsuccessful IVF cycles. In most cases, couples accessing IVF treatment through their GP will be referred to an assisted conception unit. They will be sent an information pack which will contain forms for them to complete about their history.

Some people may find it harder than others to access treatment. Historically it has been harder for gay and lesbian couples to access fertility treatment, but over the last few years more clinics are treating male and female same-sex couples and the law around supportive parenting has also changed to give equal rights to same-sex couples. Some clinics will not treat anyone who is positive for HIV, hepatitis B or hepatitis C. All couples going through IVF are screened to assess the risk of contamination. If you are found to be positive, there are only a few clinics that have the appropriate laboratory storage facilities so your clinic choice may be restricted.

Choosing a Clinic

The Human Fertilisation and Embryology Authority (HFEA) regulates all clinics carrying out IVF and other assisted fertility treatments, under the Human Fertilisation and Embryology Act of 1990. Clinics must have an HFEA licence in order to store gametes (egg and sperm), create embryos or perform any form of assisted conception, or pre-implantation screening (see Chapter 12 for more information on these techniques). The HFEA website (www.hfea.gov.uk) provides very comprehensive information on all aspects of assisted fertility and a search facility to choose a clinic.

IVF forums and chat rooms, such as Fertility Friends, Infertility Network UK and IVF Connections, can help you find out about other people's experiences. I believe you should really do your research before embarking on IVF, especially if you are paying for your own treatment.

It is a good idea to attend open evenings at one or more clinics. This will give you a feel of the place and enable you to find out if it meets your individual needs. Generally, couples taking their first steps on the IVF route are a bit vague in terms of their expectations. Many of my clients say to me, 'If only I had known then what I know now.' At the Zita West Clinic we asked 100 women how they chose their clinic.

Satellite Clinics

Many large IVF clinics have links with individual doctors or affiliations with smaller fertility clinics. These 'satellite clinics' will usually monitor the woman's cycle, with scans and blood tests and then at the appropriate time the couple go to the main IVF unit with laboratory facilities for creating embryos. The egg collection, and embryo transfer, is performed at the main IVF centre.

Their approaches included:

- following the recommendation of their doctor or our clinic
- asking friends who had been through IVF
- viewing the HFEA website
- searching the internet

Zita's Top Tips on Choosing a Clinic

If you are doing an NHS cycle, then your choice of clinic is likely to be limited, but rest assured there are many very good NHS clinics offering increasingly good services. If you are paying for your treatment privately, then you can choose your clinic carefully and even visit more than one clinic or get a second opinion. The choice will be yours, but sometimes having seemingly endless options can feel overwhelming.

Consider its Location

It is more practical and less stressful to visit a local clinic. Think about how much time and money you are able to spend travelling there and back. However, if you have had several unsuccessful IVF cycles, you may want to spread your wings and try another clinic further afield. If you opt for a clinic further away, you may be able to have your scans and blood tests at a more local satellite clinic (see Chapter 14).

You Cannot Compare Like for Like

Look for a clinic that has the expertise to deal with your particular problem. For example, check out clinics that are used to dealing with older women, or that cater for those who have had previous unsuccessful IVF cycles.

If You Are on Your Fourth or Fifth IVF Cycle...

Think about what your next steps are going to be. Sometimes I advise couples in this situation to have initial consultations at two separate clinics. You need to find out what your next clinic can do for you that is different from the previous one. After the consultation you should feel you have been listened to and that your situation is understood.

We asked women at the Zita West Clinic if there was anything, in hindsight, they would do differently going through an IVF cycle. Many said they would have:

- had acupuncture earlier in order to de-stress in the month leading up to IVF
- rested a bit more
- asked more questions
- done more research
- paid a few hundred pounds for private blood tests as these took about 10 months on the NHS
- given more consideration to their emotional and psychological needs
- not proceeded unless they felt 100 per cent healthy
- budgeted better
- gone to another clinic
- started sooner
- lost weight
- taken more time off work
- gone to counselling earlier
- done a bit less travelling

Find out How Much Treatment Costs

The HFEA does not regulate treatment costs, so they can vary significantly from clinic to clinic. More expensive treatment doesn't necessarily increase your chances of success. Clinics will explain their charges upfront but ask about 'hidden costs', such as extra tests that may be needed, and ensure you have budgeted for all possibilities (see also page 296).

If You Are Unhappy, Move

Don't feel you have to stay at a clinic if you are unhappy. So many of my clients feel they have to stay where they are because the clinic has their frozen embryos or sperm. However, most clinics are happy to help you transfer frozen gametes and embryos. The logistics are not that overwhelming.

Use the Internet

Message boards and IVF chat rooms can be invaluable. Log on if you can and look up different women's experiences, and even chat to them on line.

IVF Success Rates

It is difficult to choose a clinic on its success rates because they are based on many factors. For example, older women have a lower success rate than younger women. Success rates vary up and down the UK. Be careful not to confuse success rates with your chances of conception. Clinics believe that success is based on looking at couples as individuals, not treating them on a one-size-fits-all basis.

The HFEA website provides information on success rates of clinics (www.hfea.gov.uk). All clinics are obliged to give you their statistics based on the data gathered from the clients they have treated. Please

IVF works best for:

- Women under 35
- Women who have had no previous IVF treatment or a previous success
- Women who have had a previous spontaneous pregnancy
- Women with a body mass index (BMI) of below 30

IVF is more difficult for:

- Women over 35
- Women who have had several attempts at IVF
- Women who have had no previous pregnancies
- Women with a BMI of above 30
- Women with severe endometriosis
- Couples who have been trying for five years or more

I don't want anyone to read the above and think IVF is not going to work for them. There are many factors involved in IVF and there is a lot that can be done to help it succeed (see Chapter 12).

note that the pregnancy rate is very different from the live birth rate. A live birth rate is also called the 'take home baby' rate.

Interview with Debra Bloor, Head of Inspection, Compliance, Human Fertilisation and Embryology Authority (HFEA)

How does the HFEA monitor the standards of fertility clinics?
The HFEA inspects clinics on a regular basis to ensure they meet the standards set out in our Code of Practice. Fertility clinics can't operate in the UK without an HFEA licence which ensures that they are able to

deliver a safe, high quality service for patients. This is a compliant sector with clinics working hard to continually improve their practice. Incidents are rare. In 2008–9, eight major incidents were reported out of over 52,000 cycles of fertility treatment. When incidents do happen, however, we work closely with the clinic involved to learn from the incident and to try and ensure it does not happen again.

The Cost of IVF

About 25 per cent of IVF treatments in the UK are funded by the NHS but, as we have already discussed, there are still gaps in NHS service provision for IVF. Where couples are paying for their treatment, IVF is usually offered as a standard package. This can include a consultation with a doctor, ultrasound scanning, blood tests, egg collection, sperm preparation, laboratory work and embryo transfer. It may also include a pregnancy scan and a free follow-up review, but it generally does not include the price of drugs. At the time of writing, the standard cost of such a package is £3,500 upwards, but it could be considerably more and can vary in terms of what is included. Sometimes more blood tests and scans will be required and, as a result, the costs will increase. If it is not an all-inclusive package, make sure you get a fully costed treatment plan ahead of your treatment. You will also have to pay a small HFEA fee.

If you are paying for your treatment, it is essential to have a clear idea of your budget as the costs can spiral out of control. I often ask couples how they are going to fund their treatment. Many do it using their credit cards, which I find worrying, and some will say they don't even think about the money they are spending, because if they did they wouldn't sleep at night. Others use their savings or have help from family members. I have seen couples who have been trying for six to ten years and have spent up to £60,000 on IVF.

The Initial Consultation

Once you decide to have IVF treatment and have chosen your clinic, the next step is to visit the clinic for an initial consultation. Many couples who go along for this expect to come away feeling absolutely fantastic. Without a doubt some do, but others leave feeling very disappointed. I see it from both sides, and I have sat in on consultations at IVF clinics. No matter which clinic you attend there is an awful lot of paperwork that has to be completed before even getting into a consultation. The doctor then focuses on the medical side to be able to assess the type of treatment that is beneficial to you. Predictably, it is often hard to cover emotional and psychological factors as well, such as how anxious you may be feeling about starting IVF treatment. That is why a holistic approach is so important.

Consent Issues

In the initial consultation, you will be asked to sign lots of consent forms. This is standard practice and includes consent forms for your treatment; consent to disclose information; consent to the use and storage of sperm, eggs and embryos; and consent to parenthood. The clinic also has to consider the welfare of any child born as a result of the assisted fertility treatment – this includes the child's right for supportive parenting and to ensure that the child would not be at risk of significant harm or neglect. A centre has the right to refuse treatment in certain circumstances, in which case the couple are notified in writing including how the centre might reconsider its decision.

In signing consent for the use of egg and sperm and the creation of embryos, you will need to think about issues such as the legal situation in the event of your death, or if in the future you are no longer able to give consent for some reason for the use of your gametes (eggs or sperm) or embryos. You will both have to decide if you want to have the embryos frozen and stored for future use, or to donate them for medical research. You may find the legal aspects rather overwhelming. For more information see the HFEA website (www.hfea.gov.uk).

Your Medical History

Your medical history is looked at, especially if this is your first IVF cycle, and any further tests that you may need are arranged. If applicable, it may be useful to take any results you have from previous IVF cycles. You will be asked about past medical events, such as if you have ever had a pregnancy, and any medical conditions such as thyroid problems, high blood pressure, diabetes, epilepsy, or anything else that might be affecting your ability to conceive. Your doctor will ask you if you have had any pelvic infections and if you have been on any long-term medication.

An ultrasound scan is always done to check for any abnormalities such as cysts and fibroids, and to see if any further investigations may be needed. This is usually a trans-vaginal scan (TVS) where a probe is put into the vagina (see page 261). Blood tests will be done to look at the menstrual cycle and to measure hormonal levels (see 'The AMH Test', page 300, and page 48). The man will be asked to produce semen for analysis. You will also be asked to be screened for hepatitis B, hepatitis C and HIV. These tests are valid for one year so you shouldn't have to repeat them. If you are found to be positive for any of these, especially HIV, you may not be able to receive treatment at your chosen clinic (see page 291).

Once the initial results come back the doctors will review them and formulate a plan of action. They will decide which drug regime suits you and which protocol to put you on (see Chapter 12). Whether you use IVF or ICSI (see page 336) will depend on what the semen analysis is like on the day the eggs are collected. If the sperm is poor at the initial consultation then a repeat sample may be required.

Baseline Tests for Ovarian Reserve: FSH, AMH and Antral Follicle Count

There are two key hormones which IVF doctors look at, along with your chronological age, when assessing your suitability for IVF: FSH and AMH. The AMH test is a relatively new test and is not used by all clinics. Some clinics may also use antral follicle count to help decide the most suitable IVF protocol.

The FSH Test

Almost all clinics will use the FSH test as a predictor of IVF response. The FSH level increases with age as the egg follicles are becoming less responsive in the years leading up to the menopause. The FSH is trying to get the response from the ovaries so the higher the FSH level, the more it is a sign that your ovaries are struggling to respond (getting deafer to the message). It is not quite as simple as just measuring the FSH, it is really about the relationship between FSH and oestradiol (a form of oestrogen) levels. At times the FSH may be relatively low, but the oestradiol is too high – so essentially the high oestradiol level has convinced the FSH it can turn down its production. This can occur, for example, if there is an ovarian cyst which would be producing an excess of oestrogen and this would confuse the picture. Sometimes the high oestradiol itself indicates a problem with egg reserve. (Ideally the oestradiol should be below 150 pmol/l.) There is often so much focus on the idea of 'getting your FSH down' that the whole concept of this hormonal dance is lost – so essentially it is about having your FSH and oestradiol in balance.

An FSH test is done between Days 1 and 4 of your period. If your level is less than 10, you can generally expect a good response (the lower the better). If your FSH level is over 20, the response is likely to be very poor. As ever, individual clinics will have differing figures and success rates. Some clinics will not treat women with an FSH level above a certain number (often 10) and may wait for the level to settle. Although some IVF doctors feel this is of benefit and may achieve good success rates by waiting; other doctors feel there is no proven benefit to waiting for the perfect 10.

Indeed, some clinics specialise in the treatment of women with reduced ovarian reserve and have much higher FSH cut-offs. Generally it is regarded that your ovarian reserve is only as good as your 'worst FSH', so if your FSH level is swinging around a bit – say, as high as 18 one cycle, and then drops to 9.5 – you would be treated as if you have ovarian reserve issues as you would be expected to respond and have the chances of success related to the higher reading. Rest assured that some of the clinics that specialise in older women and egg reserve issues can achieve some good results when confronted by some of these more challenging situations.

The AMH Test

Anti-mullerian hormone (AMH) is produced by the small resting (antral) follicles in the ovaries, so the AMH level correlates strongly with the number of antral follicles (the egg reserve). AMH cannot measure the actual number or the quality of the eggs. The introduction of the AMH test over the last few years has helped doctors decide how well women will respond to IVF treatment. Although it does not provide any information on the quality of the eggs, it gives a very good indication of how well a woman is likely to respond to IVF drugs and how many eggs she is likely to produce. The test is measured in numbers from 0–45 pmol/l: the higher the number the better.

Although this test is not available in every IVF clinic, more and more clinics are starting to use it. Women with lower AMH levels and antral follicular counts produce significantly fewer eggs compared with women with higher levels.

The AMH test may not be accurate for women with polycystic ovaries. Due to a hormone imbalance, women with PCOS have two to three times the number of antral follicles. This is reflected in higher AMH levels.

It can be very difficult to come to terms with a low AMH level and there is very clear research showing a poor response to ovarian stimulation. However, laboratory tests are there to give guidelines and I have seen women with very low AMH levels get pregnant – both naturally and also with IVF – so it is not always the be-all and end-all.

Facts about AMH

- The AMH test can be done on any day of the cycle.
- The AMH test can be used alongside an antral follicle count done by ultrasound (see below and page 49).
- Some IVF clinics require an AMH level above a certain limit to do IVF.
- Many clinics are now using AMH as an indicator rather than the standard Day 1–3 FSH test (see page 299) because you can have a normal FSH reading but still have a low AMH.

Antral Follicle Count

Antral follicles are small follicles about 2–8mm diameter which can be seen, measured and counted on ultrasound. These are often referred to as 'resting' follicles. It is presumed that the number of antral follicles that are visible on ultrasound gives an indication of the relative number of microscopic (sound asleep) primordial follicles remaining in the ovary. Each primordial follicle contains an immature egg and could potentially develop in the future. So the antral follicle count (AFC) is a representation of the number of eggs left – not an absolute number.

The number of antral (resting) follicles will depend largely on the woman's chronological age and also her 'ovarian age'. There is a correlation between AFC and IVF success. The AFC generally gives a good prediction of the number of mature follicles expected following ovarian stimulation, and IVF success correlates strongly with the number of eggs collected. A woman who has an average or high number of antral follicles will tend to get a good response to IVF stimulation and therefore a high chance of pregnancy. A woman with very few antral follicles will generally get a poorer response to ovarian stimulation with few mature follicles, so a low pregnancy rate and a high chance of a cancelled cycle due to poor response will be anticipated. The image on page 404 shows this clearly.

As ever, chronological age still plays a key part, so younger women will tend to have a higher pregnancy rate, even if they have a low AFC, whereas the pregnancy rate may not be good for women over 35 who have few antral follicles. Women with a very high AFC may have polycystic ovaries, or they may respond in a similar fashion – being ultra-sensitive to the drugs and so at risk of ovarian hyperstimulation syndrome (see page 371). The highest chance of a successful pregnancy following IVF is for women with an AFC of more than 15, but even women with counts of around 2 may still be able to achieve successful pregnancies.

A woman's age, AFC, and often blood levels of hormones such as FSH and AMH, will influence the doctor's choice of drug regime, dosage and IVF protocol.

Common Questions

I have asked many nurses in IVF clinics what are the most common questions that couples ask at the initial consultation. Two seem to come out on top:

1. 'Will it work?' This is the most common question of all. However, this is very difficult to answer as nobody can guarantee a pregnancy or a baby.
2. 'How often do I have to come here?' The number of times you attend a clinic will depend on that clinic's protocol for monitoring with scans and blood tests. You may find that a satellite clinic will do a lot of the monitoring (see page 291), but you will go to a main IVF centre for the egg collection and embryo transfer.

At the initial consultation you can discuss when you can start treatment. Having taken a while to get to this stage, many women are often really surprised by how soon they can start treatment. Depending on where you are in your menstrual cycle, there may be situations where you can start almost immediately and some couples are not ready for this.

Zita's Top Tips on the Initial Consultation

Think About What You Want from the Consultation

It is worth familiarising yourself with, and understanding, the names and terms that will be used. Make a list of the questions you want to ask. Look through the clinic's website and information brochure before your consultation. If there is anything you don't understand, make a note and then get clarification at the time of your visit. Ask who you need to contact if you have questions, whether there is an email address you could have or a contact number for emergencies.

Take Control of the Situation

Many couples we see hand over the complete control of their fertility to the IVF clinic once they get there. While this is helpful to a certain extent, and it is essential to trust the clinic team, it is worth trying to maintain some influence. It is a combination of letting go at one level, knowing that you are doing as much as you can to make this work – just going with the flow – while at the same time maintaining an understanding of the challenges imposed along the way. This is where a supportive partner can really help, if he has an understanding of all the different stages and what to expect. You can then relinquish some of the control. You both need to have a certain level of knowledge about your situation so that you can ask relevant questions. I realise this is more difficult when you are going through the process for the first time. Doctors have told me that they like to work with well-informed and motivated clients and you will get more out of a consultation.

Tell the Clinic if You Are Unhappy

If you are unhappy with any aspect of the initial consultation, tell the doctor, one of the nurses or the clinic manager about it. If you don't communicate how you feel, they cannot help you. Many clients worry that if they complain about the service it will affect their treatment; this is not the case at all.

Go with Your Partner

It will be difficult to remember everything that is said during the consultation. You will be given an awful lot of information in those early days. Having your partner there will help you remember as much as possible and to question areas of uncertainty.

Tell the Doctor if You Have Any Concerns

If you have any specific fears or anxieties about treatment or how you are as an individual, tell the doctor. For example, your doctor should know if you have a fear of needles, if you are anxious about internal examinations or if you are worried about a general anaesthetic or sedation.

Questions to Ask at the Initial Consultation

- What are the chances of success with this treatment?
- How does this compare with our chances of natural conception (or other treatments)?
- Are there any short- or longer-term risks associated with the IVF procedures or the drugs used?
- Are there any risks to the baby associated with the proposed techniques?
- What is the time commitment involved?
- Is the clinic open at weekends?
- Do you have set days for egg collection and embryo transfer?
- Are there likely to be any extra costs?
- What if this treatment is unsuccessful?
- If the IVF is unsuccessful, how long will it be before a review takes place?
- How many older women do you treat and how many have gone on successfully to have babies?

After your consultation, whether this is your first consultation, or a review, you and your partner will want to discuss your feelings about the proposed treatment. Consider the following:

- Does the treatment feel appropriate for you?
- Any risks to your physical or psychological health.
- The impact on your relationship and any ways to cope with this.

- Whether you have any religious or ethical concerns about the treatment plan.
- Whether anything has changed since your last cycle (if you have had a previous cycle).
- Whether you feel confident with the clinic and the staff.
- Whether you ask for a second opinion at another clinic.
- See a fertility counsellor to help you look at all options.
- Not having this treatment or discontinuing treatment altogether.

As always with decision-making, it is a good idea to write down why you are choosing to go down the proposed route as you are unlikely to remember why you made the decision if you look back later on.

The Emotional Roller Coaster Ride

Once you have started an IVF cycle, you will probably feel optimistic and excited, especially if this is your first attempt. If it is, say, your fourth attempt, however, you are more likely to feel negative about the whole situation. It is easier to deal with IVF if you understand what is happening and are aware of the hurdles and pitfalls you may face.

There is a difference between positive encouragement and being given false hope, such as about the likely success of a treatment. You need to sit down and have a rational discussion with a specialist to consider your realistic chances of success based on your specific situation and the clinic's statistics. This will help you decide whether you want to put yourself through a process that may have a very low chance of success.

If you decide to go ahead with a treatment with a very low success rate, let's say 5 per cent, it helps to believe that you will be one of those five women in a hundred who will have a baby – and why shouldn't you? Women often say that they don't dare to feel positive because if the cycle fails they will have 'further to fall'. You will be hurt however far you fall, so not daring to feel positive can only give you the sense that maybe you somehow didn't give it your best shot, and that you were holding back on some level. So once your decision is made rationally (and you have both discussed the realistic chances) just go for it – believe in yourself and you can do it! Men can help by encouraging their partner to stay positive.

Women start IVF in all sorts of different emotional states. I am a big believer in managing your mindset to get through IVF; this takes time and practice but is well worth the effort. If a woman has a very busy life then she must consider making time for herself to go through IVF, otherwise she can end up angry and frustrated. Everything becomes a crisis and she can be a nightmare to be around. There are many underlying reasons for this. Some women I see simply don't want to be doing IVF so they fight it every step of the way. A much better approach is to schedule in time for yourself; perhaps reduce your workload or even consider taking unpaid leave, if at all feasible. I am not suggesting that every woman who reads this book gives up work (that can often be the worst scenario), but do look at ways of making sure you manage your mental and emotional wellbeing. The key is to feel as relaxed as possible about the whole process, to be flexible, accepting and go with the flow, and some research shows that women who are able to let go have higher success rates.

Although I believe in preparing your body and mind for IVF for at least three months if possible (see Part 2), I am also a realist. If you have had many cycles, you can feel as if your life is on hold, dominated by the whole business of IVF. My advice to such couples is to try and lead a fulfilling life between cycles, to relax and enjoy themselves.

Some women who go through IVF spend a lot of time getting stressed and anxious throughout the whole process. They are angry with themselves or their partner for having to go through IVF, and they tend to focus their anger on everyone and everything around them.

Case Study

Louise, aged 40, had recently lost her parents and was quite devastated by this. She was also newly married but, because of her age, was anxious about the fact that she hadn't got pregnant immediately. She thought she might have missed the boat. Her blood tests were very good and her AMH (see pages 48, 300) was good for her age, but despite this she still ended up having to go down the IVF route, and this made her very frustrated and angry. She found she was venting all her negativity on the people around her: on the nurses and doctors at the clinic, her partner and everybody she came into contact with.

It was easy to see that the root of her frustration was the fact that she was having IVF when she always thought she would conceive naturally. She was also in a high-powered job and permanently attached to her PDA. Louise was resisting IVF at every level, virtually kicking and screaming inside, fighting the thought and the process. She was also frightened by the prospect of the IVF not working for her, and busy thinking about what she was going to do next if it didn't work before giving it a chance. I thought she was creating blocks and obstacles for herself at every single step of the way. She was using up so much energy worrying and trying to second-guess what was going to happen next with the treatment. She also admitted to feeling out of control. Her partner told me she could become so angry and frustrated that they were arguing more than ever before.

I challenged her on her feelings and explained why I thought she felt the way she did. I am a great believer in affirmation: when your mind believes it can conceive, your body will follow. Louise's problem was that she didn't believe she could conceive. Her main emotion was anger – she was looking for fights with everyone she met along the way, which wasn't benefiting her on any level. She agreed to do some specific work on managing her mind to help her get through the IVF process. I wanted her to learn to go with the flow and to be flexible. For example, she needed to understand that although a scan appointment might be booked for 8am, she might not be seen until 9am or later. She learnt techniques she could use to disassociate herself from her negativity when she was actually in the clinic so that she would avoid getting stressed and angry.

Here are some of the negative thoughts that many couples experience while going through fertility treatment and IVF:

- 'Why is this happening to me? I don't deserve it.'
- 'We are letting everybody down.'
- 'What if it never happens to me?'
- 'I hate everything being so clinical and I am fed up with being prodded and probed.'
- 'All of these investigations, tests and results have left me feeling battered.'
- 'I no longer feel feminine or attractive.'
- 'My moods sometimes really scare me because I am so unpredictable in the way I am thinking. I'm irrational.'

Zita's Top Tips for Coping with IVF

Make Sure You Are in this Together

Men and women tend to approach IVF differently. As I said earlier, when a woman decides she is going to have IVF, she is likely to commit to it fully. Within a week, she will know 20 times more than her partner about the process. However, it is important to be there for each other at this time. It is worth sitting down and spending some time talking about how you are both feeling.

Prepare Your Mind for IVF

You will benefit from preparing yourself mentally and emotionally for IVF. See Chapter 5 for tips on preparing your mind and for stress-reduction techniques. Understanding the IVF process will also be of great value.

Manage Your Time

This is so difficult when you are working. I see how stressed women can get because they already have so many demands on their time, and an IVF appointment in their busy schedule adds extra pressure. When you can, try and find ways of reducing those demands. Manage your partner's time carefully as well: don't expect him to attend absolutely every scan appointment with you.

Allow for Some Setbacks

Things don't always go smoothly. There will be times when you don't have a good scan or your blood test is not as it should be. All of these things and more can make you highly anxious. Very often these anxieties can be resolved with a good night's sleep.

Optimise Your Nutrition

Make sure you are getting all the nutrients you need to help you cope well with the IVF process, both mentally and physically (see

At the Zita West Clinic, we asked men and women about their experiences of IVF. Here are some of their responses.

What Men Say about Women Going through IVF:
- 'She talks about IVF all the time, never anything else.'
- 'The whole focus of our relationship has become IVF.'
- 'She blows the tiniest things out of proportion.'
- 'I don't know what to say, and when I do say anything it's wrong.'
- 'I can't reach her.'
- 'She is constantly on internet chat rooms.'
- 'It's not that I'm not interested in what she's going through, it's just that she's far more advanced in this whole area than I can ever be.'
- 'I hate the business of her having to go through all this and me doing nothing. It makes me feel really bad.'
- 'I try not to get irritated but she pushes me to the limit.'
- 'We just chug along together but are not connecting.'
- 'I hate the quiet, sulky moods on a daily basis. She lashes out for the littlest thing – if I am late home or want to go and play football or do something else, it doesn't fit in.'

What Women Say They Want Their Men to Do:
- 'I need him to be there for me, even if he doesn't understand my emotions or what's going on.'
- 'I need more cuddles.'
- 'I want him to be patient about me going over the same thing again and again.'
- 'I don't want him to push me away or get ratty with me.'
- 'I need him to understand that every part of the process I've been through is important, and that I have real up and down days.'

- 'I need to feel special.'
- 'I'd like him to do little things like empty the dishwasher.'
- 'I need him to encourage me to rest.'
- 'I want him to tell me it will all be fine.'

Please remember that you are both on the same side.

Chapter 7). Try to ensure you are within the optimal BMI range – so lose or gain weight if needed.

Fertility Counselling (by Jane Knight, Fertility Counsellor)

Fertility counselling is a process through which individuals and couples have the opportunity to explore their thoughts, feelings and beliefs in order to come to a greater understanding of themselves and their situation. It also provides support and can help you to clarify your life goals.

If you are going through assisted fertility treatment, then your licensed IVF clinic must offer you access to counselling in line with the HFEA Code of Practice. Many couples are put off counselling as they feel they don't have a problem. However, it can be useful to talk things through at any stage, from first discovering difficulties in conceiving to IVF and beyond. It is common for couples going through assisted conception to feel that their private life has been invaded. The intimacy is lost – what was once a private and special part of your relationship has suddenly become public; you are being told when to have sex by a complete stranger. If you are having a monitored cycle or a fertility drug such as clomiphene, it is likely that the ultrasonographer will be the one who dictates when you should have sex – spontaneity is out of the window. If you need to move on to IUI (see page 243), things suddenly take another turn; you need to schedule things around producing the sperm sample at the optimum time. This in itself causes pressures for many men. Many couples report that this loss of intimacy places huge pressure on their relationship. Fertility support counselling can help you to discuss some of these issues and find new ways to manage your situation if this is creating tension.

There are so many decisions to be made throughout IVF – from choosing the right clinic to considering how many embryos to have put back. For couples who are lucky enough to have embryos of good quality to freeze, it can be hard to make the decision to have the embryos put back, particularly if this is your last remaining chance of pregnancy. While the embryos are still in the freezer, it can seem as if time and hope are frozen. Going for that last cycle or using the frozen embryos can feel very frightening as it may mean facing the devastating reality of failure yet again.

Do take up the offer of fertility counselling, even if you feel you are coping. So many people think that they won't go for counselling because 'it's not that bad'. You don't have to be at crisis point to feel the value of a counselling session. In many ways it is preferable to get some support at an earlier stage, rather than wait for things to get really bad.

Fear of IVF

Fear can be a crippling emotion – it is probably the most powerful emotion of all – and a normal emotional response to a perceived threat. Women have many fears associated with IVF. These include:

- Going through the IVF process
- The drugs they will be putting into their systems

- The amount of time they have to take off from work for scans and other investigations
- Giving themselves injections
- The emotional roller coaster

The overriding fear for most women around the whole issue of fertility is fear that it won't work and it is this uncertainty that is a major cause of anxiety and worry. So the combination of fear and anxiety can be even more difficult to manage. Do not allow the uncertainty to paralyse you – if there is something that you can usefully do to change something then do it, but otherwise accept that you are doing as much as you can and distract yourself.

Most of the women we see tell us that the thought of doing IVF is always much worse than actually doing it. As with everything, once you have started IVF and you understand more of what is going on, it's never as bad as you imagined. The drugs used now are very pure, and doctors will use fewer rather than more whenever possible.

When you are going through IVF in a busy clinic, there will be times where there is a breakdown in communication. If you don't understand the process or what is going on, you can feel isolated, irritated and anxious, causing stress hormones to surge through the body. Please communicate with the clinic staff – they are not against you; they do want to help you. If you don't feel you are coping well ask for help talking it through. You must also learn to adapt and be flexible, as IVF clinics are very busy places. Many clients tell me they are too nervous to say anything to the staff in case it affects their IVF. That is not the case: the nurses and doctors are there to help you, but you must be able to deal with the highs and lows of the IVF cycle, which I promise you will be present. The way you deal with these emotions will make a big difference to how you will feel when you finally come to the end of the cycle.

I honestly believe that if you are mentally, emotionally and psychologically prepared, you will be better equipped when going through IVF. A positive attitude is important. Learning stress management techniques that you can practise will help you enormously (see Chapter 5).

Preparing for IVF

How you prepare for IVF will depend on how many times you have been through the procedure. Preparation for IVF means looking at your life physically, mentally and emotionally. We use four key areas at the Zita West Clinic. Remember that you are laying down a foundation for the best possible eggs and sperm to be produced, and also ensuring that when you do get pregnant your body's nutritional stores can support the developing foetus.

Step One: Your Diet

- Begin with getting rid of bad habits in your diet (see Chapter 7).
- Try to cut out alcohol for four to six weeks before starting IVF.
- Avoid alcohol completely when going through IVF.
- Take a multi-vitamin and mineral supplement containing folic acid.
- Remember to drink plenty of water.

Step Two: Exercise

You can continue to exercise prior to IVF. Exercise increases blood flow to the organs, including the womb. It releases endorphins, improving your mood, making you feel in control and reducing stress. I am a great believer in doing some exercise you enjoy in the lead-up to IVF but you need to strike the correct balance. Walking, jogging, cycling, Pilates, certain types of yoga and swimming are all excellent forms of exercise and will help with your fitness levels. However, if you are doing intensive aerobic exercise – up to 10 hours a week – it may adversely affect your hormones. During an IVF cycle, I don't believe women should exercise, and advise gentle walking only.

Step Three: Your Mindset

Before you start IVF, spend some time looking at your relationship. Are there any areas of stress? It is useful to deal with these before IVF as the treatment is likely to magnify any difficulties. A mind workout (see Chapter 5) can be beneficial for both partners before treatment begins.

Step Four: Acupuncture

Having acupuncture in the lead-up to IVF can be very beneficial. For more information on this and other complementary therapies, see Chapter 8.

Preparing for IVF means sorting out the logistics – the practical stuff – and feeling good and positive. You will slip up occasionally, perhaps by having a glass of wine, but that is okay. Don't beat yourself up about this as it's important for you to feel as relaxed as possible before treatment begins. You will now have done everything in your power to help make it a success.

Chapter 12

The IVF Process

This chapter takes you through each stage of the in-vitro fertilisation (IVF) process: the drugs used to stimulate the development of multiple follicles; egg collection; sperm preparation; the creation of embryos and embryo transfer. Having a clear idea of what is happening at every stage will help you deal positively with the process. It is also important to look after yourself while going through IVF, so there are tips on relaxation and coping strategies including tips for coping with the two-week wait to see if you are pregnant.

The main aim of an IVF cycle is to create enough good-quality embryos to be able to transfer one or two embryos during the IVF cycle and hopefully to be able to freeze any additional embryos for future use. In order to do this, the ovaries are stimulated by a range of different drugs to create as many eggs (oocytes) as can be produced safely. A woman is monitored closely during this process with scans and often blood tests to ensure her ovaries are responding appropriately, while minimising any risk to her health.

Essentially, there are five key steps to IVF:

1. Ovarian stimulation
2. Egg collection
3. Sperm collection and preparation
4. Fertilisation by IVF or ICSI to create embryos
5. Embryo transfer

Before an IVF cycle starts, a decision has to be made about the right protocol for the individual woman. It is not just about getting eggs, but using the right combination of drugs to produce good-quality, mature eggs that will make good-quality embryos. The assessment is made prior to the IVF cycle by checking baseline hormone levels of FSH, LH and oestradiol between Days 1–4 of the cycle. An AMH level and antral follicle count may also be done to see how you are likely to respond to the ovarian stimulation. Not all clinics will do all of these tests – this can be quite varied. The choice of protocol and drug dosages will also be decided based on your age and how you may have responded in any previous IVF cycles. Women with polcys- tic ovaries tend to respond excessively to ovarian stimulation, so this is also taken into consideration and careful monitoring is required.

When you are told which protocol (drug regime) you will be on, you will also be told about the required monitoring by ultrasound scans and blood tests to see how you are responding to the drugs. You will be monitored from the start of any drugs. Some women will require drugs for a week or two to shut down (down-regulate) their normal menstrual cycle first before they can start ovarian stimulation – known as **a long protocol**; whereas other women will be able to start the stimulation phase without prior suppression – **a short proto- col,** so the overall length of an IVF cycle will vary.

The aims of the drugs given in an IVF protocol are to:

- 'Down-regulate' or suppress your menstrual cycle (if needed)
- Stimulate the growth of follicles containing eggs (while at the same time preventing a natural LH surge and premature ovulation)
- Trigger the maturation of eggs in preparation for egg collection
- Build up the womb lining

The hormones used in an IVF cycle actually mimic what happens hormonally in a woman's normal menstrual cycle, but with IVF

Time-line Comparing a Normal Menstrual Cycle with an IVF Cycle

Time-line	Normal menstrual cycle	IVF cycle
Day 21 of menstrual cycle (luteal phase). [Some women on contraceptive pill to schedule IVF cycle.]	The corpus luteum is producing progesterone to build up the endometrium and sustain a pregnancy. It is possible for pregnancy to occur at this time prior to the start of IVF stimulation.	**Start of the 'Long Protocol'** **The down-regulation phase** Lasts about 10–14 days. An LHRH agonist e.g. buserelin (nasal spray) suppresses pituitary production of FSH and LH to shut down the normal menstrual cycle, prevent spontaneous ovulation, and thin the endometrium. A 'short protocol' omits this stage and starts with ovarian stimulation (see below).
Day 1	Start of period.	Start of period – inform the clinic to book scan.
Day 3–4 of cycle	The endometrium (womb lining) is shed during the period. A pool of over 20 immature eggs in each ovary is ready to be stimulated. Very low oestrogen levels so there is a sensation of dryness with no cervical secretions.	**'Baseline Scan' and Blood Test** To assess ovaries are ready to be stimulated. Monitors effect of down-regulation drugs. Scan shows inactive ovaries, no cysts and a thin endometrium. Oestradiol levels are low. A FSH blood test may be used to determine whether it is a good cycle to start stimulation.

Time-line	Normal menstrual cycle	IVF cycle
Day 3–4	The hypothalamus releases gonadotrophin-releasing hormone (GnRH) to stimulate the pituitary gland to produce follicle stimulating hormone (FSH). FSH starts to do just as its name implies – stimulates the immature follicles in the ovaries.	***Start of stimulation phase*** Lasts for 9–14 days. Injections of FSH-based drug to stimulate multiple follicles. Long protocol: LHRH (GnRH) agonist continues right through stimulation until hCG injection – to suppress LH surge and premature ovulation. Dose may be reduced. ***Start of the 'Short Protocol'*** Stimulation of FSH drug as above, with inclusion of a faster-acting LHRH (GnRH) antagonist starting Day 6 – to suppress LH surge and premature ovulation.
Day 5 onwards	The growing follicles produce increasing amounts of oestrogen. This effect is observable as cervical secretions become more 'sperm friendly' – sticky white then wet, clear and stretchy.	***Monitoring with scans and blood tests*** As multiple follicles grow, they produce higher and higher levels of oestradiol (oestrogen). Scans monitor the number and size of follicles. Blood tests measure increasing oestradiol levels.
Day 13–14	When oestrogen reaches a critical level (with one dominant follicle) the pituitary releases a surge of LH to mature the egg.	When scan shows at least 2 or 3 follicles about 18mm size an **injection of hCG** (LH substitute) given to mature the eggs.

Time-line	Normal menstrual cycle	IVF cycle
Day 15	LH surge triggers release of egg (ovulation) about 36 hours later. The collapsed egg follicle (corpus luteum) starts producing progesterone to support implantation of the embryo.	**The eggs are collected** about 36 hours after the hCG 'trigger' injection. **Progesterone pessaries** are usually started the day of egg collection to support implantation of the embryo(s).
Day 16	The woman's cervix has a role in 'sperm sorting' – the strongest, fastest swimmers will be the ones to win the 'great sperm race'.	Your partner produces a fresh sample of sperm on the morning of egg collection. **The sperm are prepared** in the laboratory to separate out the best sperm **for fertilisation using IVF or ICSI.**
Day 18–21	If successful, the fertilised egg starts to implant several days later.	**The embryo(s) are transferred back** into the uterus between 2–5 days after egg collection.
Around Day 28	A pregnancy test would show positive around 14 days after ovulation.	A woman is usually asked to do a **pregnancy test** 14–16 days after egg collection.

everything is scaled up, physically (and often emotionally too). As we have discussed earlier, a woman's normal menstrual cycle is around 28 days but can be very varied, with a single egg being released at ovulation about 14 days before the next period. The aim of the IVF drug regime, however, is for the doctors to take over the complete control of your menstrual cycle, to ensure there is no chance you could ovulate spontaneously (and prematurely). The target is to stimulate the ovaries to produce around 8–12 follicles. The table on pages 319–321 compares the sequence of events during a normal menstrual cycle with an IVF cycle. This provides a generic overview of an IVF cycle and an approximate time-line, but there are many variations on this theme.

IVF Protocols

An IVF protocol is a regime of drugs and procedures used during an IVF treatment cycle. Protocols can vary from clinic to clinic. For example, some clinics may put you on the contraceptive pill before starting an IVF cycle. This helps to schedule the timing of your IVF cycle. It is important to get the protocol right to ensure your ovaries receive optimal stimulation and you produce mature eggs and good-quality embryos.

Many women are concerned about the drugs they will be prescribed. As IVF improves, so do the drug protocols, and there has been a lot of research behind fertility drugs and dosages required. The amount of drugs given varies from woman to woman. Some will need only a very small dose to get follicles growing, while others will require higher doses. In many cases IVF doctors try to give the minimum stimulation dose to begin with and increase it according to how you respond. The frequent scans and blood tests will show you how well you are responding, and how many follicles are growing. The aim is to get enough follicles of a similar size. As the follicles increase in size, they are producing increasing amounts of oestrogen and there is always a chance that this could trigger a natural surge in LH (the ovulation trigger hormone), so a principal aim with all IVF protocols is to ensure that a woman's natural LH surge is suppressed to prevent spontaneous ovulation.

If this was allowed to occur while the ovaries are being stimulated, then it could be dangerous (risk of high-order multiple pregnancy). So all women undergoing IVF will be given some form of LH suppression to prevent ovulation.

This bit is quite complex and there is no reason for you to remember it all, but you will often hear or see terms used, so this explanation is included. In a normal menstrual cycle, the hypothalamus (major control centre in the brain) produces gonadotrophin-releasing hormone (GnRH) – also known as luteinising hormone releasing hormone (LHRH) to complicate things further! This regulates the production of the gonadotrophins FSH and LH by the pituitary gland and their release into the bloodstream.

In an IVF cycle your natural LH is suppressed with the use of a gonadotrophin-releasing hormone (GnRH) analogue, sometimes known as an LHRH analogue. A GnRH analogue is a synthetic drug modelled on human GnRH. It interacts with the GnRH receptors and modifies the release of FSH and LH. There are two types of GnRH analogues: agonists and antagonists. A GnRH agonist, such as buserelin, has a very brief stimulating effect on FSH and LH but then after about two to five days has a suppressing effect on FSH and LH, so is used over a length of time to 'down-regulate' the cycle (long protocol). The other type of GnRH analogue is known as an antagonist, such as cetrorelix acetate, and this has an immediate blocking effect on GnRH receptors in the pituitary gland resulting in a rapid drop in FSH and LH secretion so this faster-acting form is used in the short protocol.

So, the two main types of protocol are:

1. A long (Day 21) protocol
2. A short protocol

See also diagram in Appendix 2 (page 484).

The Long Protocol – Down-regulation

A long protocol begins with 'down-regulation' about seven days before your expected period – so around Day 21 of the menstrual cycle before you start ovarian stimulation. The down-regulation drugs are usually a GnRH agonist, such as naferelin nasal spray or buserelin by nasal spray, or an injection under the skin. This effectively suppresses the production of FSH and LH in the pituitary gland, switching off your natural hormones. The IVF doctors are hoping to dampen down your ovaries prior to the start of your IVF cycle. This gives them a clean slate, so to speak, when it comes to stimulating your ovaries.

Side Effects of Down-regulation Drugs

Some women experience side effects usually associated with the menopause such as headaches, hot flushes and sleep disturbance and may feel emotionally fragile at this time, while others have no side effects at all.

I feel it is important to take it easy even at this stage while you are going through the down-regulating as for some women it can seem like quite a hormonal upheaval. Avoid exercise, and rest when you are tired.

Some women can be on down-regulation drugs, waiting for their period to start, and discover that they are pregnant. Don't panic – this does happen. There are different schools of thought around whether it is okay to have sex in the cycle you are down-regulating as there is the potential for the suppression drugs to prevent implantation of a natural pregnancy which was just starting out. Pregnancies occurring at this time are not that unusual. You can rest assured that there does not appear to be any adverse consequences. I think of them as little miracle babies.

Blood Tests and Monitoring for the Long Protocol

After about seven days of down-regulation you should get your period. Once this happens you need to call your clinic. You will usually have a scan and a blood test between Days 3 and 5 of your period to ensure the down-regulation drugs have had the desired effect. Your oestradiol level should be low (usually less than 100 pg/ml) and your scan should show that your ovaries are very calm with no sign of follicular activity or cysts. The endometrium (womb lining) should be mostly shed and appear thin.

If you do not get a period at the expected time, this may be because your cycle has not been sufficiently down-regulated so you may be given a progesterone-containing drug to induce a period. It is only natural that all women want their IVF cycle to go like clock-work, but if it doesn't then this might be the first hurdle you have to deal with (see page 369).

A woman with specific problems, such as polycystic ovaries (PCO) will need extra monitoring and possibly a different mix of hormones to produce mature eggs. Women with PCO may over-respond to IVF drugs and are at an increased risk of ovarian hyperstimulation syndrome (OHSS) if not monitored closely (see page 371).

Ovarian Stimulation

After Day 3–5 of your period, you will start the stimulation drugs provided your scan and blood test confirm it is safe to continue. The fertility drugs used to stimulate the ovaries are the same hormones that the body naturally produces to encourage eggs to develop in the ovaries (FSH and LH). When going through IVF these hormones are given (added back in) in larger doses than a woman would produce naturally to increase the number of growing follicles. The ovaries are stimulated with an FSH-based drug sometimes combined with LH activity. The brand name and dose of the FSH-based drug will vary according to your circumstances and the doctor's preference. The dose is likely to be adjusted as the cycle progresses. You will usually continue your down-regulation medication alongside the stimulation drugs although you may be advised to reduce its dose. Although this may seem strange to be stimulating and suppressing at the same time, remember the continued suppression of your natural LH is to ensure that you do not ovulate spontaneously.

During the first half of the IVF cycle as the follicles grow, they produce increasing amounts of oestradiol (oestrogen). Regular ultrasound scans monitor the number and size of the follicles and blood tests check the oestradiol levels. The process of stimulation usually takes about 9–12 days or until the measurements of the follicles and the oestradiol levels look optimal. The aim is to get at least three follicles (ideally 8–12) with diameters of about 17–20 mm. The peak oestradiol level will usually reach between 1,000 to 4,000 pg/ml. When instructed you will give yourself the injection of hCG – a similar drug to LH – to mature the eggs. This is often a late-night injection (around midnight) and you will have your egg collection about 36 hours later. Clearly the timing of this is all quite critical.

The Short Protocol

The short protocol may be used in preference to the long protocol for older women who may have previously responded poorly to IVF stimulation or for women with raised FSH levels. It bypasses the lengthy down-regulation phase (used in the long protocol) and begins by stimulating the ovaries, usually starting on Days 3–4 of your cycle using the same stimulation drugs as the long protocol. After a few days of stimulation as the follicles are starting to grow and produce more oestrogen, a fast-acting GnRH antagonist is added to the regime to prevent a natural LH surge and spontaneous ovulation. This is continued through until the hCG injection is given.

The Stimulation Stage

As with the stimulation phase during the long protocol, this involves daily injections administered by yourself or your partner (see 'Injections', page 329). Usually you have these injections for about 9–14 days. The doctors want to see that you are producing a reasonable number of follicles, that they are growing at a similar rate and your endometrium is starting to thicken – in other words, that you are responding to the treatment. You will therefore have regular ultrasound scans to look at the number and size of the growing follicles and blood tests to monitor your oestradiol (oestrogen) levels. The level of monitoring varies from clinic to clinic.

Your doctor may increase or decrease the level of drugs, depending on how you are responding. If your ovaries are not responding or are slow to respond, your stimulation drugs are likely to be increased up to a certain limit. Your cycle may be stopped and either cancelled or converted to an IUI cycle (page 243) if you are not getting an appropriate response when you reach the maximum drug dosage.

Conversely, if your ovaries are over-responding to the drugs there is a danger of OHSS (see page 371) so your cycle may be coasted (see page 372) or stopped. Some clinics will offer a refund, depending on how far you have got in the treatment. You will need to check your clinic's policy on this.

Drugs Used for Ovarian Stimulation

It is possible that you will have already experienced some form of ovarian stimulation before proceeding to IVF as this is used to promote the growth of one or more follicles in the treatment of ovulation disorders (see page 238) and also in intrauterine insemination (IUI, see page 243).

Ovarian stimulation is sometimes referred to as controlled ovarian hyperstimulation or 'super-ovulation'. Most of the IVF protocols (both long and short protocols) use injections of a drug containing the gonadotrophin FSH with or without LH. There are basically two forms of these gonadotrophins: urinary FSH with LH which is extracted from the urine of post-menopausal women; and recombinant FSH which uses DNA technology for large-scale production of FSH.

Zita's Tips

The hardest thing for a woman going through IVF is the feeling that she has lost control. There will be so many questions that you want to have answered so you can schedule and plan what you are doing. You will want to know exactly how long your IVF cycle is going to take, and whether it is the long protocol or the short one. You will also want to know when the egg collection will occur and when the transfer will take place. However, you have to be flexible at all times. Nobody can tell you exactly when the egg collection will happen or when you are going to have embryo transfer because different things happen along the way. It might take longer to regulate your hormones than you thought. Your ovaries might not respond to stimulation as well as you expected. Your hormone (oestradiol) levels might go very high, which may delay things for a few more days. I think you can feel confident in a clinic that really seems to be working with you as an individual, closely monitoring you and making sure all the timings are right for collecting the eggs and transferring your embryo(s).

Urinary FSH or human menopausal gonadotrophin (HMG) (also known as menotrophin) is actually a combination of FSH and hCG with LH-like activity extracted and highly purified from the urine of post-menopausal and pregnant women, respectively. HMG was first developed in the late 1940s and for many years this was the only source of gonadotrophin for ovarian stimulation.

Recombinant FSH (rFSH) is a synthetic form of FSH produced by genetically engineered Chinese hamster ovary cells. These chemically engineered products are very pure and batch-consistent, so may give more reliable results, but they may be more expensive than urinary derived FSH (HMG).

Injections

One of the biggest fears that many women have before starting IVF is giving themselves injections. Nurses at the fertility clinic will show you how to do this. If at first you don't take in the drug information that is given to you, please go back and get clarification. All the drug companies have websites containing information about drugs and how to give the injection, and some offer explanatory CDs.

Many of the drugs are easier to give nowadays because they come in a pen applicator. The best place to give the drug is in your thigh or your abdomen. However, if you are prescribed some other additional injections that don't come in a pen applicator, such as heparin (Clexane) then warm the area you are going to inject by rubbing it with your hands first. If you still find the idea of injecting yourself abhorrent, your partner might be willing to give these injections. Men can sometimes be very squeamish and terrified of doing this, however, so please be patient with one another. You will both need patience and understanding. Make sure you discuss this openly before you start.

Some women feel that, as they are having to go through the process, their partner should do the injections. Don't start a war here as it will only lead to resentment.

Some of the medications you take will be by using a nasal spray; others will be subcutaneous, which means injected just under the skin; and others will need to be injected a bit deeper into the muscle. One of the most important things is to feel organised when doing this. Make sure you wash your hands before administering the injection. The first injection is always the worst. If you are very nervous about injections, you can buy a special anaesthetic cream that will numb the injection site. Ask your doctor or nurse about this. So, for that first injection, be calm, be still and be quiet. You may find it easiest to have the injection while lying down or sitting. After the injection, have a nice warm bath and relax.

Women are sometimes concerned when they see a little leakage from the injection site and fear they are not getting enough of the drug. However, this is quite normal and nothing to worry about. Similarly you may get a slight bruising where the injection was given and that is fine. If you have any concerns, discuss them with one of the IVF nurses who can go over the injection technique with you. It's a good idea to chat to other women who are in a similar situation because they can offer you a lot of support and answer questions you may have been too shy to ask the doctors.

Preparing for Egg Collection

If everything is progressing well, and your scans and blood tests are showing good follicular development and appropriate hormone levels, the doctors will check to see that the leading follicles have reached 18mm or more, and your womb lining is around 8mm thick, which will mean that you are ready for egg collection and you will be told to stop the stimulating drugs.

The hCG Injection

When your scan shows that two or three of your growing follicles have reached about 18mm in size you will give yourself an injection containing the pregnancy hormone human chorionic gonadotrophin, or hCG, which is a substitute for the natural LH surge. The hCG injection matures the eggs in preparation for egg collection about 36 hours later. It is important to have this injection at the correct time – you may need to set your alarm and get up in the middle of the night. If you miss the trigger injection you must let your clinic know as it will affect the date and time your eggs will be collected.

Many women express concern that they might ovulate before their eggs can be collected, but, remember, this is where your GnRH analogue (your suppressant – usually a nasal spray) is playing its part. Whether it is a long- or short-acting drug you are on, this is preventing a surge of LH and therefore preventing you from releasing any eggs spontaneously. Once you have had the hCG injection you usually stop all of your fertility drugs – so are drug-free for a day or two.

Another concern for many women at this stage is how many eggs will be collected. However, it is the quality and maturity of the eggs, and not necessarily the quantity, that is important here.

Egg Collection (or Egg Retrieval)

Egg collection day is a big day for you and your partner. You will have an idea about how many eggs may be collected based on the number of follicles you have, but remember that not every follicle will contain an egg. For the procedure, you will be given either adequate sedation or a light anaesthetic, depending on the hospital's policy and sometimes your choice. The eggs are normally collected vaginally. Although it may not look like it from 2D diagrams, the ovaries actually lie very close in proximity to the top of the vagina, so can normally be reached very easily through the vaginal wall. The egg collection procedure is usually done by guided ultrasound. The gynaecologist and embryologist work very closely together at this stage. The gynaecologist carefully aspirates the fluid (hopefully containing the egg) from each follicle into a test tube and hands this straight to the embryologist who immediately checks (under a microscope) to see if there is an egg. Eggs are tiny – only 0.1mm in diameter, which is smaller than a full stop. Sometimes the gynaecologist may flush out the follicle in search of an egg. Each follicle is aspirated in this way from both ovaries until all the eggs have been collected.

The whole process takes around 20–30 minutes, and you will then be given about an hour or two to recover. How you feel afterwards and the pain you may experience will vary. You may get very slight bleeding from the small needle puncture points at the top of the vagina. Many women feel rather bruised, particularly if their ovaries responded very well and a lot of eggs have been retrieved. You may be given antibiotics as there is a slight risk of infection.

I generally encourage women to rest after egg collection as they can feel quite groggy and tired for a while. It really helps to get a few early nights and practise some visualisation in order to build yourself up for the next stage of the process. It is fantastic that you have got this far and the eggs have been collected.

Progesterone Supplementation

Alas, you do not remain drug-free for long, because after egg collection you will be advised to start progesterone supplementation. This is usually given in the form of vaginal pessaries, but other injectable forms of progesterone are also available if there are problems with absorption.

The word progesterone, as its name implies (pro = for; gestation = pregnancy), is a hormone designed to support pregnancy. If we consider again what happens in a natural menstrual cycle: once an egg is released, the follicle collapses and forms the corpus luteum – this 'yellow body' secretes progesterone to sustain the pregnancy. In an IVF cycle during egg collection when the follicles are aspirated, this inadvertently removes quite a lot of the progesterone-producing cells. Also, the drugs used to suppress the natural LH surge reduce the production of progesterone after egg collection. Progesterone supplementation is therefore started after egg collection.

Side Effects of Progesterone

Progesterone pessaries can usually be used vaginally or rectally as you prefer or as your clinic suggests. As you may get slight leakage, you may want to wear a panty liner. Side effects of progesterone supplements include: gastro-intestinal disturbance, such as nausea, flatulence and constipation, bloated tummy, sore breasts and irritable mood.

The Number of Eggs

Women inevitably compare their progress – whether this is in the waiting room at the clinic, tales from friends or online chat. It can be very hard not to panic when you hear of one woman having 20 eggs and another having 10, if you only have a few. You may feel that a low number of eggs reduces your chance of getting pregnant, but you need to try and lose that notion – erase it from your brain. It is so important that you remain positive, and once again I remind you that it is quality rather than quantity. I have seen many women who only manage to produce one or two embryos who have been successful with their IVF, and that is what you need to hold on to.

Producing a Semen Sample

Men are asked to abstain from intercourse and masturbation for two to five days before giving a sample, and are told not to use any soaps or lubricants because they can be toxic to the sperm. They then have to ejaculate into a sterile container. Most men are fine about producing a sample, but for some it can be difficult. Men can feel self-conscious and embarrassed about having to perform this very private act in a clinical environment, often with lots of noise from people milling around outside the room. Occasionally, a man will be too stressed to produce a sample.

There is nothing worse than dreading the whole business or worrying about not being able to do it. Clinic staff are used to dealing with these issues so there is no need to be embarrassed. If you want your partner to come into the room with you, ask at the clinic, but a lot of these rooms are very small so it may be difficult. If you feel anxious that you may have difficulties on the day of egg collection, it is a good idea to talk to the doctor and voice your concerns. You may be able to arrange to produce a sample ahead of time which can then be frozen. You can then attempt to produce a fresh sample on the day, but if this is not successful, the frozen sample can be used. Clinics generally prefer to use a fresh sperm sample as fertilisation rates tend to be slightly higher than with a frozen-thawed sample, but with modern freezing techniques this is less of a problem.

Sometimes women are elated to get, for example, 14 eggs, but can come crashing down when maybe only six are mature enough to fertilise. You have to build in realistic expectations – not all follicles will contain a mature egg. It is only when the eggs get to the lab and the embryologist is able to grade them that you will know which ones are mature.

You must try not to be anxious, difficult as it is, about only having a few eggs, and don't worry now about the next steps. The situation is as it is and nothing is going to change it. You are using up valuable energy worrying when you only need one good egg. Instead, use your energy visualising a nice thick womb lining, and go to bed early, putting a well-padded hot water bottle on your tummy to keep the area warm. The heat can feel very relaxing at this stage, but don't use additional heat after embryo transfer. I also suggest having some acupuncture or indulging in some relaxation therapy if possible.

Creating an Embryo

Once the eggs have been collected and the sperm has been given to the laboratory, the embryology comes into play. I spent an afternoon in the lab at the Lister Hospital in London with the embryologist. It is incredible to observe the process from start to finish and to see embryos being graded. Embryologists do an amazing job and have a big role to play, not only on the scientific side, but also in talking to couples and letting them know how their embryos are developing.

The eggs are put into a medium – a liquid environment – which nourishes the eggs and embryos, ready to be graded. What the embryologist has to assess by a scoring system is how many of these eggs are mature enough to make an embryo. The embryologist will have an idea of what the sperm are like from the sample and will make a decision as to whether to do IVF or ICSI.

IVF (literally 'in-glass fertilisation') is where the egg and sperm are put in a Petri dish and the sperm swim to the egg by themselves. The embryologist places a drop of seminal fluid containing tens of thousands of specially prepared sperm into the medium containing the eggs. After a couple of hours, the winning sperm normally penetrates the egg and fuses (fertilisation). The eggs are checked the morning after they have been collected and then the embryologist will call you to tell you how many eggs have fertilised. To achieve fertilisation by straight IVF at least half a million progressively motile sperm are usually required in total. Quite amazingly 50,000–100,000 sperm are mixed with each egg to optimise fertilisation.

ICSI (intracytoplasmic sperm injection) is when the sperm is injected directly into the cytoplasm in the middle of the egg. ICSI is

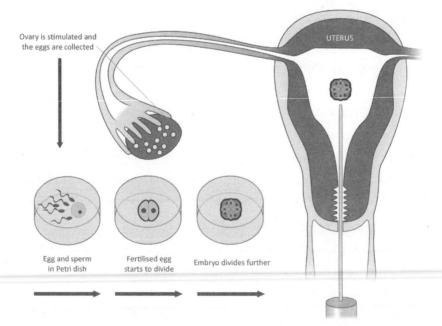

Ovary is stimulated and the eggs are collected

UTERUS

Egg and sperm in Petri dish

Fertilised egg starts to divide

Embryo divides further

performed under a microscope using micromanipulation equipment. This is a very delicate procedure requiring great precision. ICSI may be appropriate if the sperm are poor quality and may not be able to fertilise the egg by themselves. Reasons for this may include:

- Very low sperm count
- A very high percentage of abnormally shaped sperm
- A high level of anti-sperm antibodies
- If none or less than 50 per cent of eggs have been fertilised in previous cycles

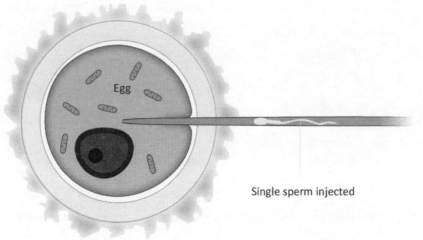

Single sperm injected

The fertilisation rate is higher for ICSI than straight IVF. ICSI is now used in about 44 per cent of all IVF treatments in the UK, and this number is growing. Some clinics will have a higher rate of ICSI than others, to optimise fertilisation rates.

If a man has very few sperm in his semen sample it is usually possible to do ICSI. If there are no sperm present in the ejaculate, then it may be possible to retrieve sperm surgically from the testicles or epididymis. ICSI is then performed with the surgically retrieved sperm. The development of ICSI has therefore revolutionised male infertility for men who would otherwise not have been able to father their own genetic child.

Embryo Development

The freshly fertilised egg has two pronuclei, one derived from each parent. The pronuclei contains the genetic material (23 chromosomes from each parent). The two sets of chromosomes then pair up to form 23 pairs. By the end of Day 1, it should have divided into two identical daughter cells (cell division is called cleavage); by Day 2,

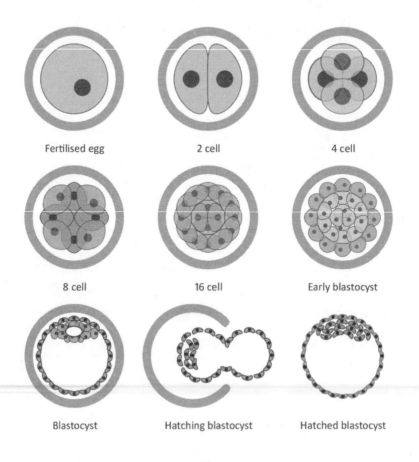

Fertilised egg	2 cell	4 cell
8 cell	16 cell	Early blastocyst
Blastocyst	Hatching blastocyst	Hatched blastocyst

four cells; by Day 3, six to eight cells. Up until Day 3 all of the cells are identical and embryonic development is controlled by the maternal genes in the egg. When there are about eight cells, the potential for further development comes under the control of the embryo itself.

The Blastocyst Stage

By Day 5, the embryo will be at blastocyst stage with as many as 100–1,000 cells. Not all embryos will get to blastocyst stage; some will stop dividing along the way. The more embryos you have to begin with, the better chance you have of getting to this stage. The cells of the blastocyst start to differentiate into specific types, each with a specialised function. The outer cells will become the placenta and foetal membrane; the fluid in the middle, the blastocoele, will become the amniotic fluid; and specialised cells on the inner surface of the blastocyst, or the inner cell mass, will develop into the foetus. As the cavity fills up with fluid, the blastocyst expands and eventually hatches from the zona pellucida, which is the shell surrounding the embryo. In a natural cycle the hatched blastocyst will then implant into the endometrium six to seven days after ovulation. Similarly, in an IVF cycle, implantation starts one to two days after the blastocyst is transferred into the uterus.

Getting good-quality blastocysts is associated with a higher pregnancy rate. Clinics are moving towards elective single embryo transfer to reduce the risks of multiple births, so are aiming to put one good-quality embryo back, preferably at the blastocyst stage. It is not unusual, however, to start off with a lot of embryos and end up with only two or three blastocysts. Not everybody will have enough embryos for there to be any advantage in culturing them to the blastocyst stage. Some embryos will be put back sooner – around Day 3. I don't want you to feel disappointed if you haven't got a blastocyst. Pregnancy can still happen so long as the embryo quality is good. The best-quality embryo(s) will always be the one which is put back at embryo transfer.

Embryo Grading

All of the embryos are assessed or graded by the embryologist about two days after collection, but there are many grading systems, so you need to understand whether a low number grade indicates the best or worst embryo. The grading is complex, but is mostly done on

Freezing Embryos

The embryologist will assess how many of your remaining embryos (if any) are of good-enough quality for freezing (cryo-preservation) and at what stage. Only the top-quality embryos are likely to survive the freeze-thaw process. The main problem with freezing is the formation of ice crystals as this can destroy the cells. Vitrification is a new fast-freezing (with dehydration) tech-nique which has a very good freeze-thaw rate. Although it can be very disappointing not to have any surplus embryos for freezing, it is better not to be given false hope.

Frozen-thawed embryos can be used for a later IVF cycle if needed which means you would not need to go through the stim-ulation phase of the cycle again.

Couples often express concern about the use of hi-tech proce-dures such as embryo freezing, and it is always important to discuss any concerns with your doctor. There are many long-term studies observing the development of babies born following IVF, ICSI and freezing techniques. It seems that babies born from frozen embryos do not appear to suffer at all: in fact there is some evidence that these babies may actually be healthier as they are less likely to be born prematurely or underweight.

appearance – it includes looking at the number of cells and whether the cells are dividing at the expected rate; the cells need to be equal in size and with little or no fragmentation (where portions of the embryo's cells have broken off). Each cell of the embryo should only have one nucleus (containing the 23 pairs of chromosomes). It is understandable to be hoping for the highest-grade embryos, but this is still a subjective process and normal pregnancies will still result from apparently poor-quality embryos.

Screening of Embryos

Up until recently the embryologist relied on the naked eye (and a microscope) to select good-quality embryos for transfer or freezing. As technology improves there are ways of looking at the embryo and being able to screen for chromosomal abnormalities. An embryo with a normal chromosome complement is 'euploid' and an embryo with an abnormal number of chromosomes (extra or missing chromosome) is 'aneuploid'. Specialised screening techniques are used in specific circumstances, for example for couples with a family history of genetic disorders. There is currently much debate about the technology used to screen for chromosomally normal embryos (see page 350).

Embryo Transfer

The embryo transfer will be done between two and five days after the eggs are collected. The precise timing will depend on the number of embryos you have and how they are progressing. This can be quite an exciting, but tense day. It is great that you have got this far – you have already got through so many hurdles and your hopes and expectations will be mounting. The next big thing is to hear how your embryos are progressing, before they are transferred inside you.

You will be awake for the transfer and your partner is usually with you. You will normally see your embryo(s) on the screen or photographed before the transfer, which can be very exciting. Depending on the position of your womb, you may be asked to have a full bladder to allow for an easier transfer, so this can feel rather uncomfortable.

Nowadays, most embryo transfers are done under ultrasound guidance. A soft narrow catheter is inserted through the cervix into the womb and the embryo(s) are slowly and gently replaced. The skill and dexterity of the person doing the transfer is important. Different IVF doctors take different approaches to this. Some take a long time over transferring the embryos back, while others will do it over a shorter time.

Self-help Measures

Try and keep as still and relaxed as possible, breathing deeply and slowly and be as positive as you can as the embryos are going back. Many of the hormones that are released at times of stress – including adrenaline and cortisol – may cause the womb to contract. So, if you can, try to do any visualisation techniques you have learned, because I think it can really help. I encourage women to try and disassociate themselves from what is happening. Listening to music can help (I have put together a relaxation CD for before and after embryo transfer. See page 486).

Pre- and Post-acupuncture Treatments

If possible try and have an acupuncture treatment before and after embryo transfer (on the same day). Many women cannot manage both, but if you can manage one, it will be very beneficial. I believe you should avoid too much interference or complementary therapies, such as reflexology, abdominal massage or anything similar, in the early days after transfer and I would not encourage acupuncture on a daily basis. I feel you have to be very careful at this time. I also suggest you avoid heat, so no hot baths or hot water bottles on your abdomen after embryo transfer.

Activity after Transfer – Where Is the Evidence?

Women often feel anxious about getting up and moving around immediately after embryo transfer – feeling that the embryos may 'fall out'. The natural instinct is to want to rest for a while after the procedure and this makes complete sense – you need to follow your own hunch and what your body dictates. Many women like to go home and have a good snooze after an emotionally exhausting day. There is no research evidence to support my thoughts around rest and relaxation at this time – this is based on common sense and hearing over the years from so many women who regret having 'overdone it'.

Researchers have looked at this whole issue. One research study compared two groups of women – the first group rested for 30 minutes after transfer, while the second group got up and moved around immediately. They found no significant difference in pregnancy rates between the two groups. Similarly research shows that more prolonged bed rest (24 hours) does not significantly affect the pregnancy rate. So, I think you can rest assured that getting up, moving around, leaving the IVF clinic, going for a relaxing post-transfer acupuncture treatment, or quietly getting on with life is all quite safe and will not jeopardise your chances of success. The key issue here is to follow your instincts.

How Many Embryos to Put Back?

Currently up to 30 per cent of IVF pregnancies are twin pregnancies or higher.

Although the idea of twins may conjure up wonderful images of cute smiling babies, sadly the reality can be very different in terms of the medical risks for the mother and potential health consequences for the babies, who are more likely to be born prematurely. Multiple pregnancies are considered the most serious complication of assisted conception.

For many years it has been common practice to put two or more embryos back, so clearly a double embryo transfer (DET) could result in non-identical or fraternal twins. However, clinics are now moving towards elective single embryo transfer (eSET) because it reduces the risk of multiple births. It is understandable that some women want two or more embryos put back to increase their chances of a successful singleton pregnancy or even twins, but this is something which you need to discuss with your doctor. The decision about how many embryos to replace depends on many factors – the principal ones being the woman's age, embryo quality and past experience of IVF.

Recent studies in the UK have shown that if you have a single embryo transferred it may be about a third less successful than replacing two embryos, but if the spare embryo is frozen and used in another cycle then the success rate is equal to replacing two. Putting it another way, you can think of the success rate as an equation: 1 DET = 1 SET + 1 frozen SET. So, provided of course the option of freezing is available, the policy of eSET is a good one. I would rather plan to have one healthy baby and then do a frozen transfer for my next pregnancy.

It is important to remember that embryos can still split into two after they have been transferred back into the uterus. Recent research from Japan has used computer software to record the blastocyst essentially collapsing and splitting the genetic material in half resulting in identical twins, so replacing a single embryo still does not rule out the possibility of twins.

Selecting the best-quality embryo has become easier with extended blastocyst culture. If you manage to get as far as blastocyst stage, the chances of success will always be higher than if the embryo is replaced at the two to three-day stage, but as ever success rates will vary from clinic to clinic and this is why it is important to discuss this with your doctor.

In 2006 Guy's and St Thomas' Assisted Conception Unit (ACU) started a programme advising couples of the risks of multiple pregnancy and the advantages of transferring a single blastocyst. In a three-year study (2,451 fresh IVF cycles) where single blastocyst transfer was used in a selected group of women, the clinical pregnancy rate increased from 27 to 32 per cent and the multiple pregnancy rate was reduced from 32 to 17 per cent. So, the overall success rate was improved while reducing the risks for mother and baby associated with multiple pregnancy.

The Human Fertilisation and Embryology Authority (HFEA) is heading up a National Strategy to reduce multiple births to a rate of 10 per cent over a staged interval. More information on eSET can be found on the One at a Time website: www.oneatatime.org.uk

Difficult Transfers

A difficult embryo transfer is sometimes associated with a lower pregnancy rate. For this reason some clinics will do a 'mock' transfer either just before your real transfer or in the cycle preceding your treatment cycle (a monitoring cycle). This can be really helpful in ensuring the doctor is aware of the direction of your cervix and uterus and effectively mapping things out with a trial run. In my experience, women who find embryo transfer more difficult tend to be women with vaginismus, or with slight structural malformations of the cervix. A mock transfer can be reassuring for everyone concerned. If you have any concerns about embryo transfer or have had bad experiences in the past, such as sexual abuse, or you find smears and vaginal examinations difficult, do discuss this with the doctor or one of the nurses before you get to this stage. A 'mock' transfer would help you to know what the whole experience is going to be like. It is also possible to do embryo transfer under sedation if necessary which you may find very reassuring.

Many women can feel quite daunted by the prospect of having their very precious embryos replaced, feeling a real sense of responsibility for their ongoing development and the success of the cycle. It generally helps if you feel that you have done as much as you can to try and make it work – reducing your workload, eating well,

Assisted Hatching

As an embryo develops further it has to 'hatch' or escape from the zona pellucida (the gelatinous egg coat). In some women, particularly older women, the egg coat may be particularly thick or tough and the embryo may be helped out by 'assisted hatching'. This lab technique involves thinning or making an opening in the zona pellucida to help the embryo hatch out. If implantation has previously failed despite good-quality embryos, assisted hatching may be discussed as a way to improve the chances of successful implantation. This is done less frequently now as it has not been clearly shown to improve pregnancy rates.

plenty of rest and so on – but the key here with embryo transfer, as ever, is to simply try and let go and rest assured that you are doing all within your power to make it work. Some women can be quite superstitious about the whole transfer procedure even carrying lucky charms. I know you may feel very vulnerable at this stage, but be as strong as you can. This is where the support and understanding from your partner is crucial. If you have any concerns, talk to one of the clinic nurses.

What Happens When an Embryo is Put Back?

This depends precisely on the stage at which the embryo is put back. If a blastocyst is replaced, then this has a head-start in the uterine cavity. If the embryo is put back two to three days after fertilisation, it will continue to divide for another two to three days going through the blastocyst stage and eventually bursting (hatching) out of its outer coat or shell. This shedding of the outer shell now allows the blastocyst to increase rapidly in size while being in exactly the right place to start to implant into the lining of the womb, deriving nourishment from the secretions of the endometrial glands.

The hatched blastocyst goes through several phases of implantation. First it must make contact with the womb lining, then start to glue itself in place with special adhesion molecules, and finally penetrate the endometrium, eventually connecting to the mother's blood vessels to form the placenta. In order to do this, the outer layer of the blastocyst (trophoblast) proliferates rapidly, forming finger-like projections which burrow in and embed in the womb lining by the end of the first week. The blastocyst is now superficially implanted.

Interview with Eleanor Wharf, Senior Embryologist at Guy's Hospital, London

What makes a good embryo?

What's important is the rate of its development according to what is expected on a given day. So, for example, we look for four cells on Day 2, eight cells on Day 3 and blastocyst stage on Day 5. We also look at the quality of the cells.

What do couples worry about most when it comes to embryos?

There is a strong trend towards blastocyst culture at the moment and many women feel if we don't keep their embryos in culture until Day 5, when healthy embryos will develop to the blastocyst stage, they haven't as good a chance of getting pregnant. The data seem to show this, but the reality is that most women having blastocyst stage embryo transfer are the ones who are the younger patients with a greater number of embryos to choose from. Blastocyst culture is basically a tool to give us the option of transferring one embryo in patients who are at risk of having a multiple pregnancy, yet without reducing the chances of them becoming pregnant. Culturing the embryos in the laboratory until Day 5 of development won't improve the inherent quality of the embryos, so if it is possible to select the best embryos from how they appear when we look down the microscope on Day 2 or Day 3, we feel it is better to transfer them into the womb sooner rather than later. If they are good quality, there is still a good chance of pregnancy.

Couples are also very anxious about having enough embryos to have some available to freeze. We will freeze any embryos that we feel have potential to develop into a pregnancy, but our primary concern is to have good-quality fresh embryos for transfer.

How do you grade a blastocyst?
You look at the degree of expansion – how much it has grown in size – and the number and quality of cells. The better the grade, the more likely you are to get a pregnancy, although a good grade doesn't equal a baby. Embryos can sometimes change, and embryos that aren't particularly good on Day 2 or 3 occasionally catch up in development by Day 5. We don't know why this happens.

What happens when an embryo is fragmented?
Nobody understands what fragments are or why they form. All we know is that in some embryos, instead of dividing from one cell into two, a cell can form lots of little blebs that we call fragments. A small amount of fragmentation is unlikely to stop the embryo from continuing in development, but if more than half of the embryo's cells fragment it is less likely that the embryo will be able to develop into a pregnancy.

Which patients tend to make good embryos?
The woman's age is probably the single biggest factor affecting embryo quality. If the infertility is caused by low sperm count or poor motility of the sperm, ICSI can overcome the problem and we may still achieve good-quality embryos.

What stops an egg being fertilised?
Sometimes we just don't know. Even where the eggs are injected with sperm in ICSI cases, they don't necessarily fertilise. With IVF, there may be a problem with the interaction between the egg and the sperm.

Do you do assisted hatching?
Assisted hatching, where you make a hole in the outer protective coating of the embryo, usually at about the 8-cell stage to help it to hatch

out and implant into the lining of the womb, was more common a couple of years ago. Now that we have better culture conditions and are able to culture embryos to the blastocyst stage, there is less call for assisted hatching, although some studies have suggested that it may be beneficial for older women. We don't hatch blastocysts for the simple reason that there are so many cells – making a hole in the shell might damage the cells at any point.

How many embryos are put back?

This depends on the age of the woman, the quality of the embryos and how many good quality embryos there are to choose from. The embryologist will discuss this with the patient, explaining the quality and quantity of the embryos and how they are developing. Most clinics will put two embryos back. However, for younger patients with good-quality embryos on Day 5, transferring more than one poses an unacceptable risk of multiple pregnancy. In these circumstances we would therefore recommend transferring one embryo – this shouldn't reduce the chances of achieving a pregnancy.

Screening of Embryos

Many couples ask if there is any way to do more advanced screening than the standard embryo grading and you will see from the next section and the interviews with some of the top doctors in this field that this is an area of huge interest. So, the challenge is to test an embryo to identify any chromosomally abnormal (aneuploid) embryos and then replace only chromosomally normal (euploid) embryos, without adversely affecting the embryo in the short or longer term, in order to increase the chances of a successful pregnancy.

Pre-implantation Genetic Screening

Pre-implantation genetic screening (PGS) is a technique that has been used particularly for older women (who have a high percentage of aneuploid eggs) or women with a history of recurrent miscarriage or repeated implantation failure. Unfortunately, the results of PGS rely on the assessment of a single cell, and this has inherent limitations as the cell tested may not be representative of the embryo and its future potential. Studies have shown that live birth rates following PGS are not improved. In fact, there is some concern that the biopsy may actually lower the success rates, so this form of PGS has largely been abandoned. A much more sophisticated form of PGS known as Array CGH is now being pioneered in Nottingham by Professor Simon Fishel (see overleaf).

Sex Selection

Although it is technically possible to preselect the sex of an embryo, sex selection purely for social reasons, such as family balancing, is not permitted in the UK. Some couples go overseas for this procedure.

Sperm Sorting

Sperm-sorting techniques are essentially a way of spinning sperm to separate male and female sperm. The sperm of the appropriate gender are then used for IUI, IVF or ICSI to produce an embryo of the desired sex. This technique is being researched at The Genetics and IVF Clinic in Fairfax, Virginia, USA. However, there are concerns among health professionals about the lack of published data on this technique.

Pre-implantation Genetic Diagnosis (PGD)

Pre-implantation genetic diagnosis (PGD) involves taking a single cell at an early stage of development to look at the chromosomes. This can be done to test for specific genetic disorders usually for couples with a family history of genetic problems. The sex of the embryo can also be determined to avoid the transmission of specific sex-linked disorders. The Human Fertilisation and Embryology Authority (HFEA) currently allows sex selection only for couples who carry a genetic condition which would otherwise be passed on to their child.

Array CGH

Array CGH, or Comparative Genomic Hybridisation, is a complex molecular biology technique which takes a single cell and detects chromosomal imbalances, particularly any gains or losses of DNA in the whole DNA of a cell. It is now possible to test eggs and embryos during an IVF cycle to evaluate all their chromosomes to identify the most viable embryos. The latest array CGH detects changes in multiple copies of the chromosomes with results available within 48 hours.

The area that is being biopsied with array CGH is actually quite independent of the area that will form the future embryo. This is because at the time when the egg is going through the process of meiosos, where it halves its chromosome numbers (from 46 chromosomes to 23), it extrudes a tiny amount of cytoplasm and half of its chromosomes into an area known as the polar body. So, the polar body can be removed, and the chromosomes tested without damaging the egg.

Interview with Alan Thornhill, Scientific Director at the London Bridge Fertility, Gynaeoclogy and Genetics Centre, London

What do you think makes a good embryo?

The most important things are the raw materials – eggs and sperm. The egg contains all of the chemical goodies to kick-start embryo development and it is easy to think of the sperm as just providing half of the genes. However, we are starting to learn a lot more about sperm – its chance of fertilising an egg, how it can affect embryo quality and whether or not a healthy baby will result. We also know that the quality of eggs declines as a woman gets older as well as the number.

How do you grade embryos?

Since embryos are tiny and would fit on a pin-head, we use microscopes to examine them carefully to identify those which appear to have the best chance of further development. To do this reliably, we use a standardised grading system in our laboratory.

Why grade embryos?

Current methods of IVF generally require us to produce more embryos than are needed for transfer. We do this because we are trying to maximise the chances of getting enough good-quality eggs and later embryos to produce one or more babies. By having multiple embryos we have the chance to let them 'self-select' in our culture fluid. A relatively new blood test, AMH (Anti-mullerian Hormone) is now available for women which quite accurately predicts how many eggs they have in their ovaries and are likely to have at egg collection. A low AMH result usually means that few eggs are available regardless of a woman's age. However, a woman's age is still the best predictor of egg quality.

Are there any other embryo factors that affect the chance of IVF success?
Right now, almost all laboratories worldwide make decisions about
'good' and 'bad' quality embryos based only on their appearance under
the microscope. However, we can't tell whether an embryo has genetic
problems just by looking at it, so we have developed tests to examine
a single cell from an embryo to do this. These tests are collectively
known as PGD or preimplantation genetic diagnosis. One method
called FISH, allowed us to look at up to 12 chromosomes in an embryo.
The chromosomes tested for were those most commonly seen in miscarriage and babies with a chromosome imbalance. Recently another
technique, known as CGH (Comparative Genomic Hybridisation), is
replacing the FISH test because it allows us to simultaneously test for
all 24 chromosomes (22 autosomes plus the two sex chromosomes X
and Y) in the same cell. In this way, we can detect all the problems we
could using FISH and others we would have otherwise missed.

What other developments are in the pipeline?
We will soon be looking at metabolites (or the 'waste' products
produced by embryos as they grow in culture fluid). By examining
the profile of metabolites found in this fluid, we can determine
embryo quality, likelihood of successful implantation and possibly, in
the future, detect genetic problems. The real benefit of this technique
is that it costs the embryo nothing – no cells or materials are taken
from the embryo itself, only the growth medium in which it was previously cultured. If this were to become mainstream and an accessible
technology in all laboratories, it might replace or at least complement
the visual embryo selection methods commonly used.

What should patients' realistic expectations be?
It is entirely understandable that women should form attachments to
embryos but it is important to remember that they are not yet babies

– they only have the potential to become babies. Most fertilised eggs (or embryos) conceived during a woman's natural cycle never implant or continue to develop to become a baby and this fact becomes more apparent as a woman's age increases. The IVF process provides more embryos in one cycle but doesn't change this unfortunate reality. Generally, if an embryo is chosen to be transferred to the womb and is considered 'good enough for transfer' there must be some hope. But we think it is important to manage expectations without giving false hope by providing both statistical information and information specific to each patient coming through treatment. Ultimately, the embryo is only part of the puzzle and many other factors, such as the womb lining, need to be optimal as well.

I was very interested in Alan's explanation of designer babies – this has generated mass media attention over the years. Could there ever be a 'designer baby'?
This term is provocative, wholly media-generated and I don't like it. It suggests that we can design a baby with each and every desirable genetic trait a parent could wish for, presumably to give the resulting child the best possible start and advantages in life. The reality is that, for most of us, our choice of partner is the closest we will get to designing babies.

The technology associated with producing 'designer babies' is already with us. Using pre-implantation genetic diagnosis (or PGD), we can avoid the birth of children with serious genetic disease in families with a history of the disease. PGD is a very early form of genetic testing on embryos produced using IVF techniques. By testing embryos and selecting those free from specific genetic diseases, couples hope to have a child free from the disease that plagues their family. PGD has been used to help thousands of families with hundreds of different genetic problems that would, if ignored, lead to enormous suffering in children.

Instead of trying to prevent an undesirable disease, however, what if we tried to select for a trait generally regarded as desirable, such as intelligence? Let's pretend that we know there are only five genes responsible for intelligence (in reality there is no single gene for intelligence and there are probably over a hundred). We might see the high-performance version of each gene in only one in every four children. To get the desired combination of high-performance versions for all five genes in the same child, we would need 1,000 children. In terms of success with PGD this would mean having over 5,000 embryos. It would take one woman 40 years to complete enough IVF cycles to generate this number of embryos. If you use a more realistic number of genes, say 50, then using the same calculation, the chance of getting the desired combination for all 50 genes in the same embryo is a number with 30 zeros after it. Designing a baby using genetic selection from what is already present in the parents for traits as complex as intelligence is not a reality.

You need a lot of embryos and the 'right' raw materials to able to create a designer baby. Some traits are purely down to nature (genetic), some nurture, but most of what we think of as desirable in children is a complex mixture of the two.

The Two-week Wait

Having got this far is a great achievement. Many of you will be feeling elated that you have good embryos, but some of you will not have had such positive news. It is not unusual to feel a bit isolated and insecure because, after all those tests and scans, suddenly there is nothing more to do. Make your mind up now to put your energy into being positive no matter what. What have you got to lose?

As a general rule, women feel optimistic and hopeful for the first three to four days. I think the worst time is often around Day 6 or 7 when you may be hypersensitive to everything that is going on. Clients often come back to the clinic around this time for a session of hypnotherapy with positive visualisation or breathing/relaxation (qigong). You may find the second week absolutely drags by and your mind plays tricks with you. The best thing to do is try to distract yourself; perhaps go to the cinema and watch a happy film. Just try and do whatever you can to keep yourself occupied.

Tips for Looking after Yourself

1. **Make sure you rest.** My opinion is that you should go to bed after the transfer, or at least lie on the sofa with your feet up and relax – watch a film, read a book, listen to music or do some visualisation. I realise there is no evidence to support what I am saying, and many doctors do challenge me on this point, but I stick by it. I would never make any woman feel bad about going back to work immediately, but a day's rest may do you some good. I am asking you to look after yourself and give yourself a bit of nurturing, which is something most women are so poor at doing. I accept that what works for one woman may not work for another, but in those early days rest as much as you can.

2. Having **support,** either from your partner, a friend or someone in your family who is optimistic and positive, can be a great help. Many of the IVF internet forums also offer support and hope.

3. **Have acupuncture before and after transfer if you can.** Some of the research on acupuncture has been done with women having acupuncture 25 minutes before and after embryo transfer, but this is next to impossible to achieve unless your

IVF clinic offers acupuncture or you are able to take your acupuncturist to the IVF unit. We do acupuncture on the day of transfer. Some women have both pre- and post-transfer treatments; other women have one – either before or after to fit in comfortably with the timing of their transfer.

4. **Don't have hot baths.** Excessive heat may damage the embryo, and warmth and moisture may increase your risk of infection. Stick to showers until the pregnancy test.

Dos and Don'ts after Transfer

- Don't lift heavy objects.
- Don't drink caffeine.
- Don't drink alcohol.
- Don't have sex (see page 360).
- Don't exercise excessively: gentle walking is fine.
- Do play some uplifting music and laugh – get some of those feel-good hormones circulating.
- Don't listen to anyone who has a bad IVF story – block your ears, or before they start their tale, ask them if it has a positive ending – if not, don't listen.
- Do think carefully about work. Many women say that work is a huge distraction for them, so easier to be immersed in work. It really depends on your job, any travel involved and how you feel as an individual and whether work are aware and supportive.

Remember, it's not over until it's over – many women convince themselves that the cycle hasn't worked because they have had a bleed. They stop taking progesterone and then find they have a positive pregnancy test. At this stage please do not rely totally on your gut feeling.

Even if the signs are not positive, keep taking the drugs until you have confirmation or have at least spoken to the clinic.

Frequently Asked Questions

- *Can the embryos fall out?*
No. Many women are concerned about this, especially if they have been exerting themselves, but the embryos can't fall out (see page 343).

- *Is it okay to have a cup of tea the day after embryo transfer?*
Avoid tea and coffee if you can because of the caffeine. I also recommend that women drink no alcohol at all after transfer.

- *Can complementary therapies help during my two-week wait?*
You need to be cautious about how many treatments you have. This is a very anxious time, and if you have any doubts at all about any treatment, the best thing is to do nothing. However, anything that helps you relax, reduces your stress levels and makes you feel positive is good.

- *Can I exercise after IVF?*
I would not recommend exercise during the two-week wait.

- *Can I fly during, as well as after, IVF?*
Many women who fly regularly worry about this when they are going through IVF. Certainly, many aspects of air travel are difficult and tiring, such as giving yourself injections while travelling and coping with different time zones. Although many doctors feel there is no evidence to ban flying during or after IVF, many women feel instinctively that it is not right to fly at this time. I don't encourage long-haul flying as I feel women have gone through so much already that it is not worth the risk. Obviously, flying is necessary if you have had egg

donation overseas, but I usually encourage such women to try and stay a little longer after the embryos have been put back.

● *Is bleeding and slight cramping normal after embryo transfer?*
Yes, it is. Some women are more prone to bleeding. Rest as much as you can and if you have any concerns at all about whether the symptoms you are experiencing are normal, call your IVF unit.

● *Am I allowed to swim post transfer?*
I don't think you should swim after embryo transfer. There is no evidence to support this but I just feel it is best to avoid the chemicals in the water. The same applies to jacuzzis, saunas and baths. If you are going to have a massage, that's fine, but avoid the tummy area.

● *What about having sex after IVF?*
I think it is best to wait until you get your pregnancy test results. Sometimes the ovaries are quite swollen so it may be a bit uncomfortable, but as always individual circumstances vary and it is best to be guided by your IVF clinic.

Coping Strategies for Each Day

During these two weeks, women are very aware of any changes in their body. Just because you have period-type pain it doesn't mean your period is going to come. Being bloated can be a good sign, or it can be because of the progesterone. Having tender or sore breasts can be a good sign too, but it can also be due to the drugs you are on. I think the most important thing during these two weeks is to feel you have done everything you possibly can.

In my research for this book, I asked 50 women who were attending the Zita West Clinic for IVF support to complete diaries during their two-week wait. They were asked to write down their thoughts and feelings, scoring each day from 1 to 10 to reflect how they felt physically and emotionally: the higher the score, the better they felt. I also asked them to reflect on what helped them get through each stage along the way. The diaries were terribly moving. It almost felt as if you were looking into somebody's soul while they were going through an intensely emotional experience. I am indebted to all the couples who shared their intimate thoughts.

Day 1 – Transfer Day

The diary scores on these days are really high, between 8 and 10. Most women feel very positive, elated to have got this far, especially those who were told they had good embryos. Physically, many women feel a bit fat; 'bloated' is a common expression in the diaries.

The Ugly Side of IVF

Women imagine that they will be fussed over and nurtured by their partner and family during the two-week wait. Sometimes, however, the reality is very different. I have seen women in floods of tears because they have had a row with their partner on transfer day and feel that this has caused it not to work. It is so often a matter of the tension building between the two of you as this is a very anxious time for everyone. This process challenges every aspect of your relationship.

- 'Feeling nervous but excited. Slight niggly pains in the evening. I'm hoping this is the norm.'
- 'Felt really disappointed when I found out that embryos had died overnight and I only had two to put back. Named my embryos silly names so I can talk to them and encourage them to grow.'

- 'Elated as I had a hatching expanding blastocyst put back.'
- 'Third attempt. I hope it works this time. Was anxious going in today but all three embryos were grade one.'
- 'We only produced one egg but decided to go ahead anyway.'
- 'Too emotional – feel like I have just finished an exam. Relieved it is done but slightly flat.'
- 'Had a big row with my husband about attending a family gathering when I wanted to rest. Feel emotionally unsupported and worried I haven't got off to the best start.'

Day 2

The scores are still high. At this stage, I feel that listening to music and doing some relaxation and visualisation helps women remain positive. Many women feel much more tired on Day 2 because they start to relax after being on an intense emotional high. Remember, we are all different. If you are going stir crazy by being on bed rest, get up and have a gentle amble.

- 'Physically bloated. Loose stools – I think this is due to the progesterone.'
- 'Have taken the week off – looking forward to indulging myself.'
- 'I have been visualising my embryos. I cried when I read a supportive email from a friend.'
- 'Feel very tired today. Thought I would be bored at home but slept a lot.'

Day 3

The scores are still high. Some women are getting ready to go back to work. Many are wondering what their embryos are doing at this point so I suggest trying to visualise them. Others report feeling cramps and looking for signs that the IVF is working, especially if they have had a blastocyst transfer.

- 'Slight cramping in my tummy. Still really tired.'
- 'Busy doing my visualisation CD.'
- 'Low energy today – couldn't relax properly.'
- 'Had a bad night's sleep – woke at 4am.'

Day 4

The scores are still high. A lot of women have gone back to work and are grateful for the distraction. They are still feeling positive and are starting to believe it might happen for them.

- 'Feel I want to be with people today.'
- 'Back to work today. Ran for the bus. God, I hope that doesn't mean it hasn't worked.'
- 'Didn't sleep well – kept thinking about what I'll do if it doesn't work.'
- 'Feel I have a bit more energy.'

Days 5, 6 and 7

The scores now drop significantly. The average score during this time is 4–5. Most women find it difficult to sleep at this point. They worry about whether or not the IVF has worked. They become aware of every ache and pain, and try to work out if these are associated with a pregnancy. Many women feel very weepy and emotional.

When you are feeling like this it is important to seek help. Think about who could support you at this time. It could be your partner, a family member or a close friend. You need to be able to talk to someone. Think about your partner as well. Tell him how you are feeling; otherwise he may misinterpret your moods, which can cause acrimony. He needs to stay positive, too. Many women are aware that they are very snappy and miserable at this point, and nothing anyone does seems to make them feel better. You may benefit from a relaxation therapy such as hypnotherapy or massage (avoiding the tummy area). Fun distractions are usually helpful; talking, socialising and laughing are great therapy. Do anything that helps you change your mindset and feel a bit more positive because dealing with the uncertainty at this point is very difficult indeed.

- 'My body feels slightly different. I feel good emotionally.'
- 'Saw family – it definitely lifted my spirits. Feel cramp-like pains – please don't tell me it hasn't worked.'
- 'Not good today – crying over silly things.'
- 'Not sleeping – so confused as to whether I am pregnant or not.'
- 'Went to church and prayed – felt better.'

Days 8, 9, 10 and 11

On these days the scores for the majority continue to drop down. Many women are trying to be as positive as they can. I have to stay positive as well, to support my clients. Nowadays women are testing for pregnancy much earlier because there are tests on the market that can show early pregnancy. Scores remain high for those who found they were pregnant, but come crashing down for those who tested negative.

Those who did get pregnant:
- 'I do the test and it flashes positive before I even come out of the bathroom. I can't believe it so I do another brand. It's true – we have got a big fat positive!'
- 'We both stood in the bathroom looking at the line. My partner started to cry which really shocked me as I had never seen him like that before.'
- 'Oh my God, I'm pregnant. After five attempts I never thought I would say the word "pregnant".'

Those who did not get pregnant:

- 'I am so used to being disappointed. I just feel numb.'
- 'Started my period today, went for a blood test. Had a cry with the nurse and consultant I had seen on and off for the last seven years.'
- 'A third negative test but still no period. I have to accept the game is over for me.'

The diary scores reflecting women's mood during the two-week wait showed a similar curve to some of the work done by Dr Jacky Boivin at Cardiff University. She has done a lot of research on the psychological impact of IVF including levels of anxiety, depression and positive effect during an IVF cycle. The psychological impact of IVF is of increasing concern for IVF clinics due to the high drop-out rate after unsuccessful attempts.

The Male Perspective on IVF

I was interested in how men coped with their partner during an IVF cycle so I did a short questionnaire survey of 50 men attending the Zita West Clinic. Many men said their partner found the IVF process painful and depressing but had great stores of patience. The men themselves said they coped with support from their partner, but some did find it difficult to handle the mental stress. A lot of the men said it was the small things that upset their partner. The physical side of their relationship seemed to be okay.

I asked the men what support they felt they were able to give their partner. Many said it was hard to give the support needed because they felt they were being completely pushed out, and they felt guilty that their partner was having to go through all the discomfort and emotional drama. At times they felt they were being punished, almost as if it was all their fault, especially when it was a male fertility issue. Some felt that they were supportive by being positive, providing constant companionship, accompanying their partner to IVF appointments, administering the injections, giving encouragement, doing jobs around the house and listening when she wanted to talk. Practical support seemed to be the biggest thing men felt able to offer. Some said they found emotional support much harder because they couldn't fix the problem and didn't know how to do or say the right thing.

I asked the men what emotional support they felt they needed when their partner was going through IVF. Some said they felt it would help to talk, but they found it difficult to talk to friends about it. They felt neglected because so much of the emphasis was on the woman. For the most part, they were devoted to their partner, and they felt guilty and disloyal if they ever sounded off to somebody else about their feelings and emotions. Others felt they just needed to support each other.

For the majority of men the most difficult part of the IVF cycle was clearly the uncertainty. Many men found the two-week wait almost impossible to bear. They felt they were walking on eggshells, not knowing what to do or say. For others it was not being able to see friends and family because their partner would get very resentful. One man had written, 'I find it most difficult having friends and family I no longer see because my wife gets so upset and angry. I feel we have no friends to talk to; the world has completely narrowed down. I don't know what to say that is right. I feel my wife has become very difficult to deal with at all times, and years of infertility have left her very bitter. I can understand the sadness and grief when results are negative, but the attitude to the rest of the world I can't agree with.'

There are always two sides to everything so take stock from reading some of these opinions from men. Think about your relationship, and ways that you can improve things. Look after your man as well while you are going through IVF. Communication is so important so don't forget to talk to one another and express your feelings.

Testing for Pregnancy

Your IVF clinic will give you a date when you should go in to have a pregnancy test done: this is usually 14–16 days after egg collection. However, I don't know any woman who sticks to these dates. Generally, women are so anxious leading up to the pregnancy testing date that many of them test themselves with the new kits which can detect the pregnancy hormone very early. However, they can be quite misleading. Different clinics will ask you to test at different times, which can be frustrating, especially if you have a friend at another clinic who has been told to do a test at a different time.

The Quantitive Beta hCG Blood Test

On about the 14th day after egg collection, most clinics will ask you to do a urine test. Some will also do a blood test, both of which can diagnose whether you are pregnant. This identifies the presence of the hormone hCG, which is produced in small amounts in early pregnancy. This test will usually be repeated two days later to see if that level has doubled. If it has, it is a good indication that the pregnancy is starting to implant.

The clinic will probably keep you on your progesterone supplements (e.g cylogest pessaries or progesterone injections) for around two to eight weeks or more following the confirmation of pregnancy. As the pregnancy progresses, the placenta takes over the production of progesterone, but medical opinion is currently divided on the optimum time to continue progesterone supplementation. For some

Some Early Signs of Pregnancy

There are many signs and symptoms of early pregnancy, including:

- Lower abdominal cramps
- Tiredness
- Breast tenderness
- Metallic taste in mouth
- Nausea
- Dizziness and fatigue
- Fainting spells
- Aversion to certain smells and foods

women this can be a highly anxious time, especially if they have previously miscarried. Although they might be expected to be elated after spending so much of their lives having fertility issues, often they are surprised by the result and start to experience a new level of anxiety.

A small degree of vaginal blood spotting is not uncommon when women are pregnant. This can be caused by a variety of factors:

- The embryo is embedding into the endometrium (the so-called 'implantation bleed').
- It may be a miscarriage or an ectopic pregnancy (see page 375).

There is no way of knowing what causes the spotting in these early stages, and it is hard to isolate the problem. Many women that have very slight bleeds are convinced that it is the end, that they are no longer pregnant. I have heard numerous women tell me this, when it turns out that they are still pregnant. It is very important to keep having the blood tests done so that you can see whether the hCG level has slowed down, dropped or is continuing to rise.

> ## Case Study
>
> Beth had a positive pregnancy test following IVF but started to bleed over a weekend and was convinced it was over. She stopped taking her progesterone and spent the weekend in bed in tears. She had a scan on Monday morning and was still pregnant. She had been pregnant with twins but had lost one.

Possible Difficulties Occurring During an IVF Cycle

Things don't always go to plan, which can be demoralising. Difficulties can occur at each stage of the IVF process from down-regulation through to ovarian stimulation and beyond:

Problems with the Endometrium

Just as in a natural menstrual cycle, the womb lining is under the influence of oestrogen and progesterone. The lining should be very thin after the period, increasing in depth during the stimulation phase as the follicles produce oestrogen and then becoming much thicker under the influence of progesterone – ready to receive the embryo.

Down-regulation Phase: Lining Still Too Thick or No Bleed

Some women will not get a bleed at the expected time or find that when they go for their scan to confirm that the down-regulation drugs have been effective, their womb lining hasn't thinned enough for the stimulation phase to be started. After excluding the presence of a pregnancy, they may be given a progesterone-based drug to encourage a bleed. If this happens there may be quite a delay until you can start stimulation, so the whole cycle can seem a lot longer. I generally suggest that a woman has some acupuncture alongside the progesterone supplementation to help induce a period.

Lining Not Thickening During Stimulation

If the lining isn't thick enough, then it will be harder for the embryo to implant and grow successfully. There are a number of possible causes for a thin womb lining, including inflammation, infection, scarring and fibroids. These things may irritate the endometrium and prevent the development of a thick, lush womb lining. Some of these causes can be ruled out prior to the cycle starting based on the tests and investigations that have already been done. Sometimes your doctor may suggest a hysteroscopy to take a closer look at the womb lining and exclude problems.

If I have a client whose lining has not been thick enough in one cycle, I will often recommend that she has acupuncture to try and boost the uterine blood flow. Some doctors may try using aspirin or additional oestrogen therapy prior to stimulation, to improve the receptivity of the endometrium, but success is limited. Some clinics use the drug Viagra, which is usually given to enhance male sexual performance. In women it can be used in tablet or suppository form to try to increase the blood flow to the womb, but this is highly controversial. Not all clinics use it because they feel the evidence is not strong enough to support its use.

Formation of Cysts

Other women may find that ovarian cysts have formed. These enlarged, fluid-filled follicles, which are detected on scan, may be left over from a previous cycle. A cyst raises oestrogen levels, causing a hormonal imbalance and this keeps the womb lining thick at a time it should have thinned. The doctors will decide how best to treat a cyst, depending upon its size. Some cysts will disappear in a few days; others may need to be aspirated, and this will help the oestrogen level to fall. Some doctors use the contraceptive pill to try and suppress the development of cysts.

Ovarian Hyperstimulation Syndrome (OHSS)

Ovarian hyperstimulation syndrome (OHSS) is a complication of ovarian stimulation. It is thought that the stimulated ovaries release chemical substances which make blood vessels more porous. Fluid leaks out of these small blood vessels leading to dehydration. The fluid accumulates in the abdominal cavity or, in more severe cases, around the lungs or even the heart.

The severity varies from mild to severe. About 3–10 per cent of women going through IVF will suffer mild hyperstimulation. OHSS develops when the ovaries respond too highly to the medication. This might occur in the lead-up to egg collection once the hCG trigger has been given or after the eggs have been retrieved. Many women going through an IVF cycle will have some degree of overstimulation because this is what IVF is all about; however, some women will be more susceptible to more serious problems. Traditionally, women who produce more than 20 follicles greater than 14mm in diameter, and whose oestradiol level is higher than 4,000 pmol/l on the day of the hCG injection, have an increased risk of developing severe ovarian hyperstimulation syndrome (OHSS). In severe cases the ovaries may become so enlarged (with cysts up to 5cm) that there is a danger of twisting or rupture. There is also a serious risk of thrombosis (blood clots) and kidney problems (and even death). At times urgent hospitalisation is required. Symptoms include:

- abdominal distension (bloating) due to fluid collecting in the abdomen
- weight gain
- abdominal pain
- nausea
- vomiting
- backache

In severe OHSS, symptoms also include:

- dark-coloured urine and less in amount
- extreme thirst
- marked abdominal bloating and pain (including fluid in the abdominal cavity)
- difficulty breathing (due to fluid in the chest cavity)
- pain in the calf
- chest pains

If there is a risk of OHSS, doctors might use 'coasting'. This is where a woman stops FSH injections and is left for a number of days (usually 1–4) until her oestradiol levels have come down. The difficulty about this condition is that women often do not know they have it, or are unaware of the potentially serious implications. You are more at risk if you are young, slim or have PCOS and a high level of AMH. If you develop any of the above symptoms, seek medical help immediately. If you do end up in A&E, it's very important to tell your doctor that you are going through fertility treatment.

If embryos have been created when OHSS happens, doctors may decide not to transfer them back, depending on the severity of the condition. It may be preferable and safer to let the swelling go down and the body get back to normal. The embryos may be frozen and transferred on another cycle and then have a good chance of successful implantation.

Potential Risk of Cancer

Women often express concern about cancer risks related to ovarian induction or IVF. There have been some concerns about the potential increased risk of breast and ovarian cancer, but the current research shows no increased risk of these cancers in women who had undergone IVF compared with other women with fertility problems who had not had ovarian stimulation. There is a possible increased risk of endometrial cancer but this has also been observed in women with fertility problems who have not undergone ovarian stimulation.

If a woman has had an oestrogen-dependent cancer, such as breast cancer, she may still be able to undergo ovarian stimulation within a clear time-frame, provided her oncologist and gynaecologist have both agreed to this and have outlined any potential increased risk to her future health.

When You Are Not Responding to the Drugs

Some women will find that their ovaries do not respond well or sometimes completely fail to respond to the stimulation drugs. This can be due to a number of factors:

- age – older women will not respond so well
- hormonal imbalance where the FSH level is high at the start of the cycle
- a diminished ovarian reserve (low AMH or antral follicle count) in younger women

- lack of monitoring: the stimulation drugs were not increased when perhaps they should have been to help with the stimulation
- the womb lining didn't thicken as it should

Any of these factors can be very demoralising. A decision needs to be made as to whether to carry on with an IVF cycle in the hope that the one egg that is needed will be good quality. Very often the doctors advise against doing this because having to go through a surgical procedure and anaesthetic just to get one egg which might be immature or not fertilise is not always a good thing to do. Also, if it is your first IVF cycle doctors don't know how you are going to respond, so another cycle will give them a chance to look at doing something different. Just because you haven't responded in one cycle doesn't mean you won't on another one.

At this point some clinics will offer to do IUI (intrauterine insemination) instead of IVF (see page 243). If this happens then I usually suggest my clients have more frequent acupuncture, and use visualisation techniques. In some cases it has made a difference in terms of the number of eggs produced and some women have felt convinced that the acupuncture and the positivity engendered helped to bring about a successful outcome.

Complications of IVF

There are complications to everything in life. For most people who go through IVF, everything is fine, but serious complications can occur, such as ovarian hyperstimulation syndrome (see page 371) and ectopic pregnancies (see below). Infections and bleeding can also occur at the time of egg collection. The main complication of IVF is multiple pregnancy, so this is where eSET has such a strong role to play. If a woman is attending a private fertility clinic and has serious complications, she will be transferred to an NHS hospital.

Ectopic Pregnancy

An ectopic pregnancy is a devastating event for a woman, whether she becomes pregnant naturally or following IVF. This life-threatening condition occurs in 1 per cent of natural pregnancies and results from the fertilised egg implanting outside the cavity of the womb, usually in the tube. As it grows, it causes bleeding and pain. If not treated it can rupture the tube and cause abdominal bleeding, potentially placing the mother's life in danger.

Case Study

Julie had a negative pregnancy test and had started to bleed so she convinced herself she was not pregnant. She had a pain on her left side which she thought was down to the fact that she had lots of follicles on that side. A week after taking her test she collapsed on the train to work and was taken to hospital where they discovered she had had an ectopic pregnancy.

Risk factors for an ectopic pregnancy are:

- previous ectopic pregnancies
- endometriosis (see pages 178, 254)
- pelvic (lower abdominal) surgery
- damage to the fallopian tubes due to pelvic inflammatory disease
- hydrosalpinx (collection of fluid in the tube, see page 256)
- smoking: women who smoke 20 cigarettes a day are thought to have four times the risk of an ectopic pregnancy, which is a very good reason to give up smoking

- IVF (see below)
- age: older women are thought to be at higher risk of having an ectopic pregnancy

The risk of an ectopic pregnancy following IVF is about 3 per cent. This can happen if some of the fluid containing the embryo(s) leaks into one of the fallopian tubes. Sometimes, the transferred embryo(s) float around in the womb cavity and find their way up into one of the fallopian tubes.

An early diagnosis of an ectopic pregnancy is important as this can be a surgical emergency. In some cases, an ectopic pregnancy happens very early and is absorbed by the body: there are no symptoms and no treatment is required. Otherwise what happens is the fertilised egg (which usually takes four to five days to travel along the tube into the womb) gets stuck and starts to implant either in the tube or somewhere else outside the womb.

After around seven days, the woman may feel a sudden pain on one side of the lower abdomen, or this may be felt as a referred pain in the tip of the shoulder. There may be dark bleeding from the vagina, and pain when passing urine or having a bowel movement. A blood test is done to diagnose an ectopic pregnancy. It measures the pregnancy hormone Beta hCG to see if the levels are rising. A trans-vaginal ultrasound scan will also be performed, and may need to be repeated. The risk of a further ectopic pregnancy is around 7–10 per cent.

Ectopic pregnancies are generally treated surgically and a woman may lose her tube along with the pregnancy. She will then need time to recover from the anaesthetic and the impact of the surgery. The drug Metothrexate has made non-surgical treatment possible. The drug disrupts the growth of the developing embryo, thus causing the pregnancy to end. Metothrexate is administered by injection in a specialist unit. As this is a powerful drug, women will be given very strict instructions regarding alcohol, folic acid and other drugs and will need to avoid sex for as long as the doctor advises. Beta hCG will be measured seven days after injections, and in most cases will start to decline. This will be monitored until the pregnancy hormone level reaches zero, which can take four to five weeks. If the hormone level plateaus, then another injection may be administered or surgery (dilatation and curettage, or D & C) may be needed.

Women can find it difficult to come to terms with having had an ectopic pregnancy. After the initial shock, there is the realisation that they have had a potentially life-threatening condition. If they have had a tube removed they may worry about future pregnancies. Although it is devastating to lose a tube, women can go on to conceive naturally. Provided the other fallopian tube is patent (open) and mobile (not tethered by scar tissue) there is good evidence that the 'good tube' can move around quite freely and even pick up an egg from the opposite ovary. So losing a tube does not necessarily reduce your chances of a natural conception by half. Women who have had tubes removed generally respond well to IVF treatment if everything else is working normally. For further information on ectopic pregnancy contact the Ectopic Pregnancy Trust (see Resources).

It can be very difficult to cope emotionally after an ectopic pregnancy. So often it is not possible to grieve in the way you would normally following miscarriage, due to the seriousness of the condition and all the emergency medical intervention. Many women experience a delayed grief reaction once the medical side has been sorted and can then feel quite devastated by the whole experience. Fertility counselling may help (see page 115).

Other Forms of Assisted Conception

Natural IVF

In natural IVF, one egg is collected from the woman's ovary in a natural menstrual cycle, using no drugs or medication. The advantage of this approach is that you do not need to have 'resting' cycles between treatment cycles. The success rate for this is very low. You have to remember that it is still an invasive procedure as the doctor has to go in and collect the egg. You can find yourself going to a clinic to do this month after month and ending up having conventional IVF.

Mild IVF

There is now a move towards women having milder drug stimulation. The side effects of the IVF drugs are reduced, as is the cost to the client, and there are very minimal risks of multiple pregnancies. Mild IVF is usually used on younger women. During the luteal phase, support is given in the form of progesterone. The aim is to collect between two and seven eggs, whereas in conventional IVF doctors try to get as many eggs as is safely possible, usually eight or more.

IVM

A new approach to assisted conception is to collect immature eggs and then mature them in the laboratory. This technique does not require the woman to have her ovaries stimulated so may be a safer option for some women – particularly younger women with polycystic ovaries.

Interview with Tim Child MA MD MRCOG, Consultant Gynaecologist at the University of Oxford and Director of the Oxford Fertility Unit

Tim has done a lot of work in the field of IVM. This type of treatment is still in its infancy but holds promise and hope for many women.

What is IVM?

It stands for egg in-vitro maturation (literally, maturing eggs 'in-glass'). During standard IVF, daily injections are given for around two weeks to stimulate the growth of multiple follicles. The eggs mature inside the follicles, are then collected, and IVF or ICSI is performed. The downside of IVF is that the two weeks of injection drugs are very expensive and are associated with a risk of developing ovarian hyper-stimulation syndrome (OHSS).

During IVM no ovarian stimulation is used at all. The immature eggs are collected, using the standard IVF egg-collection technique, from the tiny resting follicles present within ovaries (called 'antral follicles'). The immature eggs are matured in the laboratory ('in-vitro') for 24–48 hours and, when mature, are fertilised using ICSI. We need to use ICSI routinely because the egg shells harden during IVM. Once fertilisation has taken place one or two embryos are put back into the body the same as in IVF, and women are given oestrogen and progesterone tablets and pessaries until 10 weeks of pregnancy.

IVM eliminates the risk of OHSS and can be done whether or not you are ovulating. It is safer, simpler and cheaper than IVF, but it is less successful.

Which patients are suitable for this?

We decide who is suitable for this treatment by doing an antral follicle count (AFC), which is more important than testing the blood hormone levels. It's most successful in women aged 35 or below who have an AFC of at least 20. Women with polycystic ovaries, who have many antral follicles on scan, are particularly suitable for IVM. Around one in four IVM cycles will result in a clinical pregnancy with a heartbeat.

Where do you think IVF is going over the next five years?
We are trying to minimise the risk of multiple pregnancy so need to be improving the way we culture and choose the best fertilised egg for single embryo transfer.

Chapter 13

When IVF Works – A Positive Pregnancy

Any woman who has had difficulties conceiving or gone through IVF longs to be able to say, 'I'm pregnant.' It may seem incredible but, in practice, pregnancy often causes such women a great deal of anxiety. Many have been trying for a long time, have had previous miscarriages or had unsuccessful IVF cycles, and so they didn't really expect ever to be pregnant. For many women the happiness of finding out that they are pregnant is all too often quickly overtaken by a roller coaster of fear and elation during the first trimester. Fear that there won't be a heartbeat at the six to seven-week scan, elation when there is; fear that you might miscarry before 12 weeks, joy when you don't; and finally fear that there may be something wrong with the baby when you have your 12-week Down's syndrome scan, and sheer relief when you get past that point and all is well. At this stage you really must close the chapter on your infertility history as you have now reached an important goal. You are now a normal, pregnant, healthy woman and you must start seeing yourself as such, as the risk of miscarriage drops to less than 1 per cent once you reach 12 weeks.

I believe that emotional and psychological support is vital throughout this stage. Research shows that women who feel supported, and who have regular access to a midwife or practice nurse, have a much better chance of their pregnancy continuing. At the clinic we provide support for women from the moment they discover that they are pregnant and there are also many excellent early pregnancy units (EPU) in the NHS that provide such a service.

How Many Weeks Pregnant?

A natural pregnancy is usually calculated to be 40 weeks from the first day of your last menstrual period. However, when calculating how many weeks pregnant you are after an IVF cycle, you start to count two weeks prior to your egg collection so that by the time the result is positive you will be just over four weeks pregnant.

Managing Your Mind during Pregnancy

Early pregnancy can be an anxious time – largely due to 'fear of the unknown'. For many women at this stage they know everything about infertility, about IVF, even about recurrent miscarriage, but they have a very limited knowledge of what to expect when they actually do get pregnant. Most of the first trimester – 12 weeks – is spent waiting to have tests to see if all is normal. You are likely to focus on every little twinge and change in your body. Pregnancy symptoms vary from day to day and from woman to woman, and in the early days you will be adjusting to the changes that are taking place in your body. The common symptoms are tiredness, breast tenderness, nausea and vomiting. Women who experience unpleasant symptoms, such as morning sickness, sometimes feel guilty because they are not as happy as they think they should be.

One of the most important things you can do for yourself is to learn techniques to manage stress levels. This takes as little as 20 minutes a day. Maternal stress has been shown to have an impact on pregnancy. Some studies show an adverse effect on the environment in the womb when a mother's cortisol – the stress hormone – part of the fight or flight response, is raised. It is known that cortisol crosses the placenta. Isolated periods of stress are unlikely to be harmful, but prolonged stress which affects your everyday life and sleep patterns has been linked to increased anxiety in children.

There are many ways to release stress – it is a question of finding what works best for you. The main aim is to get your body into a state of physical and mental relaxation. When you practise relaxation techniques, both you and your baby will benefit. At the Zita West Clinic, we like to reassure women that they are doing everything right and offer them hypnotherapy and other relaxation techniques. (For more on managing your mind and complementary therapies, see Chapters 5 and 8.)

Older women can be particularly anxious during early pregnancy. They are affected by the statistics they read, for example about higher miscarriage rates in older women. Often, they have busy careers and a lot is expected of them in a working week. I advise them to embrace their pregnancy, to connect with their baby and to practise stress-reduction techniques, not to sit at home waiting in case something goes wrong.

Worries in Early Pregnancy

Spotting

If you experience blood spotting, don't panic, and don't stop taking any prescribed medication. Spotting appears to be more common in IVF pregnancies and it doesn't always mean that you are going to miscarry. Some women have a brown discharge that carries on; others experience intermittent bleeding in early pregnancy. If you are experiencing any kind of spotting or bleeding you should always contact your IVF clinic or GP so that a scan can be arranged if necessary. In some cases you may need to increase your intake of progesterone. I always advise women to rest as much as they can, avoid exercise completely and avoid sex. You may also need a lot of reassurance and support.

Case Study

Caroline, aged 40, had two unsuccessful IVF cycles before getting pregnant with her third cycle. During early pregnancy, she had some brown spotting which turned into a small red bleed. Caroline began to panic and felt convinced she was miscarrying, although she had no cramping. She contacted her IVF clinic who repeated her beta hCG test, and found it was still rising; her scan looked good and she continued her progesterone supplements. Caroline was still unconvinced and spent virtually all day in the toilet checking the bleeding. Despite the reassurance from her doctors, we had to work hard with her over the next few weeks to build her confidence, using relaxation techniques, hypnotherapy and a lot of telephone support. Her pregnancy continued successfully.

Weight Gain

Some women who have had IVF will feel bloated and may have gained more weight than expected. Some of the IVF drugs result in more weight gain and bloatedness during the early weeks. Many women are concerned about carrying extra pounds at the start of the pregnancy, as they think they will get much bigger as the pregnancy goes on. Pregnancy weight does sort itself out as the pregnancy progresses as long as you are careful about what you eat; some women are more susceptible to weight gain than others. Don't listen to stories from other women telling you that you are too big or too small. Unless you are pregnant with twins, you will not be showing until you are at least 14–16 weeks pregnant. The change you will notice early on is the rate at which your breasts are growing.

Tiredness and Sickness

Tiredness is often the first symptom that you will notice and you may well feel overwhelmingly tired during the first 12 weeks. It can be difficult to carry on with your usual routine during early pregnancy when you are feeling nauseous and tired. My advice is to rest, eat little and often and consider having acupuncture if you are feeling sick. Try and get to bed early at night and catch up with your sleep at weekends.

Work

Even if you don't want to let people know that you are pregnant until 12 weeks, it is a good idea to tell your boss or HR department as legally you have a lot of entitlements once you are pregnant. You are likely to feel exhausted at some point during the working day so this is not a time to increase your workload or take on any additional projects. It may help to spend some time during the day away from

—— Tips for Early Pregnancy ——

- Get plenty of rest.
- Take care with aerobic exercise for the first 12 weeks – your body needs time to adapt to being pregnant.
- Be careful not to increase your core body temperature as this can damage the developing foetus. Avoid electric blankets and saunas, for example.
- Don't have sex until after 12 weeks, especially if you have a high risk of miscarrying.
- Look at your work/life balance and try to reduce any stresses in your life.
- Take a multi-vitamin/mineral supplement, such as Vital Essence 1 and vital DHA (see page 149). The essential supplement to continue until 12 weeks is folic acid.
- Cut out all caffeine as it has been linked to miscarriage.
- Be cautious about flying in the first 12 weeks. Many people will tell you it's okay to fly but I don't think women with high-risk pregnancies should fly at this stage, especially long-haul. Although there is no evidence to support this, experience tells me that some women can get away with flying during early pregnancy while others can't so it's not worth taking the risk.
- Where possible, avoid toxins and pollutants that may cross the placenta (see Chapter 4).
- Don't drink unpasteurised milk or eat uncooked eggs.
- Avoid buying pre-packed food and salads or at least wash them well before eating.
- Avoid raw fish and shellfish such as prawns and mussels.
- Avoid peanuts and other nut products if you have a family history of allergies or eczema.

- Avoid liver and liver products as these contain high levels of Vitamin A.
- Avoid ripe and soft cheeses (such as Brie, Camembert, soft unpasteurised goat's cheese) and blue-veined cheeses (Bavarian blue, blue Brie, Danish blue, Dolcelatte, and so on). Stick to hard cheeses and soft, processed cheeses such as cottage cheese and cream cheese.
- Yoghurts are okay but try to choose organic brands.

your desk or work environment, for example by taking your lunch breaks outside the office if you can. Eat every two hours to stabilise your blood sugar. You may get a craving for carbohydrates such as bread, potatoes and pasta, so try to eat high-protein and low-glycaemic snacks and meals to balance this.

Look at your workload and what you have planned for the next few weeks. The most important factors are to make sure you rest and go to bed early, and that you have time to meditate, visualise (see below) and connect with your baby.

Visualisation

Some women who have had miscarriages or unsuccessful IVF cycles in the past can find it very difficult to connect to their pregnancy. They hold off, on some level, to try and protect themselves from disappointment should something go wrong. Use visualisation to make a connection with the baby each day and help you reach a state of calm and tranquillity. Try to avoid looking up things on the internet at this stage as it's only likely to cause you more stress and anxiety.

A Pregnancy Visualisation

- Make yourself comfortable – either sitting or lying.

- Imagine yourself in your perfect place – a place of peace and calm.

- Close your eyes and imagine a blue silk scarf or blue beam of light travelling down from the blue sky to your head.

- Let this blue stream pass down through your head to your forehead and on down to your cheekbones. Feel yourself relaxing more and more as the blue stream reaches your chin and jawbone.

- Release any tension from your jaw, allowing your lips to part a little and your tongue to relax in your mouth.

- Send the blue stream down through your neck and shoulders, feeling the muscles loosen and stretch as the blue stream floats on down to your arms and hands, resting for a moment.

- Allow the blue stream to circle your chest and stomach. Let your stomach go.

- Continuing on down through your body, allow the blue stream to circle your pelvic region. Feel the tension fade away as you become more and more comfortable, more and more at ease.

- Visualise your baby, growing in a calm, safe environment within you. See the womb and your baby receiving energy with every beat of your heart. You are his/her whole world; he/she has the backdrop of your heart beating rhythmically.

- Your baby feels calm when you are calm – all those 'feel-good' hormones pass through to him/her with every heartbeat, and every pulse brings him/her nourishment and helps him/her to grow and thrive.

- Focus your thoughts on your baby, on how much you love him/her and how precious he/she is to you.

- Allow the blue stream to flow onwards through your upper legs, so you feel yourself becoming more and more still and comfortable.

- Let the stream move on down, down towards your knees and lower legs. Feel your whole body relax now, relaxing into a gentle, calm state of wellbeing. Allow this wonderful feeling to continue all the way down, down through to your feet and toes.
- Rest, drift and dream. This is a moment of respite – a place of sanctuary.
- Rest for 5–15 minutes and then count up from 1 to10, ensuring you are fully awake, before you get up and move around.

Early Pregnancy Milestones

- **6–7 weeks:** A foetal heartbeat may be detected on an ultrasound scan.
- **11 weeks:** The development of your baby's organs is now under way.
- **12 weeks:** The time for Down's syndrome screening.
- **13 weeks:** The second trimester officially begins.
- **16–20 weeks:** The mother may be able to feel the first fluttering movements of the baby.

Twins

Many women are very excited when they discover they are pregnant with twins. The rate of twin pregnancies has risen due to IVF, but this should decline as clinics move towards replacing just one embryo (see page 344). A twin pregnancy carries a higher risk of premature labour, lower birth weight and maternal complications such as diabetes and high blood pressure. Some minor pregnancy ailments, such as sickness, are magnified in intensity. A twin pregnancy is also harder on the older mother. Having said all this, many women feel very well and have a good experience of twin pregnancy.

Although many women expect to be able to carry on as if they were pregnant with just one baby, expectant mothers of twins need to make lifestyle adjustments earlier and to get more rest. It's a good idea to decide early on in the pregnancy to give up work earlier, as the high risk time in twin pregnancies is around 20–28 weeks. Also, don't underestimate the impact of twins on life after pregnancy; so, as time goes on, start making necessary preparations.

At the Zita West Clinic we generally find that women need quite a lot of reassurance and hand-holding during early pregnancy but, as the weeks progress, they become more and more confident. Many women feel 'in limbo' after all the intensive monitoring of an IVF cycle – suddenly no one seems interested in them or their pregnancy achievement until 12 weeks of pregnancy. Our midwife-led Early Pregnancy Programme at the clinic is designed to fill this gap. The programme includes judicial use of acupuncture, relaxation therapies, massage and a gentle fitness programme.

For help and support in your area, talk to your GP or local midwife. There are many books, CDs and online resources providing help and support to enhance your pregnancy and your general wellbeing.

For more information on early pregnancy advice contact Tommy's Baby Charity at www.tommys.org or go to the Food Standards Agency website: www.eatwell.gov.uk

Chapter 14

When IVF is Unsuccessful

Case Study

I can't remember when I started to feel like a substandard woman. There wasn't a particular moment but a series of moments – failing to conceive after years of trying, while others fell pregnant at the drop of a hat; being asked at weddings when Andy, my partner, and I were going to have children; being prodded and invaded during various fertility tests.

In my 30s I met and fell in love with Andy, and we soon started to try and conceive. I'd had some fertility issues as a teenager and so was keen to try for a family as soon as possible. It was surprising how quickly our approach and attitudes changed, from being casual and optimistic to becoming more regimented and anxious over time. For the following four years, our mission increasingly consumed us; it was an almost constant pressure. Later on in our journey, as we were about to embark on our third round of IVF, a friend advised me to keep things in perspective, and not to let the fertility treatment take over. I bit my lip at that, and during similar 'counselling' conversations.

With each successive 'failure', talking about other people's children became more difficult. Relationships with friends and family were tested as our fertility treatment became more involved. Celebrations to mark pregnancies, weddings and children's birthdays were events to be endured and eventually avoided altogether. What should have been happy occasions, particularly with nieces and nephews, often left a bitter and empty aftertaste. There were few places to go to for support. I gradually became withdrawn and less able to talk about my unpredictable and often irrational behaviours and emotions.

The arrival of each menstrual period was devastating. It shouted out that I had failed again that month; I would then struggle to cope over the next few days – a period is not something you can ignore or hide from. I recall going to a friend's hen night and barely being able to speak because my period had arrived that day. What could I say, when all I wanted to do was cry?

After two years of trying we resigned ourselves to the fact that we probably needed fertility treatment. We had tried to avoid this for a while. First, it felt like admitting to my failure as a woman; I felt completely useless and pointless as a human being. Second, I was terrified by the idea that we would be put on 'trial' to prove that we deserved treatment (and so prove how useless I was!) I retold my infertility story to numerous doctors, nurses, fertility specialists, NHS administrators and so on. I specifically remember being told off by a young doctor for waiting until I was 34 to request fertility support (you are categorised as a 'geriatric fertility patient' at 36). We were challenged about the intimate details of our sex life. As time went on, I became more detached from these clinical discussions and learned to reduce my emotions to a mournful numbness to be endured as we spoke.

Each stage of the fertility testing process was more dehumanising than the last. My sense of femininity and attractiveness became more diminished each time. After each examination I would often head directly to the toilet and sob silently, bereft of my dignity. I felt ugly and lifeless; I couldn't cope with more disappointments and sex seemed pointless. It is ironic that the processes designed to help me fulfil my womanly functions also androgenised me.

We were presented with various options – IUI (insemination), clomiphene and IVF – but given our history and ages we were persuaded that our best option was IVF. After further tests and treatments, our IVF experience began. IVF treatment is hard and all-consuming from the moment you agree to undertake it to the moment you decide to stop. In our case this was two years. It is a common misunderstanding that IVF simply involves taking hormone supplements for a few weeks, followed by the removal of eggs and sperm and the implantation of an embryo. The physical side of this procedure is tough enough, although it varies according to doctor and individual. In our case it involved sniffing hormones at specific times (inconveniently, usually during meetings), taking tablets at fixed times up to six times a day, self-administering injections in my stomach and eventually legs, and being injected in my bottom by Andy (he assured me that it was as painful for him as me but I doubt it!) I observed others having even more gruelling experiences. Despite this, in many ways the physical side of the treatment is easier to bear; at least you feel you are positively engaged in activities that may help you become fertile and conceive.

More challenging are the months taken beforehand to prepare physically and emotionally to be 'match fit' for the clinical treatment. You never quite know whether you are doing enough, or indeed the right thing: the compass of beliefs around fertility enhancement range from the strictly scientific to superstition and witchcraft, with a healthy dose of alternative therapies in between. Without going to the absolute extremes, we changed everything: diet, lifestyle, the daily habits and activities that ultimately make us who we are. I stopped running, cycling, travelling, swimming, partying and taking hot baths. Ironically, these were replaced by rituals that you do when you are pregnant – not drinking, giving up certain foods, not 'overdoing it', drinking litres of water… Psychologically, I was encouraged to have faith that I would conceive, to imagine myself pregnant and with a baby. Logically this makes sense, and it is a philosophy that I adopt in other parts of my life – believe and it will happen; work hard and you will be rewarded. As a result, we nested; we thought of names; we discussed rooms that could be nurseries, and local schools; we considered our good and bad qualities as parents.

Then, after many months of build-up, we had an embryo implanted. We were lucky – not all couples who start IVF treatment reach this stage. Embryo transfer takes place up to five days after having the eggs removed in a minor surgical procedure. It is an agonising wait; I still remember much of each painful and long day. The transfer itself is clinical but also magical. Clinical because I was again on a bench, my legs wide apart, with cold metal implements being poked through my genitals by strangers; magical because hope and life was placed inside me and I was pregnant, if only for a few wondrous moments.

The following two weeks are another torturous wait. At this stage we changed from daily injections to suppositories – more intrusions. These weeks were the longest times of my life – and I have now endured them three times. I worried about each step, breath, change in my emotions, physical twinge or meal. I feared for anything that could bring about the loss of our precious cargo. To this day I struggle to ignore memories of things I did, decisions I took or emotional reactions that I feel might have caused the loss of our embryos.

Eventually we were able to take a pregnancy test. It is so difficult to describe the feelings immediately before and after getting these results. I have the memory of an overwhelming secret hope in one instance and drowning in grief the next. The grief in these moments was immediate, crushing and profound. I lost myself for the following days and weeks; for the first time I drifted away from Andy as we both struggled to come to terms with our individual loss. No more Fergus, Thomas… I grieved their children, my grandchildren and our future together. I knew that this sadness would be with me for ever.

Similarly overwhelming is the immediate desire to try again. It could be animal instinct, a determination not to be beaten, hope whispering through the darkest moment, a diversion from grieving. I have now responded to that impulse on two occasions; there are others who do so 10 or more times. I don't know if I am strong enough to do so again. I know this is different for every woman, man and couple.

It's now four months since the end of our last treatment and it's the first time in three years that we have stepped away from our fertility challenge and started to live our own lives again.

We've drunk red wine, run, travelled, worked, and worried about others rather than ourselves. The moment when we first had sex again, for no other reason than love and pleasure, was intense and beautiful and one that will stay with me for ever. We've started going to children's parties again; as time goes on the paralysis and grief of holding someone else's baby or being involved in parental discussions about others' children subsides. It still hurts to hear the news of another's pregnancy (I am shocked and frustrated by how powerful and painful my reaction is), but I find that the genuine joy and happiness for the friend or relative lift me more quickly each time. As a result I have genuinely enjoyed our 'release'.

After my first treatment, a friend sent us a card that said, 'You have to feel the rain to know the rainbow.' This is one of the few things that helped me make sense of our fertility journey. Andy and I have been blessed to discover the strength of the love, empathy, acceptance and support of our family and friends, and have had experiences that enable us to face our lives stronger together as a couple. I wish other women struggling with their own (in)fertility at the very least the same; at most, to become the success statistic we have yet to achieve.

When it Doesn't Work

It doesn't matter who you are – if your IVF cycle doesn't work, you will undoubtedly feel that you personally have failed and will look for reasons why. Even though some women find it hard to think positively and may not expect their IVF to succeed, the realisation that it hasn't worked still always comes as a shock.

Each of you will react in your own way and go through an array of emotions, depending on whether this is your first or subsequent attempt at IVF. It will take a while to get over the disappointment and to accept the loss, and then to move on and look ahead. You can't compare yourself to other people and their reaction when their IVF cycle doesn't work. Many women blame themselves for their IVF cycle not working, and this is a huge psychological setback. They are often unable to look forward at this point or believe that motherhood is still a possibility. So many of the women I speak to say they feel they have done something wrong for it not to have worked, but they have no idea what. Understandably, the question they ask themselves is, 'Why didn't it happen for me?' The tyranny of the 'shoulds' then come into play: 'I should have rested more', 'I shouldn't have had that extra cup of tea', 'I shouldn't have argued with my partner'. Trust me (and you know it really) – these are not the reasons why an IVF cycle didn't work.

You are likely to feel hurt, let down and betrayed. You will inevitably look for someone or something to blame. You may feel the need to lash out or punish in some way, or you may experience overwhelming feelings of jealousy that someone else's IVF worked. Some women shut down emotionally and can't be reached at this point. They remain silent and contain their feelings of anger, frustration and despair. So many women don't like who they have become and feel like a shadow of their former selves.

Much of my work and the work of my team involves supporting couples who have had an unsuccessful IVF attempt. I work with them to come up with a plan, making small changes to their lifestyle, helping with their emotional wellbeing and relationship, or finding them a clinic that is more suitable to their needs. I also help couples to move on to other options. I sit in my consulting room day after day and hear the most tragic stories. However, I am usually able to help couples feel more optimistic because there really are things that can be done to help them achieve their goal. Sometimes it will depend on how far they want to go to achieve it.

Should You Try Again?

Many couples want to know if they should try again. This depends on their circumstances. Is their relationship solid? Can they afford to pay for another cycle of treatment? Are they emotionally and mentally strong enough? Some couples re-evaluate their situation and decide they simply cannot go through the possibility of another disappointment.

Some couples give themselves a cut-off point in terms of how many cycles they are going to do: 'We are going to do three and if it doesn't work we will give up.' Doctors are often criticised for doing endless IVF cycles on women, but many women want to continue treatment at all costs, and persuade their doctors to keep going. Women, more so than men, sometimes feel that if they throw everything at the process then it will eventually work. My inclination is that something has to change – that might be to do with mindset, nutrition or lifestyle. It might be worth seeing if there is anything that can be done to improve the sperm, considering moving to another clinic or even taking a break from the whole process. For some it will mean moving on to egg donation, surrogacy, adoption, or moving on completely and coming to terms with childlessness (see Chapter 15).

Making a Decision

To help you decide whether or not to try again, work through the following plan, adapting it to your particular needs:

1. Wait at least two or three weeks before making your decision. This will give you some time to re-evaluate your
   emotions. Everybody reacts differently: some women want

to start again right away while others can't face another cycle and need a break. How long you leave it between cycles is up to you and the clinic treating you, but being strong emotionally, psychologically and mentally is all key to that decision.

2. Practise ways of changing your mindset to enable you to feel positive. Daily meditation or relaxation and visualisation will help you to feel more optimistic – this is very important at this point. Get emotional help and support if you need it.

3. Don't punish yourself – build treats into your lives. I have said so many times in this book that many of the couples I see put their lives on hold. They focus exclusively on IVF and forget to have fun. I sometimes think you just need a complete break from everything – eating whatever you like, drinking moderately – just to get a bit more fun back into your life.

4. Start to plan what you are going to do next. This could be a follow-up appointment at the clinic. Jot down a list of questions you want to ask your specialist when you next meet. Sometimes it helps to write down what happened during your last IVF cycle: what were you happy and positive about? What were the negatives? What would you do differently next time?

5. Think logically. So many women say to me, 'I am a failure' and that is not logical. You are not a failure as a person. Try listing your achievements and positive attributes (get your partner or a good friend to help you) to get the balance back.

6. Look at areas of your lifestyle where you can make improvements (see Chapter 4).

7. Don't give up on sex after IVF. I have seen many women get pregnant the month after IVF. I don't know why, but it can and does happen.

Before you decide on your plan of action, get some normality back into your lives. For weeks now your lives have been a whirlwind of appointments and preparing yourself for IVF. It is easy to lose your sense of self, and feel you are no longer the person you were. Many women ask me whether they can exercise again. I say just go off and do the things you have always enjoyed, including exercise; have a drink if you want; put recent events behind you and let go before you decide what to do next.

Doing an emotional workout and managing your mind (see Chapter 5) is key to coming to terms with an unsuccessful IVF cycle and deciding what to do next. I look at how the couple is managing emotionally and psychologically within their relationship. I want to find out what happened during their last round of IVF and look at what their plans are for the future.

To come through the rigours of IVF and to stay together afterwards is an achievement in itself for many couples. The more cycles you do, the harder it is. While some couples remain incredibly close, for others there are lots of barriers, and an emotional distance can develop. The first thing I look for is the dynamic between the two people and how they have survived the process. I give them a chance to sit down and talk about their thoughts and feelings, and get everything out in the open. I ask them how they coped and supported one another through the process, and what their differences are (see Chapter 6).

Why Does IVF Fail?

So many clients ask me, 'How can it have failed when the embryo was absolutely perfect? The cycle went like clockwork and yet it still failed.' All clinics offer a review consultation when it hasn't worked. This gives you a chance to discuss what happened in that cycle and what you want to do next. Doctors will look at the protocols you were on and may make some changes to them based on the way you responded. They will also look at the quality and number of embryos you produced. If your embryos were created using IVF and the number of eggs fertilised was fewer than expected, it may be suggested that in the next cycle ICSI is used (see Chapter 12). You may be offered further blood tests and investigations.

You need to remember that although the IVF cycle aims to get you pregnant of course, it is also the first opportunity to piece together some of the jigsaw to determine where the problem may lie – it provides an opportunity to have a close look at all stages of the process: your ovarian response, the health of the sperm, egg quality; to observe fertilisation and early embryo development microscopically and to look at the thickness of the womb lining and implantation. So it really acts as a learning curve for all – a final part of the diagnostic process.

Sadly for many couples, they have one round of IVF and feel so disillusioned by their experience that they never go back again. This often saddens me. Some couples only feel ready to attempt another IVF cycle after a number of years, by which time the biological clock could be working against them.

A number of studies have looked at the drop-out rate for assisted conception, and this varies from 12 per cent up to 62 per cent. These are not all couples who have come to the end of the road with IVF; this is mostly couples who have been told they have a good chance of a future cycle working. Similarly for most couples cost is not the issue as couples do not make full use of NHS-funded cycles and it is a similar situation internationally. Research has shown that couples find IVF psychologically stressful and many feel emotionally exhausted and that they have reached their limit.

Reasons why your IVF cycle was unsuccessful may include:

- Age and ovarian reserve (see below)
- Poor response (see page 411), the extreme form of which is ovarian failure (see page 412)
- The ability of the endometrium to receive the embryo (see page 418)
- Infections (see page 419)
- Immune system issues (see page 419)
- Male factor (see page 419)

Age and Ovarian Reserve

The main factor underlying successful IVF is the woman's age. This determines both the quantity and quality of her eggs. This can make depressing reading, but we have to remember that we are born with our full supply of eggs and chronological age is probably the single most important factor in IVF success. A woman's fertility is optimal between about 18 and 25 years (sadly this is often not an ideal time socially). Fertility levels stay fairly constant until early 30s when a gradual decline begins. By the time a woman reaches 35, the decline accelerates and, when she reaches 40, the decline becomes even more dramatic. Although assisted conception helps many couples, it is really important to realise that IVF cannot fully compensate for lost years and chances of conception.

For most women the decline in egg quality is around 37 years and it is this decline in egg quality, rather than the receptivity of the endometrium (womb lining), which affects the pregnancy rate. This is clearly demonstrated by the fact that there is a dramatically increased pregnancy rate for older women who use egg donation. With egg donation, a successful pregnancy is related to the age of the woman donating the egg and not the recipient. So although the chances of IVF success for a woman of 45 using her own eggs may be close to zero, if she were to use a donor egg, her chances of a successful pregnancy would be related to the age of the donor and in many cases approach or even exceed 50 per cent (see page 452).

As a woman gets older and towards the bottom of her egg pool, there are not only fewer eggs left, but many of the eggs will be chromosomally abnormal, so many embryos created would be aneuploid (chromosomally abnormal). It is estimated that at age 45, between 70 and 80 per cent of embryos will be chromosomally abnormal. So it is not simply a matter of getting the right mix of IVF drugs to be able to coax the development of the eggs, but the fact that if the egg is chromosomally abnormal it will either fail to fertilise, or if it does fertilise and create an embryo it may not divide properly or will later miscarry. With some chromosomal abnormalities (such as Trisomy 21 or Down's syndrome), the pregnancy may progress to full term. This is why older women are more at risk of having a baby with a chromosomal abnormality. All pregnant women are routinely offered antenatal screening and this is particularly important for older women due to the increased risk of chromosomal abnormalities.

This can be shown very simply in the image overleaf. On the left you see a representation of a sample from the ovary of a woman in her twenties, and on the right is a sample from the ovary of a woman in her forties. The younger ovary has not only a much higher number of eggs, but a very high percentage of good-quality chromosomally normal eggs (the 0s); whereas the older ovary has a very low total number of eggs left and, of the eggs that are left, there are proportionally a high number of Xs (the chromosomally abnormal eggs). So, whether the egg is released at ovulation in a normal menstrual cycle, or the ovary is stimulated with IVF drugs and a number of eggs are collected from the older ovary, there is a high chance of selecting an X, which would be less likely to fertilise or more likely to miscarry.

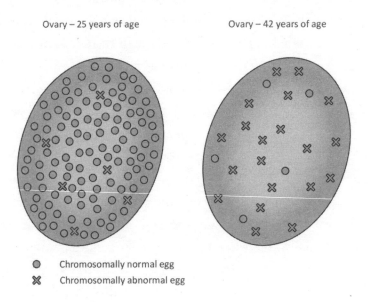

Ovary – 25 years of age   Ovary – 42 years of age

⊙   Chromosomally normal egg
✖   Chromosomally abnormal egg

A woman's chronological age is therefore the number one predictor of IVF success. A younger woman (under 35) who has a poor ovarian reserve (reduced quantity of eggs) will generally have a better prediction for IVF success than an older woman who (on paper) may have better ovarian reserve figures. This is because although a younger woman may have a reduced quantity of eggs, the quality will compensate. Remember, the younger the egg the more likely it is to be euploid (chromosomally normal). So, it is really a question of quality and not quantity.

A man's age is far less significant than a woman's age, although it seems there are some age-related changes from mid-40s onwards and this does have a minor role to play in delayed time to conception and unsuccessful IVF. As a man gets older he also has a higher chance of fathering a child with a condition such as autism (see page 180).

Ovarian Reserve Tests and IVF Predictions

There are basically three tests which are used to predict ovarian reserve: blood tests for FSH and AMH; and a scan to measure the antral follicle count (AFC). One or more of these tests will usually be done as a baseline prior to your IVF cycle to consider the most appropriate protocol (see page 299) and may be repeated if you have an unsuccessful IVF cycle. None of these tests can measure the precise number of eggs – they are simply a proxy for the number of eggs. The actual quality of the egg is much more difficult to assess.

- **FSH levels and IVF outcome** The FSH level gives an indication of the responsiveness of your ovaries. The FSH level can fluctuate, and can be linked to stress, but a higher level is never a good sign and shows your ovaries are struggling. Some clinics will be happy to observe your FSH level (and its relationship with oestradiol) at the start of each menstrual cycle and wait for the level to fall within their accepted limits to start an IVF cycle. Clearly reaching 'the perfect 10', or whatever score has been set, is likely to mean that the cycle has an improved chance of success, but these levels may never settle and therefore you could be wasting months or even years of valuable fertility time waiting for this hormone level to settle.

    If your FSH level does not settle, it may be more advantageous to move to another clinic that is happy to treat you despite the higher levels, and some clinics do get good results. Clearly your chances will never be as high as if you were within the optimum range, but if you are never allowed to start a cycle with one clinic, you will not be able to test out your chances. You may be able to go ahead with IVF with another unit which specialises in older women or higher FSH levels. As always, you need to understand your realistic chances in light of the clinic's success rates based on the woman's age and hormone levels, and make an informed decision about going ahead with treatment based on all the facts available.

- **AMH and IVF outcome** Anti-mullerian hormone (AMH) produced by the antral follicles strongly correlates with the number of antral follicles (the egg reserve). The AMH level is increasingly being used by IVF clinics as an indicator of how well you would be likely to respond to ovarian stimulation. It is possible that you may not have even been aware of the existence of this hormone and then suddenly find that if this level is low, you are being advised not to consider another IVF cycle and possibly to consider using donor eggs. It can be very difficult to hear this and it is completely understandable that you would want to consider a second opinion before giving up on having your own genetic child. The main use for AMH is as a predictor of IVF success. The lower the level, the less likely the chance of IVF success, but if natural conception is still possible, it seems that the levels of this hormone can be almost off the bottom of the scale and still natural conceptions happen (often when couples are least expecting it).

- **Antral follicle count (AFC) and IVF outcome** Small resting follicles (or antral follicles) in the ovary can be measured by ultrasound. There is a strong correlation between the number of antral follicles (see page 299) and IVF success. If a woman has a very low number of antral follicles left she will generally get a poorer response to stimulation, and few mature follicles, so a low success rate. A cycle may be cancelled or converted to IUI if there are insufficient mature follicles. Look again at the image on page 404 giving a representation of the quantity and quality of eggs – if you take a random sample from each ovary you get the idea about the number and quality of eggs.

Although this may all sound rather dire, on the brighter side there is some research that clearly shows that children born to older parents benefit from their parents' knowledge, experience and economic stability and tend to do better at school, so a biological disadvantage may be balanced to a degree by a social advantage.

I feel very strongly that while a woman still has eggs, she should be supported to do everything she can to give it her best shot. It is of course really important to sit with the doctors and hear the reality of the success rates in their clinics. You need to clearly understand how many women of your age group and with your ovarian reserve and hormone levels went on to have successful pregnancies. As ever, it is important to know the number of 'take-home babies' at the end – not positive pregnancy tests. Your goal is a healthy baby.

Many women panic about their age and the biological clock, often even before they have started trying to conceive. As I have talked about in earlier chapters, I honestly feel that although there is nothing you can do about the numbers or the genetic quality of your eggs, there is a lot you can do to improve the environment your eggs are developing in. Doctors agree that eggs can be aged by free radical damage, endocrine-disrupting chemicals and poor lifestyle choices, especially smoking (see Chapter 4). I believe that acupuncture and good nutrition with the use of antioxidants can help to improve the ovarian environment (see Chapter 8).

In our clinic programme for older women, we use relaxation techniques to help reduce anxiety levels. When a woman has been to a doctor and heard terms such as 'high FSH', 'poor egg quality' and 'menopause' all in one consultation, it will be a shock and can knock her confidence. One woman told me recently that she felt as if she had just been 'punched in the face' by a kindly but authoritarian doctor. Although I am a realist and understand the effect a woman's age has on her chances of a successful IVF outcome, most women want to feel they have done everything they can to improve their chances. When women are supported and feel more positive, I believe that they are more likely to conceive successfully. Many older women give up on IVF and then conceive naturally a while later. Older eggs may not handle so well in the laboratory yet may fertilise in their natural environment. We see this so often, particularly for couples with 'unexplained' infertility – it simply takes longer.

It is interesting talking to women who have been to America for fertility treatment. They tell me that at every step of the way everyone was so positive and said things such as, 'You've got fantastic follicles', 'Your ovaries are performing beautifully', 'We are going to get you a baby', 'You look amazing'. All these statements are a real boost to a woman, even if it doesn't happen. It is so unlike in the UK where some of the women, even before they start IVF or have had an ultrasound scan, are told, 'Your ovaries are poor', 'I doubt if it is going to work for you', 'We'll give it a go', 'You are likely to miscarry anyway'. Starting off with such negative statements discourages a woman on every single level.

I am not alone in supporting older women to try and do all that they can to have their own genetic child: some clinics specialise in this area. Mr Hossam Abdalla (see page 476) says in his interview: 'I now feel that women with reduced ovarian reserve should keep trying as long as they have eggs. I tell my patients that you can give up on me, but don't give up on treatment as long as you have eggs.' Statistics from clinics which specialise in treating low ovarian reserve reflect this – that the more attempts you make the more chance you have of luck being on your side with a good-quality egg. However, women are not simply egg-producing machines and the physical and emotional toll can be huge. You have to do what is right for you and your partner and not feel pressured in any way. Only you can know how you feel and when you are ready to move on.

DHEA

Many women are starting to enquire about supplements of DHEA (dehydroepiandrosterone) to improve egg quality. DHEA is a natural steroid hormone produced by the adrenal glands. Our bodies use DHEA to produce other hormones including testosterone and oestrogen. Levels of DHEA peak in our 20s and then decline as we get older. A synthetic form of DHEA (often dubbed 'the youth hormone') is available in tablet form and in theory should slow the ageing process.

DHEA is thought to stimulate the granulose cells in the ovary and increase the number of follicles, and therefore potentially the number of eggs. Some IVF clinics advocate its use for women with decreased ovarian reserve, while others do not. The Center for Human Reproduction in the US is conducting a large randomised study that might offer more concrete proof that DHEA can increase egg yield in older women or women with premature ovarian ageing. DHEA is available as a herbal supplement in the US, but is not available in the UK. It has to be used with extreme caution because, as it is a mild male hormone, women may experience androgenising side effects including acne, increased facial hair and hair loss. Long-term side effects are unknown, but there are concerns about increased risk of hormone-sensitive cancers such as breast cancer.

Interview with David H Barad, MD MS, Director of Assisted Reproductive Technology and Director of Research, Center for Human Reproduction (CHR); Associate Clinical Professor Departments of Epidemiology and Social Medicine & Obstetrics and Gynecology, Albert Einstein College of Medicine

Who will benefit most from DHEA treatment?
Within the ovary we can think of oocytes as existing in different stages of development: resting primary and primordial follicles; transitional stages of pre-cycle development; antral follicles and developing follicles. Most follicles are lost during the transition from resting to antral phase, a process that takes about three months. We use DHEA to help salvage more of these transitional follicles, bringing more follicles to the antral stage and thereby more follicles available to enter a treatment cycle.

Women suited to DHEA are those with evidence of decreased ovarian reserve or premature ovarian ageing. Women with premature ovarian ageing appear to have poor predictors of ovarian response relative to other women their age. We have found that women who use DHEA for 6 to 12 weeks before starting treatment will produce better-quality oocytes and embryos. As a consequence, pregnancy rates improve significantly. Furthermore, we have observed fewer miscarriages among the over-40s using DHEA but more studies need to be done.

What tests can predict the outcome of IVF?
The ovaries dictate a woman's response to IVF. Good ovarian reserve can predict IVF outcome. FSH is from the pituitary and is a secondary marker. Antral follicle count represents the follicles that will be available in a particular cycle. A relatively new test called AMH looks

at the egg reserves and is being used to predict IVF outcome in some clinics. AMH is produced by antral follicles and is a laboratory measure of how many antral follicles are present. Low AMH means few antral follicles, a high AMH means there are lots of antral follicles. However, women with a low AMH result can become pregnant, even when they have been told that there is no hope. The bottom line? Predictive tests may be used to counsel couples about the probability of success, but should not be used to prevent couples from entering treatment (see Chapter 9).

How is IVF treatment improving?

IVF treatment is a team effort. Treatment is now much more consistent throughout the world. Equipment has become more standardised, as has the training of embryologists. We are all benefiting from new communications technology, being able to speak to colleagues around the globe and share ideas.

Poor Responders

This is the term given to women whose ovaries haven't responded well to IVF stimulation. They may not have had enough follicles to get as far as egg collection, or they may not have been able to produce good-quality embryos and possibly had their cycle cancelled. It seems there are no universal definitions for 'poor responders'. Women often tell me they are 'poor responders' when in fact this is not necessarily the case. Sometimes their particular protocol was not right for them; or they may not have been monitored sufficiently closely. Simply by changing clinic, a woman will often produce good embryos and get pregnant. Fair enough, this is not always the case if the levels of FSH and AMH show a very low ovarian reserve, but a poor response in one clinic might not be the case in another. It is astonishing how one clinic can say the response was poor and suggest a move to egg donation, while another clinic may manage to get a good number of eggs from the same woman a matter of weeks later. It is a great relief to women when they realise they may not be labelled a 'poor responder' in the right setting, because they immediately feel renewed hope.

At the clinic we aim to work with women whose ovaries did not respond well to stimulation by boosting the blood flow to the pelvic region and the ovarian environment using acupuncture, reducing stress and optimising nutritional health.

Premature Ovarian Failure

Premature ovarian failure (POF), also known as premature menopause, occurs in about 1 per cent of women under the age of 40. This occurs when a woman under 40 has had four months or more without periods and has had two FSH levels in the menopausal range. The ovary can be quite unpredictable in the way it functions, and some women will still get pregnant. The cause remains a mystery. We have seen situations where a woman has been diagnosed with POF, but then finds that she is under extreme stress (possibly including rapid weight loss) and her periods stop, her FSH then goes up to try and kick-start the process – and may manage to once the stress is relieved. Clearly this diagnosis is devastating for a young woman: not only is she faced with the possibility of never having her own genetic child, but she also has to come to terms with the symptoms of menopause. Her friends are all still having periods and she feels like she is ageing rapidly. This is why it is useful to know the age your mother was when she went through the menopause – as POF may run in families. The potential for POF is being picked up earlier due to AMH testing.

Case Study

My husband and I were referred to a reproductive endocrinologist after trying to conceive for over a year. I was 33 at the time. They conducted the battery of normal tests, and my FSH came back at 34. The doctor advised me that this number, together with a low number of follicles responding to stimulation, supported his diagnosis of low ovarian reserve (or premature ovarian failure). This meant that I was low on egg reserve and the remaining eggs were [likely to be] bad. He told me it was unlikely that I would be able to get pregnant and carry a pregnancy to term. My husband and I asked what that meant in percentages. The doctor stated that they could never say 'never' because miracles happen, but that it would be a less than 1 per cent chance. I was numb and in denial. When we asked for a treatment plan we were told there were no treatments or effective plans for high FSH. IVF was not recommended and was no more successful than doing intrauterine inseminations (IUI). The doctor was willing to do a few cycles of IUI with us, but advised us that our best option would be a donor egg. He also stated that we had other family options, including not having children or adoption. My husband and I insisted on starting an IUI cycle and left to finish absorbing the information.

When the news finally sank in, I was completely devastated. Suddenly I felt that I had no purpose in life. I'm a woman. My purpose is to bear children, right? If I can't do that, then what purpose do I have? I had always envisaged myself as a mother, even when I wasn't actively pursuing it. Suddenly I had to re-evaluate myself and try to find some meaning in my life. I lost all interest in intimacy with my husband. I felt dysfunctional. If my body wasn't working properly, then why should I be sexually active? I spent days in bed crying. I then spent months scouring the internet for information. I became more and more depressed because there were no fixes I could locate. I went to see a Chinese medicine specialist and started having acupuncture twice a week and taking herbal medicines in the hope of improving my FSH. Of course, none of this was covered by health insurance. Infertility is so expensive – financially, emotionally and physically. This treatment didn't offer any definite answers but it at least gave me some hope where there was none before. I didn't see any changes in my FSH level, but I did begin to have healthier menstrual cycles.

My first round of IUI failed. Only one follicle responded. I began to search for another doctor. Every doctor's office refused to consider doing IVF with my own eggs. After about a year, I began to accept the idea of a donor. I had so many questions. Would I love a donor child as much as I would have my own biological child? How would I handle people saying the child has (or doesn't have) my eyes, hair and so on? I could never take credit for an inherited behaviour. I read many discussion boards on donor eggs that had experiences from both the donor and receiver and I finally began to feel that I was ready to pursue using a donor. However, I wanted to be sure I had tried everything first. I really wanted to try IVF, even if it was just for closure. I returned to the original diagnosing doctor's office. They agreed to 'test' my response by putting me on the injectable stimulations. They also ran the AMH test. If I responded well, they'd set me up for an IVF cycle. I responded with eight follicles! The doctor had hoped for two, expected one but was really surprised at eight. They finished the cycle as an IUI. I actually had a positive pregnancy test but there was never a heartbeat. The doctor's office advised me that this further supported what they had told me about my eggs being bad. They refused to pursue IVF, even with my better than expected response. My AMH test came back in the less than 0.1 percentage. This further supported the view that my egg supply was seriously diminished. I began to fear that I was running out of time. What if I went into full premature menopause and ruined my chances completely? I went ahead and called the donor advisor to arrange a consultation appointment. They never called me back. In the meantime, I had been reading an infertility board and learned of some clinics that were 'high FSH friendly'. I immediately called and arranged a phone consultation. I faxed my medical records and anxiously awaited the appointment.

The doctor was wonderful! During an hour-long consultation I was told that the doctors associated with this particular fertility clinic treated high-FSH women all the time with good results. They believed IVF to be the best treatment for cases like mine. My high FSH, I discovered, didn't mean I had poor-quality eggs; it just meant I had a poor response to stimulation. It also meant that the eggs might be more fragile and damaged by a higher than normal LH level that occurs with the high FSH. The clinic obtained good results by protecting the eggs from the LH. They would be willing to proceed to transfer with only one embryo (most other clinics I questioned required a minimum of eight follicles to retrieve and four embryos to transfer). Although the doctor told me I would find it more difficult to get pregnant than the average woman, it wasn't impossible. I had the right to try some IVF cycles before moving to a donor, which he agreed would be quicker and more definitive. He assured me that having IVF wouldn't ruin my chances of a future pregnancy with a donor egg. It would still be an option, even if I went into full menopause. Age is more of an indicator of success than the FSH number, and 35 was still young in the IVF world. My IVF cycle was scheduled to begin in two months. Finally, I could pursue IVF and get the answers, or closure, I felt I needed.

Only two follicles responded but the doctors were able to retrieve both, and both of them were mature eggs. Both of them fertilised. Both of them continued to grow. Both were transferred back after three days. I was ecstatic! This was wonderful news to me. I had eggs that could be fertilised and grow! Although I did not become pregnant, I wasn't ready to give up. I now had hope and was ready to go again with more confidence. We modified my protocol to include an oestrogen primer and more LH control. This time, six follicles began to respond but only two actually matured. My little girl was born in December, six months before my 37th birthday – exactly one year from the start of my first IVF cycle.

On a recent trip to visit her grandparents, I was able to see some old photos of me as a baby. I could see how much she looks like me. It then struck me that I wouldn't have had this experience if I had followed the first doctor's advice. I now know that I wasn't ready for a donor egg or embryo. I'm glad the donation advisor didn't call me back. Doctors seem to want to write us off as failures. They need to remember that although we may have a poor response and a low number of eggs, it only takes one good egg. If I was brave enough, I'd return to the first doctor and tell him how wrong he was to absolutely refuse to allow me to pursue treatment to my own satisfaction. A woman needs time to accept severing a biological link to her future children. She needs to arrive at that conclusion in her own time and in her own way, as her emotions and finances permit. Many, like me, need to know we've tried everything we possibly can. Only a woman and her partner should decide when they are ready to move on to donor or other options. This should not be forced upon them by refusal of treatment. I'm one of many on a high-FSH success board. Many of us there are biological parents, many are donor or adoptive parents, but we are all parents, no matter how we got there. [NB: This case study is from the US.]

Interview with Mr Nick Panay BSc MRCOG MFFP, Consultant Gynaecologist, Queen Charlotte's & Chelsea Hospital and Chelsea & Westminster Hospital London, and Senior Lecturer, Imperial College London

What is premature ovarian failure?

We see a lot of women with premature ovarian failure (POF). I think the name should be changed to premature ovarian dysfunction. Failure is too harsh a word for women. It implies that they have failed and nothing is possible when, in fact, 8–10 per cent of women with this condition will get pregnant. POF is often badly managed, and the diagnosis is based on one FSH measurement and no counselling. It is more common in women who have had chemotherapy treatment for cancer.

The difficulty with this is that all of the specialists you see, such as the oncologists, are keen on survival rates, so many of these women when faced with trying for a baby have to find and search out people who will help them. Some do go on to get pregnant, but there are certain tests that should be done and are not done often on the NHS, especially thyroid tests, and 10–20 per cent come back showing thyroid antibodies.

How do you treat the condition?

We treat if the individual wants treatment prior to egg donation as I feel it is important that a woman has tried before she moves on. We will do follicular tracking and use mild stimulation with gonadrophins. I don't tend to use Clomid. We may also use oestrogen patches. These women need more care and support than they are currently getting. There needs to be more awareness around. The Daisy Network (see Resources) does a good job in helping them, but clinics need to have a better understanding.

The Cavity of the Uterus

The condition of the uterine cavity is vital to allow the embryo to implant and then have a healthy, spacious environment in which to expand as the pregnancy develops. A hysteroscopy may be suggested (see page 219) to check the cavity to ensure there is nothing which could interfere with implantation. This includes congenital abnormalities and conditions which could distort the cavity, such as fibroids (see page 179). Where possible, surgery will be avoided and often things like small fibroids are of no concern at all. It is always important to weigh up the pros and cons of surgery, to have good information on any potential risks and to have time to consider your decision.

The Endometrium

The endometrium forms a sponge-like womb lining with a rich blood supply to enable the embryo to burrow in and implant. Sometimes during an IVF cycle, the endometrium does not reach an adequate thickness to allow successful implantation. It is thought that the endometrium should be at least 7mm thick to allow the embryo to implant. The endometrium might be thin for several reasons: adenomyosis – patches of endometrial tissue found in the muscle of the uterus; fibroids; Asherman's syndrome (see page 257).

Infections

Ureaplasma and mycoplasma are normally harmless bacteria found in the genital tract in up to 70 per cent of sexually active couples. There is growing evidence that couples should be tested routinely for these infections (see pages 227, 279–280). They can be present for many years without causing any symptoms, and they may not cause problems with fertility if you are trying naturally. During IVF, however, the bacteria may be pushed into the uterine cavity at embryo transfer and, as the embryo is highly vulnerable, the infection may lead to implantation failure. While the jury is still out regarding the role of ureaplasma and its effect on implantation, several studies have shown a difference in pregnancy rates among women with ureaplasma infection who were treated with antibiotics and those who were not. Other studies have not shown any difference. Treatment involves use of appropriate antibiotics and re-testing three months later.

Male Factor

Another important factor in IVF success is the integrity of the man's sperm. More and more evidence is now emerging about male fertility and the DNA abnormalities in the sperm, which may reduce implantation pregnancy rates (see Chapter 10).

Immune System Issues

There is increasing medical interest in the possibility that recurrent implantation failure may sometimes be related to problems with the immune system. So, if a good-quality embryo(s) is replaced and yet IVF cycles are repeatedly unsuccessful (taking into account the age of the woman) this may be an area to start exploring. The implantation process is a lengthy one starting from a few days after fertilisation but lasting up until at least 12 weeks of pregnancy (possibly 20 weeks). Problems can occur at every step of the way, either resulting in a delay in natural conception, an unsuccessful IVF cycle, or miscarriage. So, investigations and treatments used for many years for recurrent miscarriage may have a role to play at the very early stages of implantation. But, as with so many new developments in medicine, there are areas of debate. Some tests and treatments have good evidence to support their use and others are more controversial.

Understanding Research Evidence

Professional bodies, such as the Royal College of Obstetricians and Gynaecologists (RCOG), use standardised classifications of evidence levels when considering fertility investigations or treatments. These are ranked from A to C:

- Grade A – based on randomised controlled trials (the gold-standard)
- Grade B – based on other robust experimental or observational studies
- Grade C – based on more limited evidence but the advice relies on expert opinion and has the endorsement of respected authorities

Within each of these grades there are further classifications. This is where the whole area of reproductive immunology is lacking. Although there is strong evidence in some areas (such as clotting problems), other areas are seriously lacking in good research.

It is understandable that women who have had repeated unsuccessful attempts at IVF would be 'willing to try anything' but this puts you into a very vulnerable position, which is why it is really important to discuss any proposed tests or treatments thoroughly with your doctor and consider any potential long-term consequences as well as short-term side effects.

Blood Clotting Problems (Thrombophilia)

Thrombophilia is the general term given to the tendency of the blood to clot too quickly (forming thromboses). If a woman's blood clots too quickly, it may reduce the blood flow through the placenta to the foetus. This is a well-established cause of recurrent miscarriage, but there is increasing evidence that the factors which cause recurrent miscarriage can also cause problems with recurrent implantation failure with IVF, or may even be a factor with 'unexplained' infertility. Women with clotting problems are also more at risk of clots occurring elsewhere, such as deep vein thrombosis.

- **Antiphospholipid antibodies** Antiphospholipid antibodies are a family of 20 antibodies which, as their name implies, are directed against phospholipids – the glue molecules which help the embryo to stick. Dr Graham Hughes first described the Antiphospholipid Syndrome (APS) or 'sticky blood' in 1983. These antibodies are auto-antibodies meaning they work against your own tissues. The significant antiphospholipid antibodies are lupus anticoagulant and anticardiolipin antibodies. If a woman has lupus – an auto-immune disease affecting joints and muscles with extreme tiredness – she will inevitably test positive for lupus antibodies. However, women who don't have the lupus condition can also test positive for the antibodies.

   Women with recurrent implantation failure tend to show higher levels of these antibodies, so they are increasingly tested for in IVF clinics. If present, the woman's blood clots too quickly and the phospholipid 'glue' is weakened preventing the embryo from attaching firmly to the endometrium. This is a common cause of recurrent miscarriage and there is a very well-established treatment for this using aspirin and heparin (see below). These anti-coagulants (anti-clotting) drugs may also be used during IVF although the evidence for their use is less clear.

Use of aspirin: Aspirin stops platelets from clumping together and causing a clot to form. It improves the blood flow and circulation, including blood flow to the womb and the ovaries. Some research shows that low-dose aspirin improves the implantation rate in IVF. The use of aspirin is, however, controversial as it crosses the placenta. Some doctors believe it should be taken only when pregnancy is confirmed. Like many drugs, some people are allergic to it, and it carries a risk of stomach ulceration. It should only ever be used to thin the blood when there is a firm diagnosis of APS and under medical guidance.

Use of heparin: A second line of treatment for women with APS is with heparin (Clexane). Heparin is given as a daily injection, and generally started only when a woman is pregnant or going through an IVF cycle, but may be continued for the duration of her pregnancy. Heparin seems to bind to the antiphospholipid antibodies and help the blastocyst to implant in addition to its anticoagulant effects in later pregnancy. There is some research showing calcium depletion with long-term use of heparin, so healthy eating is important here with foods rich in calcium and vitamin D.

- **Inherited thrombophilia** Some blood clotting disorders are inherited. Factor V Leiden is the most common inherited disorder. The blood clotting protein Factor V Leiden is moderated by another substance found in the blood called Protein C. This acts as a blood thinner by combining with Protein S on the surface of blood platelets. If there is a deficiency of Protein C or Protein S it cannot do this effectively so may lead to small clots, causing problems with implantation.

In summary, if a couple are producing good-quality embryos, but they are not implanting, there is increasing evidence for routine thrombophilia screening – which includes the antiphospholipid antibodies, lupus anticoagulant and anticardiolipin, and the inherited thrombophilias (Factor V Leiden, Protein S and Protein C deficiency, and Prothrombin gene mutation).

MTHFR

Methylene-Tetra-Hydro-Folate-Reductase (MTHFR) is an enzyme that is present in our cells. This enzyme metabolises and eliminates homocysteine – a toxic amino acid. The enzyme is coded by the gene also with the same symbol. MTHFR is a genetic mutation that inhibits the production of this enzyme, thus reducing the body's ability to absorb folic acid (vitamin B9) and vitamin B12. Treatment is with high-dose folic acid (5mg).

Possible Immune Reactions to the Developing Embryo

You will remember that when an embryo is replaced, first it finds a place on the surface of the endometrium where it can stick and start to penetrate the surface. The trophoblast cells develop and will eventually become the placenta. For the union between the embryo and the maternal tissue to continue, an immunological hurdle has to be overcome. This is because the embryo is 'foreign' tissue as it contains the father's DNA as well as the mother's. When the trophoblast meets the endometrium lining it is thought that there is a dialogue through chemical messengers called cytokines. This dialogue establishes whether the embryo will continue to grow and thrive or be rejected. A woman's ability to hold on to an embryo is thought to be down to certain immunology factors. Some research suggests that during a normal pregnancy a unique type of immunity occurs that prevents a woman from rejecting the embryo. If there are problems in this immune response then the embryo may not implant or may miscarry.

Natural Killer Cells

This is where much of the controversy lies with implantation failure. Our immune system is designed to fight infection and to keep us healthy. It is made up of subsets of white blood cells. Natural killer (NK) cells are large white blood cells or lymphocytes. Although they may sound scary, they are, in fact, important as they help us to fight diseases like cancer. These NK cells are found all over the body including the uterus, but some doctors believe that if the NK cells are above a certain threshold they may cause fertility problems and implantation failure. Because the NK cells are tested using peripheral blood there are big debates about whether these levels are representative of cells in the uterus. It is also possible that the 'reaction' to taking blood can increase this immune response.

White blood cells communicate with one another via chemical messengers called cytokines. The subsets of white blood cells which may have a role in implantation failure are T-helper cells. There are two types of these: T-helper cell 1 (TH1) and T-helper cell 2 (TH2). Both have different roles within the immune system and produce their own cytokines. TH1 produces cytokines that may have a negative impact on implantation through the activation of NK cells. For implantation to take place, TH2 helper cells need to be dominant as they are more baby friendly. Certain conditions, such as auto-immune disorders, endometriosis or where there are auto-antibodies present, can trigger a response in the immune system making it become overactive and tipping the balance towards a TH1 response. Clinics that specialise in this sort of immune testing will do blood tests. These may indicate whether the NK cells are raised and the TH1/ TH2 ratio may indicate the killing capacity of the cytokines.

When the immune system becomes overactive the NK cells produce more TH1 cytokines. This happens in conditions such as rheumatoid arthritis, Crohn's disease and multiple sclerosis. Drugs that may be given to treat this condition include steroids, intravenous immunoglobulin (IVIG), humira or Intralipid. It is important to remember that testing and treatments for NK cells and other immune issues is still at the research stage and is not recommended by the RCOG.

Reading this, I don't want you to think that you automatically have immune issues because you have had an unsuccessful IVF cycle. It is difficult for doctors to decide how far to go with testing. These tests are not available on the NHS. If the tests are done privately, it is very expensive for couples. A few IVF units will be very encouraging of doing different immune tests, but as there is not always evidence to support their use in diagnosis or treatment, many doctors will advise against immune testing. Of course, not all women with implantation failure will have immune issues; it is possibly quite a low percentage.

Auto-immune Diseases

Auto-immune diseases include some forms of thyroid disease, endometriosis, lupus, rheumatoid arthritis, Crohn's disease, type 1 diabetes and Raynaud's disease. They are thought to be caused by an immune response causing inflammation and destruction of tissues by the body's own antibodies. Women who have a known auto-immune disease should possibly be tested for reproductive immune problems if they have implantation difficulties.

- **Lupus anticoagulant antibodies** This test is part of the routine screening for antiphospholipids (see page 421). These antibodies are common if a woman has lupus, but can also be present if she does not have any other symptoms of lupus or a family history of lupus.

- **Anti-thyroid antibodies** Thyroid disease in the family may increase the likelihood of you developing thyroid problems. If you have thyroid problems you should also be checked for thyroid antibodies. Thyroid auto-immunity is a very common disorder in women, affecting 5–15 per cent of the female population. It is five to ten times more common in women than in men, and can be present without thyroid dysfunction, thus remaining undiagnosed. The exact reason why thyroid antibodies can cause miscarriage or implantation failure is not yet known.

So, it will be clear that this whole topic is very complex and highly controversial. The late Dr Alan Beer, a pioneer in the field of reproductive immunology, wrote a comprehensive book called *Is Your Body Baby Friendly?* which gives very detailed information on the subject. I was very fortunate to meet him and sit in on some of his consultations in the US. His work was considered controversial in the medical establishment as Beer associated other conditions – Raynaud's disease, chronic fatigue syndrome, premature ovarian failure, adult-onset diabetes, and endometriosis – with having a higher chance of unsuccessful IVF.

This whole field is changing so fast, it is hard to know whether some tests and treatments will become standard practice in the future (as was the case with thrombophilia screening and the use of aspirin and heparin) or whether they will be consigned to the history books as ineffective or even dangerous practice. A phrase which is often heard at medical meetings and sums it up is: 'Absence of evidence is not the same as evidence of absence.'

Holistic Immune Therapy

Much of the work being done in the field of reproductive immunity is having a positive effect on the lives of many couples. It can mean the difference between having a baby or not after repeated unsuccessful IVF attempts. However, I feel it is also important that we should go back to basics and look at holistic approaches to support the immune system through diet, supplements, stress reduction and environmental factors.

Why are our immune systems overactive? Is it any wonder we are having problems when our immune systems are bombarded on a daily basis with pesticides, chemicals, cigarettes, alcohol, stress and environmental toxins? Stress alters immune function, and so does lifestyle. The body is fighting on every level. You cannot separate the immune system from any other body system: stress reduction and nutrition are all key (see Chapters 4 and 7). Trying for a baby and repeated IVF attempts take their toll on anyone. At the Zita West Clinic, our nutritional programme is fundamental to this approach. A healthy digestive system is vital. If necessary we may arrange blood tests for vitamin D levels, antioxidants and essential fatty acids. Chapter 7 contains some key elements of the immune nutrition programme.

Some women may benefit from manual lymphatic massage. The lymphatic system is a core part of the immune system and provides a highway for the white blood cells to travel to areas of conflict in the body. Manual lymphatic massage can help with the flow of lymph, so we use this on women preparing to start IVF and in between IVF cycles. Acupuncture can also be of benefit for some women (see page 192).

Case Study

Justine and Harry, both 34, had gone through four unsuccessful IVF attempts. Justine walked into my consulting room in floods of tears, saying Harry would rather buy a house in the south of France than have a baby. Harry denied this, but he felt they couldn't keep trying IVF time and time again without success. They had already spent almost £50,000 and he wasn't prepared to throw any more money at it.

Harry's sperm were excellent: the motility was slightly low but his count was 90 million. Justine had good hormone levels but she suffered from IBS and fibromyalgia and had a history of endometriosis. She was also very stressed and anxious. A blood test showed low vitamin D levels. After our discussion, her IVF doctor tested her for immune factors and she was found to have antiphospholipid antibodies and raised natural killer cell activity, and was treated with aspirin, heparin and steroids. At the clinic her nutritional programme ensured she had plenty of antioxidants and essential fatty acids in her diet. She also started on probiotics. She was to cut out processed foods and takeaways and reduce her intake of alcohol. Justine went on to conceive at the fifth IVF attempt.

I really believe that, evidence or no evidence, the work being done in this field by some doctors for a certain group of clients who are repeatedly failing at implantation is making a difference between having a baby and not. The top doctors working in the field of reproductive immunology in the UK are Mr George Ndukwe, Mr Mohamed Taranissi and Dr Yau Thum. I interviewed them to find out how a couple can increase their chances after unsuccessful IVF.

Interview with Mr George Ndukwe, Medical Director and Consultant in Reproductive Medicine

I met with George at his clinic in Nottingham, and we talked at great length about immune issues. He is one of the top doctors in the UK involved in reproductive immunology, and he has spent a lot of time working with Dr Alan Beer, the forefather of reproductive immunology and genetics. I had the pleasure of meeting Dr Beer before he died in 2006, and have unending respect for what he has done in this area of medical science.

What makes IVF successful?
There are three key areas: events pre-treatment, which include nutrition and stress relief; events during treatment, with attention to detail; and events after treatment which involves adequate support for early embryo implantation. If you optimise these three areas you are ensuring a good environment for the embryo and good foundations for a pregnancy. It takes three months for an egg to develop, so getting that right prior to a cycle is very important.

You do a lot of work in the field of reproductive immunology. Why are immune issues important?
In simple terms, an embryo is a foreign body when it enters the womb. Pregnancy is the only time something foreign enters the body and is not rejected. There is a special immunity that allows the mother to tolerate the embryo and not reject it, even though it is foreign. If anything goes wrong with this special immunity then embryo implantation can be impaired. Top doctors in this field now see implantation as the final frontier. We have seen huge improvement in every aspect other than implantation and most IVF cycles keep failing and miscarriages keep occurring. This is an area where better understanding is vital.

Which patients would you test?
I had several discussions with Dr Beer about the possibility of identifying the groups of women who might need early immune testing. We never really came to any firm decisions. However, he suggested that with a history of rheumatoid arthritis, Crohn's disease, thyroid problems, endometriosis or other immune conditions in the patient or her family, immune tests would be justified. This would, in my opinion, be a reasonable approach within the context of individual fertility history.

Should you wait for three unsuccessful IVF cycles before being tested?
Why three unsuccessful cycles? That is the convention, but that number is arbitrary. I feel that each couple or patient should be looked at individually. I often have patients who have had up to 10 failed IVF cycles, or indeed miscarriages, who I have investigated and treated with appropriate immune treatment, who have conceived straight away and had successful pregnancies. I often wonder whether they would have benefited from much earlier immune testing.

Some women aged 40–42 years who come to see me often insist on earlier tests because they do not feel they have the luxury of time to wait and see. They would rather know and deal with any issues that can improve their chances of a successful pregnancy.

For most patients, if after three transfers of good-quality embryos there is no success, one should stop, and start asking relevant questions. Offering more of the same treatment time and time again simply does not make sense to me.

Studies have shown that it is quite conventional to use aspirin and heparin, but IVIG is still viewed as controversial. I see it as being an effective treatment. What are your views?
I agree with you that intravenous immunoglobulin (IVIG) is certainly an effective treatment and, contrary to what has been said by some

doctors, there are a lot of published reports to support this. It is used widely in the USA and Canada. It is, however, a blood product and some women have reservations despite the intensive screening that takes place. I can understand this.

It is also very expensive. Having an effective treatment which only few can afford has always been an issue for me. After many years of research we are now pioneering a new treatment called Intralipid. This is a fat emulsion used in intravenous feeding and is much cheaper than IVIG. Published research says it is equivalent to IVIG but I feel it is more effective judging by the wonderful results I am getting in Nottingham. There is no reason for anyone to still be using IVIG other than in exceptional circumstances.

What about the use of Humira because, again, medical opinion is divided?

Humira is a drug used for rheumatoid arthritis and Crohn's disease where it could be taken for several years. It can be used to improve outcome in a certain type of immune condition associated with recurrent implantation failure. In my experience, in this special group of women it can be very effective. It is usually given well before IVF treatment so there should be no safety issues with it.

The problem I have with Humira is that it is very expensive and may not work in up to 20 per cent of women. Luckily, the pioneering work I am doing at the moment shows that Intralipid (see above) is also effective treatment for this.

Interview with Mr Mohamed Taranissi, Medical Director of The Assisted Reproduction & Gynaecology Centre (ARGC)

Mr Taranissi is a controversial figure in the world of IVF, but he has a proven track record when it comes to getting successful results.

What do you think makes a difference to IVF?
Every clinic does different things. At our clinic we monitor the cycle closely before IVF, which involves scans and blood tests. This is a huge commitment for the client, but it is a two-way thing, as it is a commitment from us as well. With so many monitored cycles, there are always results to give to the patient. This can be stressful at times, but we remain in regular contact with the clients throughout the process in an attempt to make it as easy as possible. This gives us a much greater understanding of the individual, allowing us to specifically tailor what we do for that person.

How do you maximise a woman's potential for successful IVF?
There are huge variations in women's cycles from month to month, with some months producing better hormones and eggs than others. We are able to draw on our experience to maximise the potential for getting better eggs. Priming the egg and harvesting a mature egg when the egg is ready to be collected are both critical.

I know that you have views on the length of time it takes to transfer the embryo. Do you think that it makes a difference to success?
The transfer, when we put the embryos back again, to me is a vital part of the process, although many people still claim it is not. It is critical to treat the embryos in a precise manner.

How important do you think immune factors are for IVF success?
Although we don't know all of the answers, in my experience immune issues are responsible for a lot of failures at the implantation stage. We will decide who to test on an individual basis. We do not make the decision based solely on a patient's history; instead we draw on our own experience, having treated hundreds of couples before.

What else can affect the IVF outcome in a woman who is repeatedly failing at IVF?
When you have been through a lot of unsuccessful IVF cycles, you need to be really careful about using up your egg reserves. Something has to change, because it is vital you are going in the right direction. The best way forward is to find out more about the implantation process and discover why embryos fail.

I think that a positive mindset helps enormously when it comes to the success of the treatment. When clients are tense and negative and leading a highly stressed lifestyle, it certainly has an impact.

Interview with Dr Yau Thum, Fertility Specialist at the Lister Fertility Clinic

What the medical profession finds hard to agree on is who should be tested for reproductive immunology. When do you think that clients should be tested for immune issues after IVF has failed?
The research phase of the immune system is happening now and there will be more data available over the next couple of years which will expand our knowledge. I think that clients or patients who may benefit are those that have had:

1. Three recurrent miscarriages.
2. Three failed IVF attempts with good-quality embryos (good quality meaning blastocysts or an embryo with eight cells).

3. If there are other auto-immune factors that are inherent in a family, such as lupus, rheumatoid arthritis, Raynaud's disease, endometriosis, etc.

What do you feel makes IVF successful in women whose IVF cycles are failing?

1. The client has to be looked at on an individual evaluation. No blanket policy.
2. You have to put effort into the consultation.
3. Every single case has a different element to it, e.g. every aspect of the protocol: the stimulation, looking at the lab quality, the nature of the embryos.
4. Peripheral testing such as immunology is also key to the success of IVF in many women who have had many failed attempts. What we are still hindered by is our lack of knowledge in terms of implantation.
5. The units that have good success rates and have good protocols in place, good fertilisation rates, good embryology and cultures, may have good results but in a certain group of clients they don't have that final piece of the puzzle, which is implantation. Doing further testing to see if there are immune issues may have an impact.

What does the future hold over the next five years?

Things are changing at a rapid pace. We will eventually have a greater understanding of implantation, and the cellular to molecular advance. Genetic studies will also be much more advanced. We will be able to select better embryos using techniques that are just developing, such as CGH, which hopefully will improve IVF outcome.

Miscarriage

A miscarriage is the loss of a pregnancy before 24 weeks – with the vast majority of these pregnancy losses occurring in the first trimester (12 weeks). Many doctors believe there is a crossover between implantation failure in IVF and recurrent miscarriage. Implantation can be thought of as a continuous process starting at the time the blastocyst starts to implant in the endometrium and completing by around 12 weeks of pregnancy when the placenta takes over the full hormonal production.

Pregnancy tests are so much more sensitive than they were a generation ago, so a test shows positive very early on when the embryo is making its first tentative attempts at implantation. So essentially the diagnosis of pregnancy is made based on the technology available to identify the hCG (pregnancy hormone) and this is getting earlier and earlier. It is known that there is an extremely high rate of pregnancy loss before a test would even show positive. Physiologically there may be little difference between a pregnancy not implanting at a matter of a few days or a couple of weeks, but once a pregnancy test has shown positive, quite understandably this tends to take on another whole meaning for women emotionally.

Many of the reasons why a woman has recurrent miscarriages are the same as for women who have recurrent implantation failure at IVF. These causes include:

- age
- genetic factors
- abnormal chromosomes in women or men
- hormonal imbalances (including PCO)
- blood clotting disorders
- auto-immune diseases

- infections
- structural abnormalities of the womb
- lifestyle factors – smoking and excess alcohol

In the UK, the cause of miscarriage isn't investigated until it occurs for a third time, which can be very difficult for women. We know enough to recognise there are factors in a family or in a woman's history that might make her more prone to miscarriage. We are very fortunate at the clinic because Dr Raj Rai provides the medical expertise for our couples with recurrent miscarriage.

Investigations for recurrent miscarriage usually start with blood tests to see if there are any hormonal imbalances. The blood clotting factors will be checked, chromosomes tested for both the woman and her partner, and a full infection screen performed.

If a pregnancy miscarries at any stage, a woman's body usually shows physical signs – bleeding or cramps – and the body goes through the physiological process of losing the pregnancy. Sometimes there may be no physical signs that the pregnancy is not progressing; the first indication of a problem may be at a scan to confirm everything is going well. To be told at that stage that there is no heartbeat or the pregnancy is not progressing as it should can be devastating – creating anger, disbelief and enormous sadness. It may seem more difficult because your body had not given you any sign of there being a problem.

Some women will miscarry naturally but at other times the miscarriage may be incomplete and an operation is required usually under general anaesthetic. This is known as an ERPC, which stands for evacuation of retained products of conception. Some people still refer to this procedure as a D & C (dilatation and curettage). There are many medical ways now to manage miscarriage, which involve the use of pills and pessaries, but the management of miscarriage will depend on many factors.

Clearly, miscarriage is a huge topic and a book such as this cannot possibly do justice to the subject. I interviewed Dr Raj Rai, an expert in recurrent miscarriage, to hear his perspective on all aspects of this problem.

Interview with Dr Raj Rai, Senior Lecturer / Consultant Obstetrician and Gynaecologist, Imperial College, St Mary's Hospital, London

Dr Rai also heads up the Recurrent Miscarriage Programme at the Zita West Clinic.

How common is miscarriage?
Miscarriage is a lot more common than people think. Of every 100 conceptions only 50 will result in a live birth. The miscarriage rate increases with age:
    Age 20–24 = 15 per cent
    Age 35–39 = 25 per cent
    Age 40+ = 51 per cent
    Age 45+ = 75 per cent

What is the high risk time for miscarriage?
The highest risk time for early miscarriage is less than 8 weeks, not 12 weeks as is commonly thought.

What are the common causes of a single miscarriage?
The most common cause for any single miscarriage is a sporadic foetal chromosome abnormality, the incidence of which increases with advancing maternal age and FSH level. When there is a chromosomal abnormality in the embryo, 90 per cent of the time it arises from the egg and 10 per cent from the sperm.

What is recurrent miscarriage (RM) and how common is it?

Recurrent miscarriage is diagnosed when a woman miscarries three times consecutively before 20 weeks' gestation. It is true that some women miscarry more often than chance alone would expect. When considering how common recurrent miscarriage actually is, we need to consider some numbers. The incidence of recurrent miscarriage in the general population is 1 per cent. Of this group 66 per cent will be found to have an underlying cause. In 33 per cent there is no cause found and this is the hardest group to work with as it is very difficult for couples to accept that chances are their recurrent miscarriage is due to random genetic errors in the pregnancy.

What are the possible causes of recurrent miscarriage?

The most common reason for miscarriage is a random genetic abnormality which is associated with age. The second most common cause (in about 15 per cent of women with RM) is Antiphospholipid Syndrome (APS). This is a family of 20 antibodies: phospholipids are the glue molecules – the two of importance in relation to RM are lupus anticoagulant and anti-cardiolipin. The APS antibodies attack the lining of the womb and attack the placenta.

Is there any treatment for APS?

Yes. If a woman has APS and is untreated she only has a 10 per cent chance of a live baby, also there is a very high risk of intrauterine growth restriction. Aspirin increases the live birth rate to 42 per cent, and aspirin in conjunction with heparin increases the live birth rate to 71 per cent, so this is a very successful treatment.

Many women ask about taking an aspirin 'as it can't hurt'. What would you say to these women?

Aspirin should only be used when there is a clear indication and should never be used before a positive pregnancy test. In fact, there is some evidence that if you give aspirin before a positive pregnancy test there is an increased risk of miscarriage so it should only be used after a positive pregnancy test. Aspirin taken during the stimulation phase of IVF may also decrease the pregnancy rate.

What are the standard tests for recurrent miscarriage?

The rationale for investigating is either to confirm or to refute the presence of an underlying treatable cause for pregnancy loss. The standard tests check for chromosomal abnormalities, hormonal problems (FSH, LH, testosterone, progesterone and AMH); Antiphospholipid Syndrome (anticardiolipin antibodies and lupus anticoagulant); Inherited Thrombophilias (Factor V Leiden, Protein S and Protein C); alongside an ultrasound scan to check for abnormalities in the uterus and polycystic ovaries.

What is the link between PCOS and miscarriage?

It is known that about 40 per cent of women who have a history of RM also have PCOS. The link is not only hormonal but also some women with PCOS appear not to break down blood clots as well as others. Many women with PCOS are also overweight with a high BMI and there is evidence to show that the rate of RM is higher among women with high BMI. A study at St Mary's Hospital, London, in 2008 looked at 696 women with unexplained recurrent miscarriage and found the risk of a further miscarriage was increased by 73 per cent if the woman was obese. Women with insulin-resistant PCOS are found to have poorer-quality embryos because of the increased level of insulin.

What is the role of progesterone supplementation in miscarriage?

The studies done on progesterone have generally been of poor quality and small numbers. Some studies have shown no benefit but at least five studies have shown a benefit. Many of these studies have been misunderstood and misinterpreted. St Mary's has now been given a £1.5 million grant to carry out a randomised controlled multi-centre trial on the use of progesterone in the treatment of miscarriage. This will include 790 women and will take place over two years. The aim of the study is to show if progesterone reduces the risk of RM. From January 2010 we are going to recruit 900 women to take part in a trial called Promise which will look to see if progesterone is effective for women who miscarry. So we hope to have some more definitive answers following this.

What are the chances of a healthy baby after recurrent miscarriage?
Many of the women that I see are quite naturally anxious if they have been experiencing recurrent miscarriages. What I try to get across to them is that if a woman is less than 39 and has had three or four miscarriages for which no treatable cause is identified she has a 65 per cent chance of a successful pregnancy. If the pregnancy gets to eight weeks there is a 98 per cent chance of the pregnancy progressing normally, and this can be very reassuring for couples to know. It is worth remembering here that when a woman reports that she had a miscarriage, e.g. at 12 weeks, this often means that it was only diagnosed at 12 weeks, but the foetus may have failed several weeks earlier.

Do you believe any lifestyle factors contribute to miscarriage?
Some research clearly shows a link with stress. Weight also plays a part here – either under- or overweight is associated with an increased risk of miscarriage.

What do you feel our integrated recurrent miscarriage programme offers?
The key difference here is that we look at both the medical side and lifestyle, diet and emotional factors of both partners. Couples cope

very differently with miscarriage and many find it hard to support one another. In the NHS most couples have to wait until they have miscarried three times, and many women particularly feel this is unbearable and want to do all they can to try and minimise the risk of it happening again. We would see couples after one miscarriage if it is at more than 10 weeks, and after two miscarriages if at less than 10 weeks. There is still a chance that there would be no cause found, but by applying these criteria it starts to tip the balance in favour of finding a treatable cause.

Most Recurrent Miscarriage clinics only focus on the woman. At the Zita West Clinic, we also offer a male programme. This includes testing for the genetic integrity of sperm. There is some evidence that if the sperm show a high DNA fragmentation index there is a higher incidence of miscarriage. Both partners are also offered a full infection screen which includes ureaplasma and mycoplasma. There may be some association here with miscarriage too. In addition to the medical side, the clinic offers a specific nutritional programme; acupuncture to reduce stress and improve blood flow; and emotional support through hypnotherapy / positive visualisation and miscarriage support counselling. We see some very positive results from this integrated approach and this is an area where we would like to focus some research in the future.

How do you feel we can minimise the risk of miscarriages in the future?

I think one of the advances we are going to see in this field in the future has to be in pre-conception care and preparing for pregnancy. Events that occur in the early weeks of pregnancy at the time of implantation lay down the foundations for the rest of the pregnancy, so early miscarriage, intrauterine growth restriction (IUGR) and pre-eclampsia all go back to implantation. In view of this, good pre-conception care is vital, yet there is very little focus on this. Therefore the work that you do at the Zita West Clinic, integrating the medical aspects alongside looking at diet, lifestyle factors, stress reduction, and emotional and psychological support, paves the way for healthy pregnancies.

Coping After a Miscarriage

(A counselling perspective by Jane Knight, Fertility Counsellor)

A miscarriage at any stage of pregnancy can be very difficult to cope with. There is a common perception that the more advanced the pregnancy, the more a woman (and man) will feel the loss. Of course, a late miscarriage or the loss of a baby around birth – either a stillbirth or the death of a young baby – is devastating and couples require a huge amount of emotional support, often for many months and even years afterwards. SANDS – the Stillbirth & Neonatal Death Charity (see Resources) – provides support for anyone affected by the death of a baby. However, even a very early pregnancy loss can be most distressing. The Miscarriage Association (see Resources) provides information and support for anyone who has lost a pregnancy.

A positive pregnancy test tends to send your emotions into orbit. Hopefully, you will feel excited beyond words. However, if you have previously experienced a miscarriage, you may have very mixed emotions, perhaps anxiety about miscarrying again – a sense of impending doom. A woman who has previously miscarried may find it difficult to bond with her unborn baby – this is often a subconscious means of self-protection. She may not feel able to look at ultrasound pictures or to feel encouraged by any reassuring words from her doctor or the ultrasonographer. The experience of miscarriage generally leaves a woman feeling wary and anxious – she is no longer able to be naively accepting of the pregnancy and the joys it will bring.

One of the most difficult things about a miscarriage – especially an early miscarriage – is coming to terms with the potential that has been lost. For this reason it can be hard for anyone to empathise with a woman who has had an early miscarriage unless they have been through it themselves. It is so important after a miscarriage – at whatever stage – to allow yourself time to grieve. Grief is really a way of working through the implications of the loss. Sometimes grief is talked about as a cycle with different stages – emotional numbness, denial, disbelief, separation, anxiety, despair, sadness and loneliness. Rather than a cycle with a logical progression, however, you may be hit by any of these emotions at any time – the emotions will often ebb and flow, but not in any structured way. Remember, grief is a very personal thing and you and your partner will be at different stages. Men often hit 'rock bottom' very quickly at times of loss and then start to resurface again fairly rapidly, throwing themselves into work or other distractions. Sometimes they are able to move on, but at other times the intense need to work or exercise is a coping strategy and the grief may remain unresolved. Men often find it hard to talk, whereas women need to do so frequently – almost incessantly – to make sense of their loss. You need time to let go of the anger and all the negative emotions and to reach a level of acceptance. A fertility counsellor can help you – either individually or as a couple – to come to terms with your loss. The old Chinese proverb about grief tells us: 'You can't stop the birds of sorrow from flying overhead, but don't let them nest in your hair.'

To help you to manage your grief, you may find it useful to put some things down on paper. Write down your feelings – an unconscious stream of thoughts – of what might have been. If you feel it appropriate, you might like to write a letter to your dream baby – your hopes for your life with that child and how those hopes have been dashed. You may wish to show it to your partner or to keep it to yourself – a very personal reminder of your loss and a way of moving forward. If you go back to that letter at a later time, you may be surprised at just how sad you were feeling.

You might wish to do something to mark your pregnancy, especially if you suffered a later miscarriage. This is also a good way to help you release some of your emotions. Consider getting a helium-filled balloon and releasing it from somewhere special to you – a beach, perhaps, or a beautiful area of the countryside. Allow yourself to feel sad as you watch it rise higher and higher into the sky and finally disappear. You may wish to attach a special note to it. This may be something you do alone or with your partner – whatever feels right for you.

After a time – which will vary from one person to another – you need to make a positive decision to turn a corner. You need to start to move forward again. Your loss will never go away, of course, but that heavy black cloud of sadness and despair should slowly give way to just the occasional wispy white cloud. Some people feel trapped in their grief and may become depressed. It is important to stay in regular contact with your GP and to recognise that there may be times when you need further help – whether that is counselling, other therapeutic support or even antidepressants – to help you process things and pick yourself up again. A short course of antidepressants in combination with a 'talking therapy' can be most beneficial if you are feeling stuck in your grief.

Ready to do IVF Again?

This is such a big question. On page 398 I discuss ways to help you make this decision, but as far as possible you both need to be in agreement about your next step. So many women arrive at our door seeing us as a 'last chance saloon'; some women are broken by their negative IVF experiences or the way that bad news has been delivered to them. We try to go out of our way to help couples to tick every box. With a new plan in place, some women will go on to do another IVF cycle or may even conceive naturally, sometimes against all the odds, but other women will need help to move on. Our overall aim is not a baby at all costs, although hopefully as many couples as possible will realise their dream of becoming parents in whatever form that takes, but for others the goal will be to move on to achieve a very fulfilling life in other ways. Organisations such as Infertility Network UK and their service 'More to Life' can be an invaluable source of information and support (see Resources).

Chapter 15

Moving On

Knowing when to move on from IVF can be one of the hardest decisions a couple has to face. You can never turn around and say, 'I am only doing IVF three times.' It is not always that cut and dried. There are other options you may want to consider, such as egg donation or surrogacy. Some couples may prefer to look towards adoption or choose to remain childless. This chapter looks at ways in which couples can review their situation and make a positive decision to move forward.

How Will We Know When to Move On?

This varies from couple to couple, depending on their circumstances. Each person in a couple will also have a different way of coping and of making decisions. Sometimes couples disagree on the next step: the woman might be adamant that she wants another attempt at IVF using her own eggs, while her partner is sure that they should stop. One of the main reasons why it can be so hard to move on, or to stop treatment altogether, is the knowledge that you can never be certain that the next cycle will not be the one which works. At times a couple may think they have reached a decision that it is time to move on, but then one of them changes their mind and wants to give it just one more try.

It may be particularly difficult for women to move on. Their desire for a baby can turn into absolute desperation. Even though their chances of success with another round of IVF might be as low as 1 per cent, they can't bear to think they might be at the end of the road. This can cause a lot of friction in a relationship. At this stage, many women need help to regain their perspective and to be able to move on if that is their choice.

Case Study

Janet, 44, had been through nine unsuccessful IVF cycles. She came to me to help her prepare for another round of IVF. Looking at the couple sitting there, I could see that Peter, 47, was absolutely resigned to the fact that he was at the end of the road with this, but because he loved and cared for Janet he was trying to indulge her. Janet, on the other hand, was enthused by the fact she was back at another IVF clinic and had been told they might use a different technique to get her pregnant.

Her hopes were really high, even though she knew the chances were slim. Peter was finding it hard to be enthusiastic or match her optimism for this final try. They agreed that if they went ahead with this treatment, it would be the last one, but Peter was concerned because he had heard this before. If this didn't work, there would still be more and more treatments Janet would read about on the internet or elsewhere.

Janet started to cry. She couldn't believe they had got to this stage after six years, and she couldn't bear to consider life without a baby.

A Fertility Counsellor's Perspective (by Jane Knight, Fertility Counsellor)

Janet and Peter's situation is a very difficult one. The first thing to consider is how long they have been trying. Six years is a long time to be trying to achieve anything; in many ways this quest has come to define who they are as a couple. Peter sounds very supportive and is clearly trying to keep Janet happy. In some situations, there may be little else left in the relationship if the focus of getting pregnant is taken away, so it is not only that there will be no baby, but one or other partner may fear that there will be no relationship.

Some couples may have been together for a long time and only been trying for a baby for a relatively short part of their relationship. It may be that one or other partner was not ready for a baby earlier, so there are resentments, regrets and guilt associated with this. It can be particularly difficult if a woman had an abortion earlier in the relationship when their future may have felt uncertain; now, because the relationship has flourished, there may be serious regrets that the 'wrong decision' was made, resulting in guilt and blame.

Couples such as Janet and Peter need to acknowledge that a huge amount of time, energy and money has gone into this fertility journey, and that it may feel like this has all been wasted if there is no baby at the end of it. It is always very hard to end on a negative note – with 'a failure'. Some couples at this stage may have lost pregnancies through miscarriage and not had appropriate support to manage their emotions at the time, however early the pregnancy loss. Being able to grieve and then let go of any past pregnancies (or hopes and dreams for successful IVF) may be an important part of acknowledging their grief related to not having their own child.

Couples also need to consider the importance of a baby in their relationship. Some women openly admit that a baby is more important than their relationship and are prepared to lose their partner in their quest for motherhood, but for other women, the relationship comes first. Other women will be anxious that not having a child will mean that her partner deserts her for a younger, fertile woman. Janet talks about 'her baby'. I would want to explore with her quite how she sees 'her baby'.

Would Janet consider egg donation? This would dramatically improve her chances of having a baby. After egg donation (which some women describe as 'adopting an egg') this would be her biological (and legal) child as she would carry the pregnancy and give birth. It would not be her genetic child, of course, so would she still see this as 'her baby'? It would be important for both Janet and Peter to consider the importance of a genetic link to the child. (For more on egg donation, see opposite.)

I often ask couples to think about what they really want and how they view the role of a parent. Do they want a little person in their lives to nurture; to do all the fun things with; to feel reconnected with family and friendship groups? Have they considered alternative ways of having a family – adoption or even fostering? How important is the genetic side – the physical characteristics of the genetic mix; the fantasy about the appearance of the child; the personality traits; the anticipated talents and so on? How do their views fit in with the wider dynamic of both extended families, or with friends?

I might suggest to this couple that they try an exercise where they 'pretend' that they have made their decision – to go ahead with another treatment – and then both live with that decision for a week and see how it feels. Then, the following week, they are asked to live with the decision not to have another treatment. This can be a very valuable exercise as it gives you time to start to experience the emotions related to the chosen route. So often you can be flitting from one possibility to the next. Living with a decision, and preferably documenting how it feels and then discussing it, can be a good way to start to sort out what you both really want. It may then be helpful to talk it through with an independent person, such as a counsellor, who will act as a sounding board and may also challenge you.

I am a great believer in writing things down. If this couple decides to go for another IVF cycle, I would suggest that they both document their agreement that this is their final cycle. I feel it would also help them to explore how life could look if the cycle is not successful. Any time you have to make significant decisions, it is good to write down your thoughts and why and how you arrived at the decision you did, with all the information available to you at the time. You will then always have that to look back on in years to come, and fully appreciate why you chose a certain course of action.

Egg Donation

Egg donation has been used as a standard form of fertility treatment since 1984 for women who, for a variety of reasons, have problems with egg quality. The egg donor is usually a younger woman (under 35). Her ovaries are stimulated to produce 10–15 eggs, which are then collected. The donor's part of this 'third-party reproduction' is now complete. The couple who are to receive the donated eggs are prepared and the two women's cycles are synchronised. The egg recipient has hormonal supplements to prepare her womb lining. The donor eggs are fertilised by her partner's sperm and the embryos are transferred into her uterus.

Many of you will have heard the words 'egg donation' mentioned at an IVF consultation. You may have been shocked by this. For some couples egg donation feels right because the male partner is genetically linked to the baby, and the woman can still experience the physical process of pregnancy, birth and breast-feeding. She still has the emotional attachment to the baby – she literally provides all the hormones, all the nourishment, everything to allow this single cell to grow and develop inside her body.

We see many couples who have had repeated unsuccessful attempts at IVF and want to discuss moving on to egg donation, how to find a suitable clinic and how best to prepare physically, mentally and emotionally. This is a major decision, but the big advantage about this stage is that you have time. So often, especially for older women, things have been moving at an alarming pace, but you can now relax; take a breather – you have plenty of time to consider your next steps. If you are contemplating moving on to egg donation you can forget your biological clock – you could soon be turning your clock back.

For a couple, especially a woman, to arrive at the point of considering egg donation is a real milestone. No one wants to give up the chance of having their own genetic child. Often, women have a gradual realisation that IVF isn't going to work for them, most commonly because of their age or repeated poor response to stimulation. Some men find it hard to accept the idea of their sperm with another woman's egg. For many individuals or couples egg donation does not feel right – they are honest with themselves and only want their own genetic child. For some couples, there may be moral, ethical or religious objections or concerns related to egg donation. They may not both share the same views or values, which may further complicate the situation. Then, of course, there are all the issues related to the donor and what you tell a child (see 'Implications Counselling', page 463).

Egg donation offers realistic hope to many couples, and has a much higher success rate than IVF if the woman's ovaries are not responding. However, even though the success rate may be relatively high (around 50 per cent), there will still be a large number of couples for whom it doesn't work. There is a long wait for egg donation in the UK, so many of the clients we see go overseas to places like Spain,

Eastern Europe or America. It is usually the woman who makes the decision and is virtually on the next plane out while the man is still mulling over what's what.

Moving to egg donation is a hard decision and never taken lightly. It is important that everything has been done to help the woman have her own genetic child before getting to this stage. Reasons for considering egg donation include:

- The woman's age
- Poor ovarian function (often linked to age)
- Premature ovarian failure (see Chapter 14)
- Repeated unsuccessful IVF despite good embryos being transferred to the womb (and where there are no immune issues)
- Risk of passing on genetic disorders
- Surgery or chemotherapy
- Recurrent miscarriage

Sadly, a woman's age does have an impact on IVF success. If a woman comes to see me at 45 or 46, she may be better off considering egg donation straight away because her chances of success with IVF will be extremely low. With IVF and diminishing egg reserve, there is a constant concern that time is limited, but with egg donation there is not the same urgency. Many women come back to me 18 months later and say, 'I wasn't ready to hear about egg donation back then but I would like to know more now.' You have time to research it and really think it through, weighing up the options and making sure you are happy with what you are doing. Remember, it is quite possible to do egg donation even if the woman's periods have completely stopped and she has gone through the menopause as it is the age of the donor egg which influences the success of the treatment. Provided the woman receiving the donor egg still has a fully functioning womb, there is no limit on age from the biological perspective. From the social and emotional side, however, you will still feel a pressure. Clinics all have an age limit for egg donation, but some clinics in the UK will treat women up to the age of 50.

Frequently Asked Questions

- *What is the situation regarding donor anonymity?*

Prior to 1 April 2005, the Human Fertilisation and Embryology Authority (HFEA) guaranteed that egg (and sperm) donors would remain anonymous. Couples receiving donated gametes received very little information about the donor and there was no identifying information available. However, since April 2005, donors no longer remain anonymous; when a donor-conceived child reaches the age of 18, they can apply to the HFEA for full identifying information about their donor. This has resulted in a shortage of donated sperm and eggs in the UK, although many steps are being taken to try and improve the situation. The change in law is a reflection of the experiences of adopted children and the importance for some children and adults of being able to find their genetic mother. Although donor-conceived children now have the same opportunities as adopted children to find their genetic parent, it is too early to know how many will want to pursue this.

- *What if I find a known donor?*

Many women approach either a friend or family member to be a donor. At times, a friend or a sister may offer to be a donor if she is aware of your situation. This can work very well, particularly with a younger sister who has completed her own family. However, there are many considerations and it is vital that all parties involved (including the partner of the donor) have given full consideration to all the implications for the future. Implications counselling helps you to explore all the issues for yourselves, the potential future child and the dynamic within the extended family (see page 463).

- *How is the egg donor screened?*

Egg donors go through a rigorous screening process before they are accepted on a donor programme. This includes a detailed medical history including family history; gynaecological screening, including blood tests to assess hormone levels and to check ovarian reserve; tests to exclude diseases (including sexually transmitted infections) and genetic abnormalities. Most clinics will not accept donors over the age of 35 due to the increased risk of chromosomal abnormalities such as Down's syndrome. It can be very reassuring for the recipient couple if the egg donor has donated previously, resulting in a successful pregnancy.

- *What are the success rates?*

For a woman using donor eggs, the chances of a successful live birth depend on the age of the eggs, not on the age of the mother. Not only are your chances of pregnancy significantly increased with donor eggs, your chances of miscarrying are greatly reduced. A woman in her early 40s, using her own eggs, has about a 7–10 per cent chance of getting pregnant with assisted conception, but if she uses a donor egg, her chance increases to 25–60 per cent. This tends to be higher than the average success rate for conventional IVF across all age groups because donor eggs are from fertile women under 35.

- *How can you decide if this treatment is right for you?*

The decision to go down the donor egg route is not an easy one. It is strongly recommended that you and your partner (if you have one) talk to an experienced fertility counsellor, and possibly to other people who have had egg donation, before making your decision to go ahead.

All HFEA-licensed clinics are obliged to offer access to implications counselling before you consent to treatment. Support groups such as Infertility Network UK and Donor Conception Network can also provide a valuable source of information and support (see Resources).

- *Can you recommend any clinics in the UK?*

In the UK, the HFEA is the central regulating body and register for licensed clinics so this is the best place to start (see Resources). Most fertility units will treat women with egg donation using a known donor, but many clinics will also have an egg donor programme recruiting anonymous donors. Some clinics also have an egg sharing programme (see page 460) where a couple going through IVF agree to share some of their eggs with the recipient and the recipient part-funds the donor's IVF cycle.

- *What about overseas clinics?*

I have heard mixed reports from couples about their experiences of egg donation overseas. Although some overseas clinics are good, there have been reports of clinics exploiting vulnerable couples and making it difficult for them to receive financial recompense when things go wrong. My advice is to do your research carefully and speak to as many different people as possible who have had the treatment over-seas. The internet is a great place to start as chat rooms and general advice are easily accessible. In most countries there is no central regis-ter such as the HFEA. Countries outside the UK may not meet clinical or ethical standards and the legal position may be confusing. The key issues to consider with overseas clinics include:

- ○ standards for testing donors for disease and inherited disorders
- ○ donor information and issues regarding anonymity (for the child)
- ○ laboratory standards

○ concerns about exploitation of donors (payment or reimbursement)
○ communication difficulties

Language barriers can make the situation more complex. In European clinics you generally do not get to choose the donor, but in clinics in the US, you will probably be able to choose the donor, although treatment may be more expensive. It is possible to arrange the whole cycle directly with an overseas clinic, but this is not always straightforward; it is generally better to find an overseas clinic that has a link with a clinic in the UK so that appropriate investigations and treatments can be done before you travel overseas for treatment. You may not have access to implications counselling if you are having treatment abroad.

Interview with Lena Korea, Senior Sister (Ovum Donation), Lister Hospital

Have you seen a change in egg donation recently?
Yes, anonymous donations have significantly dropped since 2005. We find that we are doing only three to four of them per year, whereas we have seen a marked increase in people entering the egg-sharing scheme. Referrals for recipients have not dropped. The number of altruistic donors has dropped since changes in regulations came into practice in 2005 which removed anonymity of the donor. However, within the same time period, we have seen an increase in the number of women enquiring about egg sharing.

Many women requiring egg donation are older women who have already failed to conceive using their own eggs, often stressed and anxious about time running out. Since donor availability is limited in the UK, many recipients are keen to try everything possible that might improve the outcome of their treatment cycle. Many will change their diet, take extra supplements, exercise, lose weight and some try alternative therapies, such as acupuncture or reflexology.

In your experience, how significant is attitude and mindset?
I think these things are really important.

The Egg Donor Cycle

Different clinics will use different drug protocols, but the key steps are as follows:

1. The menstrual cycles of the donor and the recipient need to be synchronised. If you (the recipient) are having periods, then you will be given drugs (either by injection or sniffing) to suppress your natural hormones and prevent ovulation. If you are no longer having cycles, then you will not go through the suppressing phase. The donor will be given drugs to down-regulate (suppress) her cycle. She will then start the stimulation phase.

2. The recipient is given oestrogen (and sometimes progesterone) tablets to prepare her womb lining.

3. When the donor has enough follicles (usually greater than 15mm) she will be given an injection to mature the eggs.

4. The eggs are retrieved from the donor 36 hours later.

5. The eggs are fertilised with your partner's sperm.

6. You will continue on progesterone (and possibly oestrogen) supplementation to further prepare your womb lining, making sure it is in the best possible condition to receive the embryo(s).

7. Between two to five days later your embryos will be transferred.

8. You will be asked to do a pregnancy test about two weeks after egg collection.

Case Study

Sam, 42, had one child whom she had conceived naturally. However, she could not conceive again and had been through three unsuccessful attempts at IVF.

Zita: 'What made you move on to egg donation?'

Sam: 'The feeling of failure was terrible. I had never failed at anything in my life. I am a high-flying Oxford graduate so why couldn't I achieve success in this part of my life? The clinic made me feel so old and that it was all my fault because I'd left it too late to get married. Initially, I thought egg donation was for desperate people. However, coming along and talking to you and your team planted a seed that made it seem accessible and manageable. Also, that weekend we were at an event with other friends and family, and of the eight couples I realised that only our child had been conceived naturally; the others were adopted or the result of egg or sperm donation. They all seemed happy. Their families seemed happy. These kids didn't have the label 'egg donor' on their backs. I began to realise that this was a regular occurrence and that it doesn't matter how you achieve your family as long as there is love there. We chose to go to the States as we wanted to choose from a bigger selection and know more about our donor. The first time we tried it didn't work. That was heartbreaking as my expectations were so high. I went out a second time and got pregnant with twins. I feel so blessed, although I do know the risks are greater with my age and a twin pregnancy.'

Zita: 'Do you have any fears about it being a donor pregnancy?'

Sam: 'My biggest fear is that my babies are very different to me and don't look like me at all. Also, I am cagey about telling people, but I think about what you have said to me – I am growing these babies. I am nourishing them and nurturing them inside me, and there are many ways to bond with them. I feel that they are mine.'

Egg Sharing

In egg sharing, a woman going through IVF agrees to share her eggs with another woman, who in return will fund (or part-fund) the sharer's IVF cycle. Both the egg sharer and the recipient receive implications counselling prior to their treatment. Egg sharing brings along other potential issues which need to be considered by all involved, for example after donating half of her eggs the egg sharer's cycle may not be successful, while the recipient goes on and has a successful pregnancy. Egg sharers tend to be younger healthy women who may not qualify for NHS treatment, for example if they have a child from a previous relationship or if the partner has had a vasectomy. So, it may offer hope to couples who would otherwise be unable to do IVF, while at the same time giving an older woman a chance of having a baby.

Donor Sperm

Male fertility has been revolutionised by the use of intracytoplasmic sperm injection (ICSI, see page 336) over the last 15 years. Men who would previously have needed to use donor sperm have been increasingly able to father their own genetic child. However, there are still circumstances where donor sperm may be needed. A man may be azoospermic (no sperm in the ejaculate) and in some cases no sperm retrievable surgically or there may be a risk of him passing on a serious genetic condition. It is also used by some single women and lesbian couples. Some couples have numerous unsuccessful ICSI cycles because of problems with the sperm and decide to go on to sperm donation. Sperm donors go through rigorous medical testing prior to being accepted on a donor programme.

If a couple is considering using donor sperm, it is important that they see a fertility counsellor. This will help them to explore the implications for each of them individually, for themselves as a couple, for a potential future child and for other significant people in their lives. Donor Conception Network provides useful information regarding sperm and egg donation, including reflections by young people born as a result of donor sperm (see Resources).

The Dangerous Hidden World of Internet Gamete Donation, by Laura Witjens, Chair of the National Gamete Donation Trust

It's a universal economic principle that every shortage leads to a market place. Depending on the legislation this can be open or underground but, in either case, there is money to be made. Eggs and sperm have joined the list of commodities as gold, copper, coffee and sugar. The combination of the promise of money, an ongoing shortage and no care for the end result, is fertile soil for dangerous practices.

The last decade saw a growing industry selling sperm on the internet which tested the legal loopholes. The supply of sperm for home insemination came within the scope of the Human Fertilisation & Embryology Act 1990 on 5 July 2007. Internet operations are required to hold a licence from the HFEA if they wish to supply sperm for home insemination. The provisions in the Act on gamete donation now also apply to donations procured by online organisations (described in the regulations as 'Non-Medical Fertility Services'). These include screening donors for infection, quarantining of donor samples and the recording of the donor's details on the HFEA's register. Effectively, this has brought an end to the supply of anonymously donated, fresh sperm for home insemination.

However, nowadays there are still many ways of finding your donor on the internet. Technically these sites operate within the law and get away with it as they don't supply the sperm but act merely as introduction agencies. It's a loophole that may be difficult to close as it could be argued it's a date with a certain outcome. Organising dates is not illegal and neither is the exchange of sperm, natural or not.

So how does it work? The recipient (couple) registers with the site. A variety of options are available, needless to say none of them for free for the recipients. It effectively works as dating sites do whereby both parties list their relevant statistics and a personal message. Both parties can contact each other either by the site-hosted personal message board or via the email address left on the profile.

The dangers of this service are many. Donors are not tested at all or not to the same standard as in UK clinics. Even if a donor produces a certificate of an STI test, which some do, it is invalid the day after the test. The recipient has no way of checking who the donor is (and therefore also if the test results are his), what his medical conditions are, anything about lifestyle or if he has other children.

From the donor's point of view, as the procedure hasn't been carried out by a UK licensed clinic, the donor is the father in the case of an unmarried couple or single woman. We have spoken to a donor of one of these services who wasn't made aware that legally he could be seen as the father. He also confirmed that he donated over a period of seven months, at least weekly, and had no idea how many children were fathered. During that period he was only tested once.

Internet egg donation services are based on the sample principle: they prey on the vulnerable, give misleading information, no clear contact information is given and are in the business to make money, not happy parents or donors.

The egg-donation process is, of course, profoundly different because the recipient and donor actually have to go through a UK licensed clinic. In theory it should therefore be easier to clamp down on but this depends on the resourcefulness of the donor and recipient and the awareness of the clinic.

We have to be mindful that as long as we have a shortage, shrewd business people and patients and donors prepared to flout the law, these practices will continue to exist. As soon as one loophole is closed, another one will appear. That's not to say we shouldn't try to tighten regulation. But this is a good reminder why we should continue to look at adjusting practices, reviewing guidelines and finding alternative ways of recruiting more donors.

Implications Counselling
(by Jane Knight)

The aim of implications counselling is to enable you to reflect upon and understand the proposed course of IVF treatment involving donation (of eggs, sperm or embryos). You will consider the implications for yourselves, your family and any children born as a result, and anyone else affected by your decision. This is also highly relevant for couples considering surrogacy (see page 465). At least one session of implications counselling is recommended before consenting to any proposed treatment.

The following issues will be discussed over one to three sessions:

- How you and your partner both feel about the proposed treatment.
- How this would affect any existing children.
- Who you will tell – the advantages and disadvantages of openness.
- The attitudes of friends and family to your proposed treatment.
- Your thoughts and concerns about a future child where one parent is not the genetic parent.
- Issues around openness, secrecy and what, when and how to tell a child.
- The short- and long-term implications of known or anonymous donation.

The counsellor will also explore legal and practical matters, such as:

- The changes in the law since 1 April 2005 removing donor anonymity.
- The legal maximum number of pregnancies for any treatment cycle.
- The Congenital Disabilities (Civil Liability) Act 1976 and information from donors.
- Reserving stock for siblings.
- Information on screening procedures and recruitment of donors.
- Information on relevant networks, support groups and further reading.
- Issues relevant to donation outside the UK. The HFEA does not regulate overseas treatment but provides useful information on the issues and potential risks.

In addition, for single women and lesbian couples, the counsellor will explore the child's need for supportive parenting (and male role models). The new parenthood laws introduced in April 2009 removed the concept of the child's right to a father and replaced this with the concept of supportive parenting. The new law relates to who can be registered as a child's legal father or the child's second parent. With a lesbian couple, the woman's female partner is automatically recognised as the child's second legal parent and can be named on the child's birth certificate. From April 2010, male couples will be able to apply to the courts for a Parental Order allowing both men to be registered as the legal parents. The HFEA (see Resources) is a good source of updated information on all aspects of IVF and parenthood issues.

Surrogacy

Surrogacy is a procedure where a couple with fertility problems (the commissioning couple or intended parents) seek the help of another woman (the surrogate or host) to carry a baby for them. The surrogate may be known to the commissioning couple, or may be introduced through a surrogacy network. Surrogacy is a comparatively simple procedure medically; however, it raises many ethical, emotional and legal issues.

Surrogacy may be suggested if a woman has problems with her womb and is unable to carry a pregnancy to term. This may be appropriate, for example, if a woman has had pelvic problems, a previous hysterectomy or was born without a womb. Some women may have had repeated unsuccessful attempts at IVF or recurrently miscarried. Health problems, such as dangerously high blood pressure, a heart condition or liver disease, may make pregnancy a serious risk for some women. There are essentially two types of surrogacy: traditional surrogacy (sometimes known as 'straight surrogacy') and gestational surrogacy (sometimes known as 'host surrogacy').

- **Traditional surrogacy** (sometimes known as 'straight surrogacy') may be appropriate if the intended mother is unable to use her own eggs. It combines the egg of the surrogate mother with the sperm of the intended father. This can be done at home using artificial insemination, but is increasingly performed in an IVF clinic. The baby is genetically that of the surrogate mother and the intended father. The intended mother has no genetic or biological link to the baby.

- **Gestational surrogacy** (sometimes known as 'host surrogacy') may be appropriate if the woman has good-quality eggs that can be

465

stimulated using IVF drugs. It uses the egg of the intended mother with her husband/partner's sperm. A baby conceived in this way will be genetically that of both intended parents. The surrogate mother who carries the intended parents' genetic child will therefore have no genetic link to the baby, but she will still be the biological (and legal) mother. If the intended father's sperm are not suitable for IVF/ICSI then donor sperm may be used. Any child born would then not be genetically linked to the intended father.

Case Study

After five unsuccessful IVF attempts, Ella felt low, despondent and desperate. She decided to explore surrogacy in America, where it is much more acceptable. Nevertheless, it is a very complicated process, full of potential pitfalls. I asked Ella about the hazards of surrogacy. She said that you have to be very careful in your choice of surrogate. She came across quite a few 'fruit loops', as well as very young girls from socially deprived backgrounds who were just looking for money. Ella's surrogacy worked and the surrogate got pregnant, but sadly the woman miscarried, so Ella made the hard decision to give up hope of becoming a mother herself. She felt it was a big leap to let go of the idea of ever becoming pregnant and accepting she would never be a mother. Since she had gained a lot of experience and insight while in America, she decided to help other women who wanted to explore surrogacy. Ella now helps many women going through surrogacy and is part of the team at the Zita West Clinic. Ella advises people to research surrogacy thoroughly before making a decision. There is a wealth of information available. She also feels that emotional support from other women is essential.

If you are considering surrogacy in the UK or abroad, surrogacy agencies such as COTS (Childlessness Overcome through Surrogacy, see Resources) provide advice and support to surrogates and intended parents. They also help you to draw up a surrogacy agreement. It is very important to be clear about the legal issues. The law around surrogacy is very complex and it is vital that you are familiar with the current law and seek legal advice from a solicitor who specialises in fertility and parenting law. Implications counselling (see page 463) is also a vital part of the surrogacy process. The surrogate mother (and her partner) and the commissioning couple need to consider all the possible implications of this complex parenting process and the clinic performing the treatment requires written reports to ensure that all parties fully understand all aspects of the process.

Considering Adoption
(by Jane Knight)

Adoption is rarely a first choice for couples planning pregnancy. It is generally a third option after natural conception and IVF, and sometimes if egg donation has been unsuccessful. By this stage many couples have already been through a long journey, often involving numerous IVF cycles, miscarriages or other pregnancy loss.

Pre-adoption counselling is very important as adoption is not a straightforward process. An adopted child may need help coming to terms with their own losses and difficulties. Adoption agencies, such as Adoption UK (see Resources), offer information and support to would-be adoptive parents, and ongoing support during and after adoption. There is a scarcity of babies for adoption in the UK and many older children have their own difficult pasts and sometimes health issues. These children can be hugely challenging, but given the right support many couples can find the experience of bringing up such a child as part of a loving family most fulfilling.

It can be harder for older couples considering adoption because of age restrictions and the need to have stopped treatments prior to starting adoption procedures. Some couples are now looking overseas for adoption. You start this process by going through your local authority (as with home adoption) or if this does not deal with inter-country adoption the national organisation is PACT (Parents and Children Together, see Resources). They will send you to the ICA (Intercountry Adoption Centre, see Resources) for an Introductory Course. Preparation Courses are mandatory, but are invaluable in helping you to think through the challenges ahead.

A fertility counsellor can also help couples to come to terms with the loss of their dream of having their own biological child and start to prepare for the challenges of adoption.

Moving on with Your Life without Children

It is important for all couples to feel that they have done as much as they could, or as much as they felt appropriate, before moving on. The decision to stop treatment can be very difficult as there will always be new possibilities around the corner. It can be hard to let go and to start moving on with your life. Fertility investigations and treatments can dominate the lives of many couples for years. In many ways, their lives have been on hold. It can be difficult for them to imagine a life without fertility treatments after all this time. It is so important for you both to be communicating well and to hear how the other is really feeling. You may need to start rebuilding your relationship after the toll the fertility journey has taken. Very often you will have almost lost sight of what attracted you to your partner when you first got together. Additionally, it can be hard to tell your family that you are moving on with your life – for parents it may mean the loss of their hopes to be grandparents.

Now you are free from the cycle of hopes and fears of each IVF treatment, you have the opportunity to broaden your horizons. You may wish to travel, to develop new interests, to consider a change of career or to take up new challenges. You might want to move house or even go and live in a new country. Infertility Network UK offers support and friendship for couples who are involuntarily childless (see Resources).

One of the most difficult things can be answering other people's questions about family. The very common and innocent question, 'Do you have any children?' can seem quite overwhelming. The advice from Infertility Network UK is to keep the answer simple – for example, 'Sadly not.' The more open you are able to be about your childlessness, the easier it will be to normalise it and find some level of acceptance. That is not to say that it is easy, because clearly you may be facing a future completely at odds with everything you had ever wished for or taken for granted since childhood. Some people feel that not having a child affects their whole sense of who they are as a person, and for other people there can be a strong sense of not fulfilling what seems like their main purpose in life – to reproduce.

'More to Life', a service provided by Infertility Network UK (see Resources), is a national support network for couples who are childless by circumstance and not by choice. This is an invaluable source of information and support, helping couples to have a fulfilling life, acknowledging that children were a wanted part of the future, but for many reasons were not possible.

Fertility counselling may help you to put some of the negative thoughts behind you and move forward with a more positive attitude.

It is not the future that either of you had hoped for, and you may prefer not to engage with other people's children for a while. However, for many couples who find the strength to move forward positively, you can spend many happy and fulfilling hours and develop special bonds with other children – nephews or nieces, friends' children, godchildren. Some people even choose to work with children or be involved in voluntary work with them.

The Future of Assisted Fertility

I asked a number of eminent doctors for their thoughts on IVF success and how they see future developments in assisted fertility. These interviews are included on page 475. The other area of increasing interest is for women whose biological needs are not in line with their social situation and they are contemplating the best way to try and preserve their fertility for the future.

Preserving Future Fertility

While some women are looking to preserve their fertility for social reasons, there is another group of people who are increasingly faced with fertility dilemmas – these are men and women who have survived cancers. As treatment for cancer has improved, it is estimated that by 2010 one in 715 adults will be a long-term survivor of childhood or adolescent cancers. Every effort is now made to preserve future fertility, before chemotherapy is started – this may involve sperm or egg freezing and then assisted fertility at a later stage.

Freezing Sperm

Sperm freezing is not new. It has been available since the 1960s with sperm banks supplying anonymous sperm for use in a variety of circumstances (see page 460). There may also be reasons why men may want to freeze sperm for personal use at a later stage. A man who has had cancer may have his sperm frozen prior to chemotherapy. In IVF and IUI, sperm can be frozen in advance for men who have problems producing samples on the day or if couples are geographically apart. Other reasons for freezing sperm include: testicular failure; erection problems; ejaculation difficulties; serious medical problems or a varied but declining semen analysis.

Sperm can be stored for an initial 10 years, but there must be written consent in place. There can be an extension, but HFEA rules state that samples cannot be stored beyond the man's 55th birthday. If you want to have your sperm stored, you must be tested for HIV and hepatitis B and C. This is to reduce the risk of cross-contamination between stored sperm samples. It is also important that you have implications counselling (see page 463).

The freeze-thaw process has a negative impact on sperm, affecting the quality and motility of the sperm, especially if the sample is weak to start with. Even healthy sperm may not do well after freezing. Very occasionally, none of the sperm will survive the procedure. Fresh sperm is obviously better than frozen, but many women get pregnant with frozen sperm. All donor sperm is frozen and quarantined for six months then retested for viruses including HIV.

Freezing Eggs

Until recently, it was possible to freeze embryos but not eggs. As technology has now improved, many centres can offer women the option of freezing their eggs. Women decide to freeze their eggs for many reasons, from women who have not yet found the right partner to those who are about to start a course of chemotherapy for cancer. The younger you are when you freeze your eggs, the better the chance that they are chromosomally normal.

It is important to realise that a frozen egg does not guarantee a baby. Egg freezing is technically more difficult than embryo freezing because the egg has a very high water content and ice crystals can damage the egg. So far only a few hundred babies have been born as a result of a frozen-thawed egg. New techniques of vitrification – a fast freezing technique – seem to be more successful and the freeze-thaw rate is higher, but it will vary between centres and not all centres have egg freezing or vitrification facilities.

To collect the eggs for freezing, a woman's ovaries are stimulated with IVF drugs in the usual way – the eggs are collected and then frozen for later use. The only way to have a child after egg freezing is using assisted conception again. The frozen-thawed eggs are mixed with the male partner's sperm and any resulting embryos will be transferred into the woman's uterus.

Anyone considering egg freezing will be counselled to consider the risks and benefits and the expected freeze-thaw rate and chance of a successful pregnancy at the end of it. Even if an egg thaws successfully, this does not necessarily mean that it will fertilise, and of course if it fertilises successfully, the embryo then has to divide and then implant – so there are many stages which need to go well.

Final Word

Scientific advances offer us an overwhelming range of possible technologies and treatments along with which come an even more baffling array of statistics, benefits and risks. Understandably, we often feel ill-equipped to make rational choices. So many couples today feel almost compelled to go on and on trying for a baby as there will always be something new around the corner. One of my biggest fears for couples is the effect the quest for a baby can have on their relationship. So many relationships can be damaged along the way.

Having worked in this field for many years and, along with my colleagues, having listened to and supported thousands of couples through the challenges of fertility investigations and treatments, the most important thing we say is 'Never say never!' The second thing is to accept that time is needed for each transition – from trying naturally to assisted conception and beyond. Take time to really talk and really listen to each other's anxieties so that you each feel connected and in harmony emotionally. Sadly, there are no easy shortcuts here and each of us has different ways of coping, but with time, no matter what stage you are at, you will get through!

In compiling this book my team and so many renowned professionals have collaborated to give you a real insight into all aspects of fertility and assisted conception. We are passionate and feel committed to helping as many couples reach their goal as possible. I hope this book and its collective wisdom helps you in some small way to understand not only the physical processes, but a little more about yourselves and how to cope at each step along the way.

Appendix 1

Interviews with Some Top Doctors

Over the years I have been privileged to get to know many of the top doctors working in the field of assisted conception. I hope the interviews throughout the book have given you some insight into all aspects of IVF. It is a complex field and each couple brings their own unique situation. This is why it is important to have an array of different techniques and approaches to address fertility problems. There is limited value in a 'one-size-fits-all' approach to IVF. I have been overwhelmed by the response and the generosity with which so many doctors have given their time to discuss some of the aspects which make a key difference in assisted conception. I have afforded the interviews in this final section no lesser or greater respect than the earlier interviews – it is purely a matter of space.

Questioning doctors about what they consider makes a difference to IVF success has given me more insight into the complex technological world of assisted conception. Talking to doctors, sitting in and lecturing at medical meetings both in the UK and internationally over the last few years, it has been interesting to observe the increased interest in the 'softer side' of IVF. Indeed, men are not sperm factories and women are not baby-making machines. As sensitive human beings with individual needs, stresses and complex human relationships, couples facing fertility dilemmas require more than a mechanistic approach to manage the additional stress imposed by assisted conception. Many doctors now acknowledge that the work that we do supporting couples nutritionally and managing psychological distress is helping to provide the missing link and that the way forward is with a more integrated approach.

Some doctors and clinics are achieving phenomenal success rates through their individualised approach and meticulous attention to detail, but there still remain wide discrepancies in success rates (as well as NHS access) across the country. Our work aims to look outside the box at the individual couple, preparing them for this technological process at every level, to help to maximise the success of assisted conception.

(The following interviews by Zita West have been reproduced in alphabetical order.)

Interview with Mr Hossam Abdalla, Consultant Gynaecologist and Clinical Director of the Lister Fertility Clinic

What makes IVF successful?
The patient. The patient. The patient! Everyone is different; some people have better success with IVF than others. If a woman has a higher FSH and blocked tubes she will have half the chance of someone with better hormone levels and unblocked tubes – but she can still go on to get pregnant.

We can now test for egg reserves using AMH, which can help assess the likely way a woman is going to respond to IVF treatment. Women are devastated when their results come back very low. What are your experiences with women with low AMH going through an IVF cycle?

Looking at a woman's egg reserves and IVF outcome, we have learnt a lot in recent years with AMH. We don't have a cut-off rate for AMH. At the Lister, out of 78 cycles done with women who have an AMH of less than 1, we've had seven live births. The difficulty is with age and fewer eggs being produced and you have to get a good one. Protocols used are generally longer protocols and the older you are, your AMH level isn't going to be as good. If your ovarian reserve is good and you are older, you still have a 40 per cent chance with a blastocyst transfer. If you are over 40 the pregnancy rate is 28–33 per cent and the live birth rate is 15–20 per cent.

What other factors improve IVF success?

Embryology and a good laboratory are fundamental. Many factors make IVF work. I think that support and a holistic approach helps relax patients through their cycles.

What do you think about immune issues?

We use reproductive immunology, but this is a controversial area and not everyone has immune issues. The difficulty is that less than 10 per cent of people have immune issues and there is no clear evidence that treatment provided is effective.

What have you changed your views about in the past five years?

I now feel that women with reduced ovarian reserve should keep trying as long as they have eggs. I tell my patients that you can give up on me but don't give up on treatment as long as you have eggs. My views about multiple births have also changed. I'd rather put one embryo back at a time. Having twins is the hardest thing for women; the success rate is higher but the divorce rate is also higher. When you put back two blastocysts you have a success rate of 60 per cent and a 50 per cent chance of having twins. With one blastocyst you have a 55 per cent success rate. I'd rather have a 55 per cent success rate with no twins.

Interview with Professor Ian Craft, Director of the London Fertility Centre

Professor Craft is one of the forefathers of IVF in the UK and has trained many doctors who now have successful clinics in the UK.

What makes IVF successful?
- Personalised care: a personal relationship between the consultant and the patient helps the best outcome.
- The stimulation regime has to be right for the individual.
- Standardised lab procedures for embryos which have changed dramatically over the years have improved results.
- Encouraging women to be as relaxed as possible through IVF. Women feel more at ease when they are offered complementary therapies.
- A positive frame of mind seems to go a long way to get better results.

I feel that success rates have reached a plateau and the way forward would be to look at genetics and maybe metabolites in the culture. Now with 40 per cent male factor, the contribution of ICSI has made a major improvement to couples who wouldn't otherwise have been able to have babies.

Interview with Mr Tarek El-Toukhy, Consultant and Honorary Lecturer in Reproductive Medicine and Surgery at Guy's and St Thomas' Hospital NHS Foundation Trust and King's College London

What do you think makes IVF successful?

Attention to detail at every single level – right from the initial consultation onwards, including examinations, ultrasound scanning, semen analysis, ovarian stimulation, egg retrieval, selection of embryos and embryo transfer. It helps significantly to address any lifestyle and weight issues with the couple before treatment starts and ensuring the patient understands the treatment process is also a great help. Doctors should have up-to-date knowledge and skills and be able to draw on their experience to give patients individualised care and the best chance of success. Regular monitoring throughout a cycle is important too, to prevent potential problems such as ovarian hyperstimulation. You also need a state-of-the-art lab and skilled embryologists. Having a good team of doctors, nurses and embryologists all working together helps patients through the treatment, allaying their fears and reducing stress.

Have your views on IVF changed in the last five years?

I believe more strongly that IVF success is influenced by lifestyle factors such as weight, smoking and alcohol consumption as there is growing evidence these factors can influence outcome.

Where do you think IVF is going? What changes do you see in the next five years?

Patients are becoming much better informed before they start treatment. This is great because it is easier to work with couples who understand the process. IVF medication will be easier to administer, further reducing the stress of treatment. I think there will be some exciting developments in embryo selection, which could improve implantation rates. There will also be better understanding about the endometrium, its immune function and blood supply, which may contribute to higher success rates.

Interview with Professor William Ledger, Professor of Obstetrics and Gynaecology and Head of Unit, University of Sheffield

What are the most important factors affecting IVF outcome?
The quality of the laboratory is important. The age of the female patient is a major factor, as is the quality of the embryo.

How can patients prepare themselves for IVF?
A positive outlook is essential. From a psychological point of view, IVF is a huge thing to go through, so if you are strong mentally and emotionally, and have the assistance of counselling, it can help enormously. Couples can prepare physically by looking at their lifestyle, addressing such issues as body weight.

What do you think about natural IVF? A lot of women are drawn towards this.
Sadly, pregnancy rates are very low. There are the same mental and physical challenges and women need the stamina to keep going back month after month with a very low result.

However, we do a lot of mild IVF in Sheffield. This is low-dose FSH and antagonist protocol, and a shorter protocol. This seems to suit women – they don't see the hyper-stimulation they did before – and they achieve a good pregnancy rate. It isn't suitable for women with severe endometriosis, or where there is a problem with the sperm. It works best for people who have had a baby in the past.

What do you see happening in IVF over the next five years?
I don't think any huge changes are on the horizon. Clinical practice has improved greatly year on year and we are getting better results. Many clinics now have success rates of over 50 per cent. Where we are failing is, as one research paper has said, that 30 per cent of IVF patients don't come back for a second round, no matter how desperate they are to have a baby, because they are so demoralised or traumatised by the whole process. What we need to do, therefore, is improve our management of women and their partners. The NHS needs to make more funding available. If you live in Sheffield, for example, you can access good clinics, but in some other parts of the country you can't.

Interview with Mr Paul Serhal, Medical Director, The Centre for Reproductive & Genetic Health (CRGH), Hon Consultant / Senior Lecturer

What do you think makes IVF successful?
There are many factors that help IVF succeed. First, I believe it's essential that each client is given full, individual attention. The key factors that contribute to the success of an IVF clinic include tailoring the drug regime to individual needs and avoiding blanket policies, a robust embryology laboratory, and utmost care during the embryo transfer process. Our pregnancy rates have improved as a result.

I think it's also important for a clinic to be open seven days a week. This enables it to offer the full range of services for egg collection and blastocyst transfer. Even at the weekend, an egg can be collected when it is ready to be harvested. You also need a seven-day facility to do Day 5 blastocysts.

How do you see IVF progressing over the next five years?
The way forward is being able to choose the right embryos to put back without invasive screening, especially at blastocyst stage.

Interview with Dr Geoffrey Sher, the Sher Institute for Reproductive Medicine, Nevada, USA

What makes IVF successful?

You have to treat clients as individuals. You can't expect every woman to respond in the same customised way. Seventy per cent of people will get pregnant with IVF that don't have any problems. But those that have issues and that fall outside of the bell curve need a much more individualised approach. You can't expect every woman to respond in the same customised way. Realising an individual approach is the factor which determines whether IVF will succeed or not. The egg has to be recruited and sent into the right environment. I always use the analogy of the seed and the soil: the egg is the seed and the womb lining the soil. Cultivating the soil and the techniques to do this is what makes a difference. Once the egg is released you have to be able to improve it. The way you mature that egg, looking at the delicate interplay of the hormones and ensuring the LH is managed well, will get you the best egg.

What improvements have been made recently?

We have seen a huge improvement in being able to look at the chromosomes in the egg. As a result we are achieving a 60 per cent birth rate with a single embryo and reducing multiple births. Many women fail to get pregnant because they can't get a good egg in order to make a good embryo. A lot of this is to do with the chromosomal normality of the egg. Until recently, all we were able to do was look at the embryo with a naked eye, and it's hard to tell if an embryo is competent by doing this. There are many grading systems and in recent years we have used pre-genetic selection (PGS) but this is quite traumatic for the embryo. CGH has changed matters. It is less traumatic to the embryo and enables us to look at the DNA of all the chromosomes.

What other factors do you think help a woman though the process?
I think the work that you do integrating stress-reduction techniques and complementary therapies helps relax and support women through the process.

Appendix 2: IVF Treatment Protocol

Showing the Key Stages of a Typical Long and Short Protocol

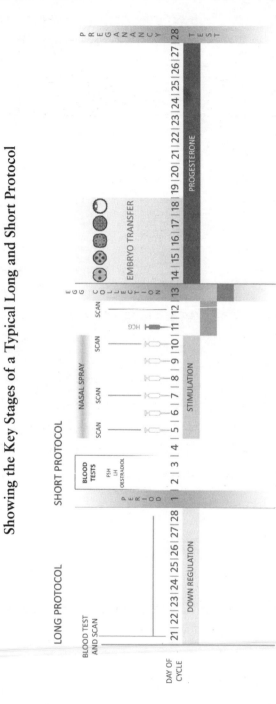

The Zita West Clinic

Following a career as a midwife in the NHS and several years in private practice as a fertility and pregnancy consultant on Harley Street, Zita founded the Zita West Clinic in Marylebone, London in 2002. It is now one of the largest integrated clinics in the UK specialising in reproductive health.

Each year, the clinic's multi-disciplinary team of specialist doctors, midwives and complementary therapists help hundreds of couples to get pregnant, both naturally and through assisted conception, with innovative programmes designed to help boost natural fertility and to improve the chances of IVF success.

Services include:

- Fertility health checks and MOTs
- Sexual health screening
- Pre-conception planning and support
- Unique male programme with comprehensive semen analysis
- IVF planning and support
- IVF failure and support
- Egg donation planning and support

- Recurrent miscarriage clinic
- Early pregnancy care and support
- Ante-natal and early-parenting training
- Post-natal care and support

Zita West Multi-vitamins

Zita has developed a comprehensive range of vitamin, mineral and essential fatty acid supplements to help support fertility, conception and pregnancy. Two new formulations have recently been added, specifically to help couples preparing for IVF.

Details of the range and further information on the clinic's services can be found at: www.zitawest.com

Zita West CDs

Zita has put together a number of CDs describing relaxation techniques which will help prospective parents cope with the stress that can sometimes make a pregnancy seem so elusive.

Details of the CDs can be found at: www.zitawest.com

Zita West Affiliated Network

There is a network of Zita West affiliated acupuncturists across the UK and the Republic of Ireland offering specialist treatment to help improve fertility and the chances of conception naturally and alongside IVF. Further information can be found at www.zitawest.com or call 020 7224 0017.

Resources

Adoption UK
www.adoptionuk.org
01295 752240
Linden House, 55 The Green
South Bar Street, Banbury
Oxfordshire OX16 9AB

**British Infertility Counselling
Association**
www.bica.net
Go to the website to find a local
counsellor who specialises in
fertility issues.

**COTS (Childlessness Overcome
through Surrogacy)**
www.surrogacy.org.uk
0844 414 0181
Moss Bank, Manse Road
Lairg IV27 4EL

The Daisy Network
www.daisynetwork.org.uk
The Daisy Network
PO Box 183
Rossendale BB4 6WZ

Donor Conception Network
www.donor-conception-
network.org
0208 245 4369
PO Box 7471
Nottingham NG3 6ZR

The Ectopic Pregnancy Trust
www.ectopic.org.uk
020 7733 2653
c/o 2nd Floor, Golden Jubilee
Wing, King's College Hospital
Denmark Hill, London SE5 9RS

Fertility UK
www.fertilityuk.org
Go to the website to find a
health professional who
specialises in fertility awareness.

**FPA (Family Planning
Association)**
www.fpa.org.uk
0845 122 8690

Food Standards Agency
www.food.gov.uk

**The Human Fertilisation and
Embryology Authority (HFEA)**
www.hfea.gov.uk
www.oneatatime.org.uk
020 7291 8200
21 Bloomsbury Street
London WC1B 3HF

Infertility Network UK (INUK)
www.infertilitynetworkuk.com
0800 008 7464
Charter House
43 St Leonards Road
Bexhill on Sea
East Sussex TN40 1JA

**Intercountry Adoption
Centre (ICA)**
www.icacentre.org.uk

The Miscarriage Association
www.miscarriageassociation.org.uk
01924 200799
The Miscarriage Association
c/o Clayton Hospital
Northgate
Wakefield
West Yorkshire WF1 3JS

**National Gamete
Donation Trust**
www.ngdt.co.uk
0845 226 9193

NHS Direct
www.nhsdirect.nhs.uk
0845 4647

The Organic Research Centre
www.efrc.com
01488 658298
Hamstead Marshall, Newbury
Berkshire RG20 0HR

PACT (Parents and Children Together)
www.pactcharity.org
0800 731 1845
Freepost (SCE6005), Reading
Berkshire RG1 4ZR

QUIT
www.quit.org.uk
0800 002200
63 St.Marys Axe
London EC3A 8AA

The Royal College of Obstetricians and Gynaecologists (RCOG)
www.rcog.org.uk
020 7772 6200
27 Sussex Place, Regent's Park
London NW1 4RG

SANDS (Stillbirth & Neonatal Death Charity)
www.uk-sands.org
020 7436 5881
28 Portland Place
London W1B 1LY

Smart Cells
www.smartcells.com
0845 604 5523
uk@smartcells.com
Smart Cells stores cord blood stem cells.

Soil Association
www.soilassociation.org
0117 314 5000
South Plaza
Marlborough Street
Bristol BS1 3NX

Tommy's
www.tommys.org
0870 777 76 76
Nicholas House
3 Laurence Pountney Hill
London EC4R 0BB

The World Wildlife Fund
www.worldwildlife.org.uk

Index